DRUGS IN CENTRAL NERVOUS SYSTEM DISORDERS

CLINICAL PHARMACOLOGY

Series Editor

MURRAY WEINER
Department of Pharmacology
University of Cincinnati
College of Medicine
Cincinnati, Ohio

Volume 1 Nicotinic Acid: Nutrient-Cofactor-Drug, *by Murray Weiner and Jan van Eys*

Volume 2 Drugs in Central Nervous System Disorders, *edited by David C. Horwell*

Other Volumes in Preparation

DRUGS IN CENTRAL NERVOUS SYSTEM DISORDERS

edited by

David C. Horwell
Parke-Davis Research Unit
Addenbrookes Hospital Site
Cambridge, England

MARCEL DEKKER, INC. New York and Basel

Library of Congress Cataloging in Publication Data
Main entry under title:

Drugs in central nervous system disorders.

(Clinical pharmacology ; v. 2)
Includes bibliographies and index.
1. Psychotropic drugs. 2. Analgesics.
3. Antidepressants. 4. Central nervous system—Diseases
—Chemotherapy. I. Horwell, David C., [date]
[DNLM: 1. Central Nervous System Diseases—drug therapy.
2. Psychopharmacology. W1 CL76H4 v.2 / QV 77 D793]
RM315.D85 1985 616.8'0461 84-26009
ISBN 0-8247-7185-0

MARCEL DEKKER, INC.
270 Madison Avenue, New York, New York 10016

Current printing (last digit):
10 9 8 7 6 5 4 3 2 1

PRINTED IN THE UNITED STATES OF AMERICA

Preface

The objective of this book is to review and update the information available from the literature on the major drugs used in the treatment of disorders of the central nervous system (CNS). Such a treatise cannot comprehensively discuss the diseases themselves, so we have focused our discussion on the drugs that are used, indicating their efficacy, major side effects, dosage, mode of action, preferred routes of administration, and the special features that affect their pharmacodynamic, pharmacokinetic, and metabolic fates. Leading references are given to enable the reader to gain a quick, in-depth investigation of these particular features of the drugs.

It is hoped that this approach, focusing on the drugs, with more general references to the disease areas where they are used, will act as a useful catalyst to the widest possible readership interested in a synopsis of the state of the art in the drug treatment of disorders of the CNS. Therefore this book should be of interest to medical and pharmacology students and pharmaceutical companies with an interest in CNS drug research.

Five chapters are devoted to major therapeutic areas concerning diseases of the CNS, the last chapter being a survey of naturally occurring drugs of ethno-origins.

Chapter 1 traces the development of centrally acting analgesics from the considerable work on chemical modification of opiate drugs to attempt to minimize their addictive and respiratory depression properties, to the milestone discovery of the enkephalins, which has further stimulated research into subclassification of endogenous opiate receptors, which may have application in the discovery of new classes of analgesics and, perhaps, antipsychotic drugs.

Chapter 2 describes the major drugs used in the treatment of depression and mania. Particular attention has been focused on the tricyclic antidepressants and the second-generation drugs with an alleged antidepressant/antianxiety profile of activity. Current research has tended to focus on the evaluation of their mode of action, particularly their ability to selectively inhibit the uptake of noradrenaline (NA, norepinephrine), or 5-hydroxytryptamine (5-HT, serotonin) and to look for drugs that have a faster onset of antidepressant activity and less anticholinergic and cardiovascular side effects than the tricyclics.

Chapter 3 describes the development of the antiepileptics, antianxiety agents and sedative-hypnotics, in which the barbiturates and related compounds with their addictive properties, lethality in overdose, and liver enzyme potentiating properties, have been superceded in many cases by the benzodiazepines. The benzodiazepines have been fine-tuned by chemical modification to produce compounds with a pharmacokinetic profile leading to short acting compounds useful as sleep inducers, and long-acting compounds used as antianxiety agents.

Chapter 4 describes the neuroleptic agents that are used mainly to treat psychotic disorders such as schizophrenia. Since the discovery of the antipsychotic effects of chlorpromazine (CPZ) in the early 1950s, emphasis in research in the 1960s has concentrated on the mode of action of such drugs, particularly their ability to block central dopamine receptors, and the ways to reduce their undesirable properties, such as the flattening of mood and extra-pyramidal side effects. The drug clozapine has created considerable interest in this regard, but its association with a high incidence of agranulocytosis has now limited its use.

Chapter 5 concentrates on the drugs that regulate the hypothalamic-pituitary axis. The dopamine stimulants such as the ergot-derived drugs bromocriptine and pergolide are of interest in this regard in that they have been shown to have use in three different therapeutic areas: Parkinson's disease, acromegaly, and hyperprolactinaemia. Drugs that selectively stimulate or inhibit secretion of other pituitary hormones may also be of value in drug therapy.

Chapter 6 is devoted to drugs derived from ethno-origins. Despite the considerable advances made in drug treatment of disorders of the CNS outlined above, the great majority of mankind still achieves relief from these disorders by self-medication with natural products derived from a bewildering array of plants and herbs. Discussion of these products is divided into three sections: those which act as psychostimulants, psychodepressants, and those which affect consciousness.

A separate chapter has not been included on CNS stimulants, as they have been used in the treatment of virtually all CNS diseases at some time, as mentioned in the appropriate chapters. However, some do appear to have an established role in the treatment of certain disorders of children and geriatrics. For example, both amphetamine and methyl phenidate are used, mainly in the United States, for treatment of hyperkinesia in children (minimal brain dysfunction, MBD), whereas the ergot alkaloid derivative, dihydroergotoxine (Hydergine), has gained widespread popularity in some European countries in the treatment of certain geriatric disorders, termed under a multitude of names such as cerebral insufficiency, senile dementia and, in the United States, Alzheimer's disease. The development of "cognition activating" drugs without the side effects of the CNS stimulants would be useful in treating such disorders which involve deficiencies in learning and memory. The drug piracetam has gained considerable interest in this regard, despite its low potency, and there is much current research interest into this type of drug therapy.

The α_2-agonist clonidine has recently found favor over the ergot alkaloids and ergot-caffeine combination in the treatment of migraine. However, much controversy exists on whether clonidine exerts its beneficial action on peripheral cerebral blood vessels or by its central properties. At present, the etiology of migraine is still unknown and further research is needed before more selective drugs can be developed.

In summary, we have tried to review the properties of the major classes of drugs that are used in the treatment of disorders of the CNS. The discussions have concentrated on the efficacy, side effects, dose regimens, mode of action, pharmacokinetic, and metabolic properties of these drugs, and indicate the areas where advances in research have been made and which hold promise for the development of new drugs for the future. We hope the book will serve as a useful introduction and reference document for a wide multidisciplinary readership interested in the drugs that are used in the treatment of disorders of the CNS.

David C. Horwell

Contents

Preface iii
Contributors ix

1 Centrally Acting Analgesics 1
Robert C. A. Frederickson and
Martin D. Hynes, III

I. Introduction 1
II. Drugs Available for Treating Pain 2
III. Limitations of Existing Analgesics 17
IV. Mode of Action 26
V. Current Trends for New Pain Treatment 32
VI. Prognosis and Applications in Other Disease Areas 46
Acknowledgments 48
References 48

2 Antidepressants 71
David C. Horwell

I. Introduction 71
II. Epidemiology of Depression 72
III. Classification of Depression 73
IV. Etiology of Depression 75
V. The Major Classes of Antidepressant Drugs 76
VI. Discussion of Some Current Trends in Research into Depression 110
VII. Summary 111
References 113

3 Benzodiazepines and Barbiturates: Drugs for the Treatment of Anxiety, Insomnia, and Seizure Disorders 123
Kelvin W. Gee and Henry I. Yamamura

I. Introduction 123
II. Benzodiazepines 124
III. Barbiturates 136
IV. Future directions 141
References 143

4 Neuroleptic Agents: Acute and Chronic Receptor Actions 149
Peter Jenner and C. David Marsden

I. Introduction 149
II. Classes of Neuroleptic Agents 152
III. Acute Pharmacological Actions of Neuroleptics on Brain Dopamine Function 157
IV. Acute Pharmacological Actions of Neuroleptic Drugs on Nondopamine Systems 173
V. Multiple Sites of Action Within the Striatal Complex 181
VI. Adaptations of Dopamine Receptor Function to Neuroleptic Drug Administration 205
VII. Discussion 245
References 249

5 Drugs Used in the Regulation of Endocrine and Motor Activity 263
James A. Clemens

I. Introduction 263
II. Drugs Used to Treat Endocrine Disturbances 263
III. Drugs Used in the CNS Regulation of Motor Activity 270
Acknowledgments 276
References 276

6 Drugs of Ethno-Origin 283
Peter J. Houghton and Norman G. Bisset

I. Introduction 283
II. Psychostimulants 285
III. Psychodepressants 296
IV. Drugs That Affect Consciousness 305
V. Therapeutic Potential of CNS-Active Plant Substances 324
References 325

Index 333

Contributors

NORMAN G. BISSET Department of Pharmacy, Chelsea College, University of London, London, England

JAMES A. CLEMENS Central Nervous System and Endocrine Research, The Lilly Research Laboratories, A Division of Eli Lilly and Company, Indianapolis, Indiana

ROBERT C. A. FREDERICKSON Central Nervous System Research, The Lilly Research Laboratories, A Division of Eli Lilly and Company, Indianapolis, Indiana

KELVIN W. GEE Department of Pharmacology, University of Arizona Health Sciences Center, Tucson, Arizona

DAVID C. HORWELL Parke-Davis Research Unit, Addenbrookes Hospital Site, Cambridge, England

PETER J. HOUGHTON Department of Pharmacy, Chelsea College, University of London, London, England

MARTIN D. HYNES, III Central Nervous System Research, The Lilly Research Laboratories, A Division of Eli Lilly and Company, Indianapolis, Indiana

PETER JENNER University Department of Neurology, Institute of Psychiatry, King's College Hospital Medical School, London, England

C. DAVID MARSDEN University Department of Neurology, Institute of Psychiatry, King's College Hospital Medical School, London England

HENRY I. YAMAMURA Department of Pharmacology, University of Arizona Health Sciences Center, Tucson, Arizona

DRUGS IN
CENTRAL NERVOUS SYSTEM
DISORDERS

1

Centrally Acting Analgesics

ROBERT C. A. FREDERICKSON and MARTIN D. HYNES, III *Central Nervous System Research, The Lilly Research Laboratories, A Division of Eli Lilly and Company, Indianapolis, Indiana*

I. INTRODUCTION

Pain is probably the earliest "disease" recognized by man, and presumably by his evolutionary predecessors as well. It is still inadequately understood in mechanistic terms, in spite of centuries of research and the fact that effective, if not ideal, treatment has been available for thousands of years. Over the last 100 years, the number of drugs available to treat pain has expanded considerably, but few of these drugs have significant advantages over morphine, the active ingredient of opium. There is still a great need to develop an effective central analgesic drug with less tolerance, physical dependence, respiratory depression, and psychotomimetic effects than existing drugs and much effort is being expended toward this goal.

A recent advance has been the development of peripherally acting analgesics with efficacy better than aspirin, although not yet comparable with that of the centrally acting agents. Such agents minimize problems with central side effects but probably are not adequate for severe pain and have their own side effects, particularly gastrointestinal and renal toxicity, which in some cases can be life-threatening. The vast array of existing centrally acting analgesics and the improvement of the peripherally acting agents nevertheless place strict criteria on the introduction of new agents to this armamenterium. Short of being the ideal analgesic (sought unsuccessfully for the last seven decades), any new agent introduced at least will need to demonstrate efficacy in moderate to severe pain and offer some significant advantage for some particular use. We will discuss examples of such situations in a later section.

The following two sections will discuss existing centrally acting analgesics available for use, their characteristics, advantages, and disadvantages, and will attempt to develop further the criteria for useful new drugs. The succeeding sections will discuss the basic background knowledge, animal model systems, and rationale available for pursuing such new agents and will subsequently discuss progress in novel research endeavors, including development of analgesic entities based on the endogenous opioid peptides. Finally, the present status and future prognosis of these efforts for producing useful new analgesics, or novel treatment in other disease areas, will be discussed.

Before going further we must define some terminology. This is not an easy task because a consistent terminology and satisfactory classification of compounds within this terminology have not been adopted uniformly by workers and writers in this field. The term "opiate" is generally accepted to designate drugs derived from opium, which among the analgesics includes only morphine and codeine and could include also semisynthetic derivatives of these alkaloids. This term has been used extensively in the literature, but very often to refer inappropriately to agents not derived from morphine. The word "opioid" has been introduced to remedy this problem and it designates compounds with properties similar to those of a substance derived from opium; practical usage has generally intended this comparator substance to be morphine, and thus opioid has become synonymous with "morphinelike." With the realization of the multiple actions of morphine, however, and the advent of compounds sharing only a subset of the actions of morphine, a problem has arisen concerning what subset is appropriate to be designated as opioid. Jaffe and Martin [1] have attempted to resolve this problen by redefining opioid as "a generic designation for all exogenous substances that bind specifically to any of several subspecies of opioid receptors and produce some agonistic actions." For the purposes of this chapter, we would like to use a modification of this definition such that opioid refers to all substances, exogenous of endogenous, that bind specifically to any of several subspecies or receptors (characterized by ability to specifically displace [^{3}H]naloxone ([^{3}H]Nx), [^{3}H]dihydromorphine ([^{3}H]DHM), [^{3}H]ethylketocyclazocine ([^{3}H]EKC), or [^{3}H]D-Ala^2-D-Leu^5-enkephalin ([^{3}H]DADL)) and produce analgesia that can be antagonized by naloxone.

II. DRUGS AVAILABLE FOR TREATING PAIN

The majority of available central analgesics can be classified as opioid agonist analgesics or opioid mixed agonist-antagonist analgesics. The opioid agonists are compounds that have affinity for one or more of the opioid receptor subtypes and have intrinsic activity (efficacy) at all the receptors for which they have affinity. They may differ in affinity and/or intrinsic activity at the different receptor subtypes, but they are not antagonists at any of these sites. Pure antagonists are compounds that may have affinity for one or more of the opioid receptor subtypes but have intrinsic activity at none, i.e., they produce no agonistic activity upon binding to any of the receptors for which they have affinity. This property is the basis for their antagonist activity, since by binding to a receptor they thereby prevent its activation. Examples of such pure antagonists are naloxone (Narcan®*), naltrexone, and diprenorphine. Mixed agonist-antagonist compounds are those which have affinity and intrinsic activity at one or more of the opioid receptor subtypes but also have antagonistic properties at at least one of the receptor subtypes. The antagonistic properties may be a reflection of true competitive antagonism at that receptor or be a reflection that they are merely partial agonists at that receptor. Such compounds exert what is called a ceiling effect, i.e., regardless of concentration or dose they cannot produce an effect equivalent to the maximum effect of a full agonist. Under the right conditions, such a compound can prevent a full agonist from achieving its maximum effect, and this appears as an antagonism. It is generally assumed that full agonist analgesics utilize μ-receptors to produce analgesia. The mixed agents are generally full or partial agonists at the K receptor and antagonists or partial agonists at the μ-receptor. These latter agents are assumed to provide analgesia at the K-receptor as well as or rather than the μ-receptor. These assumptions are not yet fully established. There is now growing evidence that agonism at the δ-receptor can also produce analgesia.

A. Opioid Agonist Analgesics

Morphine is the prototype opioid agonist analgesic and remains the standard against which new analgesics are measured. A number of other compounds are now available in this category that resemble morphine in their analgesic and other pharmacological properties. These compounds are presumed to share a similar mechanism of action with morphine while having some special property or properties differing from morphine. These compounds are listed in Table 1.1. We cannot discuss all of these compounds in detail, but rather we will concentrate on morphine, meperidine, codeine, and dextropropoxphene whose structures are given in Fig. 1.1. Abuse liability and respiratory depression will

---

*®Trademark.

TABLE 1.1 Opioid Agonist Analgesics

Name		Dose (mg)[a]		
Nonproprietary	Trade (U.S.)	Parenteral	Oral	Duration (hr)[b]
Alphaprodine	Nisentil	20-60	–	1-2
Anileridine	Leritine	75-100	25-50	2-6
Codeine	–	15-60	15-60	4-6
Dihydrocodine	Paracodine	10-30	10-30	4-6
Ethoheptazine	Zactane	–	75-150	5-6
Fentanyl	Sublimaze	0.05-0.1	–	0.5-1
Heroin	–	–	2-5	3-6
Hydrocodone	Dicodid	–	5-10	4-6
Hydromorphine	Dilaudid	1-4	1-4	4-6
Levorphanol	Levo-Dromoran	2-3	2-3	6-8
Meperidine	Demerol	50-100	50-100	3-4
Methadone	Dolophine	2-10	2-10	3-4
Metopon	Metopon	3-6	10-20	3-6
Morphine	–	7-15	–	4-5
Oxycodone	–	–	4-5	5-6
Oxymorphone	Numorphan	1	–	4-6
Pholcodine	Ethnine	–	10-15	4-5
Piminodine	Alvodine	10-20	25-50	4-6
Propoxyphene				
Hydrochloride	Darvon	–	32-65	3-4
Napsylate	Darvon-N	–	50-100	3-4

[a]Usual therapeutic dose range in nontolerant patients. The treatment of severe pain usually requires the administration of doses towards the higher level of the range.

[b]Usual duration of the analgesic effect following administration of a therapeutic dose. The duration may vary with the dose administered and intensity of pain.

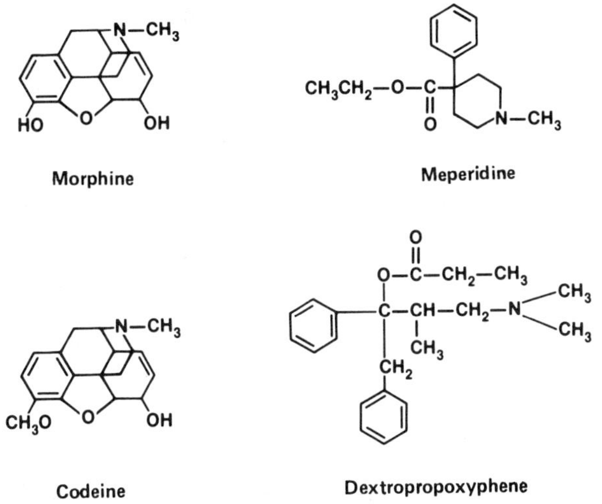

Morphine

Meperidine

Codeine

Dextropropoxyphene

FIG. 1.1 Structures of selected opioid agonist analgesics.

be discussed in the following section on limitations of existing analgesics, but we will discuss other side effects in this section.

The discussions to follow will concentrate on the analgesic efficacy of the opioid agonists in the clinic. The analgesic activity of morphine can be demonstrated in all animal model systems, although there may be species and test system differences with regard to potency. Meperidine is also very efficacious in a large array of preclinical test systems. The analgesic activity of these agents in these preclinical test systems has been well established and reviewed [2–9]. The preclinical analgesic activity and safety of codeine and dextropropoxyphene have been the subject of a number of reviews also [10–13].

1. Morphine

Morphine is the natural phenanthrene alkaloid that is responsible for the pharmacological activity of opium. The ability of opium to relieve pain has been known since ancient times. Morphine was isolated from opium as the active agent in 1803. Morphine's ability to relieve pain, particularly severe pain, is most impressive and has been attributed to an elevation of pain threshold, to an altered reaction to the painful stimuli, and even to the induction of sleep [4]. Some studies of experimental pain have shown a rise in threshold [14,15], whereas others have reported no effect on this parameter [16,17]. Many investigators have shown an increase in pain tolerance with no change in threshold [18–21]. Morphine appears to act on those systems responsible for the affective response to pain so that a patient's ability to tolerate pain is increased while the capacity to perceive the pain is not changed [1,22].

In several early studies, acceptable pain relief was achieved in 90% of the postoperative patients treated with morphine doses of 7–9 mg [23]. The mean interval between subcutaneous injection and onset of pain relief was 10 min, and the relief persisted for about 4 hr. Similar results were reported in another study [24] which showed the optimal dose of morphine to be 10 mg/70 kg. This dose provided significant relief of pain in two-thirds of the patients. Increasing the morphine dose to 15 mg provided three-fourths of the patients with pain relief for an even longer time, but this increase in dose also resulted in an increase in side effects.

A significant loss of potency is observed when morphine is administered orally. A 10-mg oral morphine dose in postoperative pain is only slightly better than placebo [25]. This marked reduction in analgesic activity has also been reported in patients with pain of malignant origin. Oral morphine was found to be one-fifteenth and one-sixteenth as potent, respectively, as parenteral morphine when compared in terms of peak effects and total analgesia [26].

The patient given morphine for pain relief sometimes experiences a state of euphoria. In the pain-free state, however, dysphoria is occasionally observed. In addition to these changes in mood, patients treated with morphine show mental clouding [27,28], reduced mental performance, and increased reaction time [29]. Nausea and vomiting are reported in volunteers and patients treated with morphine [23,24, 30,31]. These adverse effects seem to be the result of morphine stimulation of the chemoreceptor trigger zone [32] and also effects on vestibular function [33].

Morphine has very little effect on cardiovascular function, even at doses above the therapeutic range [34–36]. Postural hypotension may result, however, from peripheral vasodilation due in part to histamine release [37].

Morphine has pronounced effects on the gastrointestinal system and results in a considerable constipating effect [1]. This effect although unpleasant when not necessary, has therapeutic usefulness in the treatment of diarrhea and dysentery. Morphine administration increases the tone of the detrusor muscle of the urinary bladder, resulting in urinary urgency in some patients. On the other hand, the tone of the vesical sphincter is also increased by morphine which may make urination difficult [1]. Morphine may also have an antidiuretic effect resulting from an increased secretion of antidiuretic hormone [38].

2. Meperidine (Pethidine)

Meperidine (Demerol®*) is the ethyl ester of 1-methyl-4-phenylpiperidine-4-carboxylic acid. Meperidine was introduced in 1938 as an anticholinergic agent and has had extensive clinical use since then [39]. As an analgesic, it is effective in a wide variety of conditions, although it appears to be more effective against visceral pain than that arising from skeletal and neurologic structures [4]. The clinical analgesic activity of meperidine is dose related in the range of 25–100 mg [40]. In cancer pain, 62–79 mg meperidine was found equianalgesic to 10 mg of morphine [41]. Following parenteral administration, the onset of activity is rapid, within 10–15 min, and peak activity is reached within 45 min. The analgesic activity of 100 mg persists for 3–6 hr [4,42]. Meperidine is also orally effective, but oral meperidine is significantly less potent and reliable than parenteral meperidine.

The most frequently observed side effects with meperidine are sedation, dizziness, sweating, dryness of the mouth, nausea, and vomiting [4,43]. These adverse effects occur most frequently in ambulatory patients as opposed to those who are bedridden with severe pain. High doses of meperidine produce marked stimulatory effects on the central nervous system which are characterized by tremors, muscle twitches, seizures, and agitation [1]. Meperidine has also been reported to produce constipation, biliary tract spasms, bronchoconstriction, and urinary retention [1,3,7]. Meperidine in clinically effective doses produces as much euphoria as does morphine [43]. Euphoria occurs in up to 20% of the patients treated. A small percentage of patients, however, may experience dysphoria, hallucinations, and/or disorientation.

3. Codeine

Codeine is a natural opium alkaloid in which the phenolic hydroxyl group of morphine is replaced by a methoxy group. Well-controlled clinical studies have demonstrated the analgesic activity of codeine at doses of 60 mg or more orally in comparison to placebo [44–51]. Studies employing lower doses of codeine (30–32 mg) have been less consistent, with some showing superiority to placebo [44,45,50–54] and others no difference from placebo [25,55–57]. The parenteral efficacy of codeine has received only limited attention. Codeine, 30–120 mg intramuscularly, was found inferior to 10 mg morphine in the treatment of postoperative pain [24]. There is a general clinical

---

*®Trademark.

impression that the maximal analgesic effect of codeine, which is substantially below that of morphine, is reached at 60 mg. This perception has been substantiated in part by studying experimental pain [58]. In extensive clinical trials in cancer patients [59,60], however, evidence was obtained that the effect of codeine did not level off until doses of 180–360 mg.

Dizziness, sedation, and nausea are the most commonly observed side effects following administration of oral codeine in therapeutic doses [24,37,49,51,61–64]. As the dose of codeine is increased, more serious side effects are observed, including excitement, tremors, vomiting, flushing, and lassitude [65].

4. Dextropropoxyphene

Propoxyphene, 4-desmethylamino-1,2-diphenyl-3-methyl-2-propionoxybutane, is a centrally acting analgesic widely used for the treatment of mild to moderate pain states. Only the alpha-dextro isomer, dextropropoxyphene (Darvon®*), possesses analgesic activity [66]. In some controlled clinical studies, dextropropoxyphene at an oral dose of 32 mg was found superior to placebo [44,45,67,68], while in others it was found to be no more effective than placebo [50,53,55,56]. The majority of studies, however, showed dextropropoxyphene clearly distinguishable from placebo at doses in excess of 32 mg [44–46,48, 50,67,69,72]. Dextropropoxyphene has been found inferior to codeine at equal milligram doses in some studies [46,49,53], whereas other investigators have found them to be equieffective [44,45,48,67]. Beaver [64], after reviewing the literature, concluded that the efficacy of dextropropoxyphene in single-dose studies is one-half to two-thirds that of codeine on a milligram-for-milligram basis. In multiple-dose studies, however, the two have been found to be equipotent [70,71], which may be a result of their differing pharmacokinetic characteristics (dextropropoxyphene has a longer half-life).

Commonly reported side effects following therapeutic doses of dextropropoxyphene include sedation, anorexia, nausea, vomiting, constipation, and abdominal pain [47,49,62]. When compared with codeine in equianalgesic doses, dextropropoxyphene seemed less likely to cause nausea and vomiting but more likely to produce sedation and dizziness [64]. The Council on Drugs of the American Medical Association, on the other hand, concluded that the incidence of central nervous system and gastrointestinal disturbances (dizziness, nausea, vomiting, constipation) appear to be lower with dextropropoxyphene than with

---

*® Trademark.

equipotent doses of codeine [73]. In overdose cases, convulsions, delirium, hallucinations, and confusion are observed. Other major signs of overdose include depression of respiration, cardiac arrhythmias, and pulmonary edema [74,75]. Naloxone will antagonize the toxic effects of dextropropoxyphene.

B. Opioid Mixed Agonist-Antagonist Analgesics

The prototype agent in this category is the benzomorphan derivative pentazocine. This compound was produced as the result of an effort to provide an analgesic with little or no abuse potential and was for some time an unscheduled drug. This reduced abuse potential is one of the major intended special properties of this class of analgesics as a whole. These compounds are certainly associated with a different level of tolerance development and abuse potential than the typical opioid agonist analgesic, but the improvement is not as dramatic as originally hoped. Furthermore, they introduce problems unique to their category, such as psychotomimetic side effects. The available analgesics in this category are listed in Table 1.2. In this section we will discuss pentazocine, nalbuphine, butorphanol, and buprenorphine whose structures are given in Fig. 1.2. Abuse liability, respiratory depression, and psychotomimetic effects will be discussed in the following section on

TABLE 1.2 Opioid Mixed Agonist-Antagonist Analgesics

Name		Dose (mg)[a]		Duration (hr)[b]
Nonproprietary	Trade (U.S.)	Parenteral	Oral	
Buprenorphine	Buprenex	0.3-0.6	0.4-0.8[c]	6-8
Butorphanol	Stadol	0.5-4.0	–	3-4
Nalbuphine	Nubain	10-20	–	3-6
Pentazocine	Talwin	30-60	50-100	3-4

[a]Usual therapeutic dose range in nontolerant patients. The treatment of severe pain usually requires the administration of doses towards the higher level of the range.
[b]Usual duration of the analgesic effect following administration of a therapeutic dose. The duration may vary with the dose administered and intensity of pain.
[c]Buprenorphine is administered by the sublingual route. It is not yet available for use in the United States but is marketed in the United Kingdom under the trade name Temgesic.

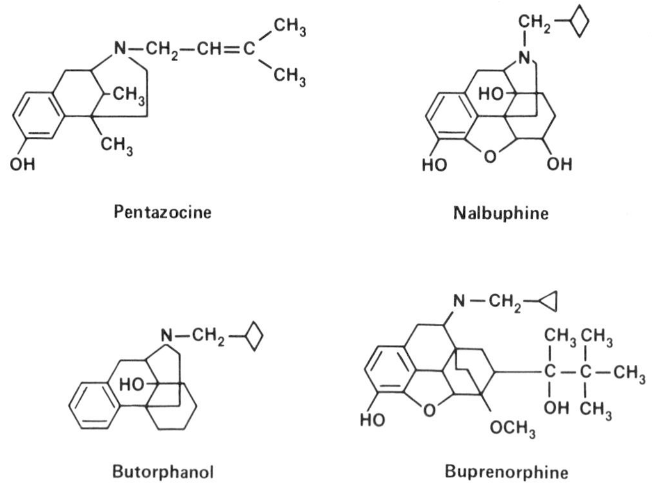

Pentazocine

Nalbuphine

Butorphanol

Buprenorphine

FIG. 1.2 Structures of opioid mixed agonist-antagonist analgesics.

limitations of existing analgesics, but we will discuss some of the other miscellaneous side effects in this section.

1. Pentazocine

Pentazocine exhibits analgesic activity in the mouse writhing test [76,77] and in the rat flinch-jump test [78] but not in the rat tail-flick or mouse hot-plate tests [79], which is typical for the opioid mixed agonist-antagonists. Weak narcotic antagonist activity can be demonstrated for pentazocine in several different test systems [76,79].

Parenteral doses of 20–30 mg pentazocine yield satisfactory pain relief in most surgical patients with moderate to severe pain. In a study involving over 1000 patients [80], 27 mg of pentazocine administered intramuscularly provided the same pain relief as 10 mg of morphine at the time of peak effect, but had a shorter duration of action. In another double-blind study utilizing 740 patients, pentazocine was evaluated with 12 other analgesics for their ability to relieve postoperative pain after parenteral administration [81]. Levorphanol was the only drug significantly superior to the reference standard meperidine, but pentazocine at 20 mg was found to be one of the most successful of the remaining drugs as measured by pain relief relative to depression of consciousness. In patients with cancer pain, 33 mg of pentazocine administered intramuscularly was equivalent to a 10-mg dose of morphine in terms of peak analgesia [82], and 60 mg was found slightly better than 10 mg of morphine in both peak and total analgesia [83]. In patients with ischemic pain from vascular disease, morphine 15 mg, pentazocine 45 mg and meperidine 100 mg were found to be equianalgesic [84]. Pentazocine has also been reported useful in the treatment of pain in burned children [85].

Pentazocine at 50 mg orally produced approximately the same degree of pain relief as codeine at 60 mg [51]. Pentazocine had a more rapid onset, but codeine had a longer duration of action. In chronic cancer pain, pentazocine orally is only about one-third as active as by the intramuscular route [86]. When nine oral analgesics were compared in cancer pain, pentazocine at a 50 mg dose was found superior to placebo and equal to aspirin 650 mg, codeine 65 mg and phenacetin 650 mg [87].

Nausea, dizziness, lightheadedness, sedation, and vomiting have been reported with an incidence of 4–8% following administration of pentazocine [88]. Autonomic effects, including sweating, hot flushes, dry mouth, transient hypertension, urinary retention, and tachycardia have also been reported, as have various dermatological effects, including discomfort at the injection site, flushing, dermatitis, and pruritis [88]. The incidence of vomiting is similar for equianalgesic doses of pentazocine, meperidine and morphine [89–91]. On the other hand, grogginess, drunken feelings, sweating and dizziness tend to occur more frequently with pentazocine than with equianalgesic doses of morphine [80,82,91–93]. The incidence of pentazocine-induced side effects appears related to the level of unmetabolized drug in the body [94].

2. Nalbuphine

Nalbuphine is a derivative of 14-hydroxy-morphine, and closely related structurally to the narcotic agonist oxymorphine and to the narcotic antagonists naloxone and naltrexone. Potent analgesic activity has been demonstrated for this substance in the writhing test in both mouse and rat but not in the mouse hot-plate assay [95]. In man, good analgesic efficacy has been demonstrated in moderate to severe pain of postoperative and malignant origin.

In both analgesic potency and duration of action, nalbuphine is about equivalent to morphine when given intramuscularly [96–98]. In postoperative pain, nalbuphine is about three or four times as potent as pentazocine and has a longer duration of action [99–102].

Following oral administration, nalbuphine is reported to be one-fourth to one-fifth as potent as when administered intramuscularly [103]. By the oral route, it was found to be about three times more potent than codeine in patients with postoperative pain of moderate to severe intensity [104].

Sedation is the most common adverse effect, occurring in 30–40% of the population treated with nalbuphine [96,97,100,105]. Nausea and vomiting occur with an incidence of about 5% which is less than for morphine, meperidine, or pentazocine. Sweaty and clammy sensations, dizziness, vertigo, dry mouth, and headaches have been observed in 5% or fewer of nalbuphine recipients.

3. Butorphanol

Butorphanol derives from a series of nitrogen-substituted 3,4-dihydroxymorphinans which possess narcotic agonist and antagonist activity. It is closely related to nalorphine, cyclazocine, and cyclorphan. Butorphanol is reported to be more effective in the mouse writhing and arthritic vocalization tests than in the rat tail flick, mouse hot-plate, or dog skin-twitch tests for analgesic activity [106,107]. Narcotic antagonist activity has been demonstrated in several animal models in which butorphanol appears less potent than naloxone but equipotent with nalorphine [106].

Butorphanol has provided satisfactory pain relief in postoperative pain [108–118] prepartum pain [119–121], chronic pain [122–124], and pain of malignant origin [100,125]. In patients with postoperative pain, butorphanol at 1.49–2.92 mg intramuscularly was comparable in analgesic potency to morphine at 10 mg; the time to peak action and duration of action were similar for these two drugs [108,112, 126]. Comparison of single intravenous doses for the treatment of postoperative pain showed 1 mg of butorphanol to be as effective as 5 mg of morphine [109], and 0.5-mg and 1-mg doses were comparable to 20 mg and 40 mg of meperidine [114]. Intramuscular doses of 0.5–4 mg of butorphanol were as active as 20–80 mg of meperidine in postoperative patients [110,111,113,127]. Equianalgesic doses produced pain relief of equal onset and duration. The relative potency of these agents is similar in labor pain [119,120,128].

By the oral route, 8 mg of butorphanol was equianalgesic with 60 mg of codeine in postepisiotomy pain, while 16 mg was superior [129,130]. A 4-mg oral dose of butorphanol produced analgesia similar to that following 50 mg of pentazocine [117], whereas by the intramuscular route, 4 mg of butorphanol was found superior to 60 mg of pentazocine [115, 116].

When administered acutely for postoperative pain, drowsiness was the most frequently observed side effect occurring in up to 88% of the patient population [110–112,131]. The next most frequently reported side effects were nausea, vomiting, hallucinations, and disorientation [100,108,110,111,114,132]. Diplopia [113], dysphoria [111], anxiety [116], euphoria [108,111] and vertigo [117] have all been reported with rare occurrence. When butorphanol was administered chronically, somnolence, confusion, delirium, and dizziness were noted [122].

4. Buprenorphine

Buprenorphine is a highly lipophilic oripavine derivative which contains a cyclopropylmethyl substitution and is a potent analgesic agent. Buprenorphine exhibits pronounced analgesic activity in a wide variety of animal antinociceptive tests such as mouse writhing [133–135], mouse hot plate [135], rat tail-flick [136,137], and rat tail pressure [133,134]. In several of these tests, the maximum response obtained is less than complete analgesia, suggesting buprenorphine is a partial agonist at the analgesic receptor. In a number of test systems, buprenorphine exhibits antagonist activity comparable to naloxone [133,134, 138].

In man, buprenorphine has analgesic efficacy similar to that of morphine, but a much longer duration of action. Analgesic efficacy has been demonstrated in postoperative pain [139–145], myocardial infarction pain [146], and pain of malignant origin [147–149]. Buprenorphine, 0.2–0.6 mg intramuscularly, was as effective as morphone, 5–15 mg, and had a longer duration of action [139,150]. Intramuscular doses of buprenorphine in the range of 2-4 μg/kg were found not to differ from 600 μg/kg of pentazocine in postoperative patients. Increasing the buprenorphine dose to 8 μg/kg resulted in significantly greater analgesia than that seen with pentazocine [140].

Following sublingual administration, 0.4 mg of buprenorphine was as effective and 0.8 mg was more effective than 50 mg of oral pentazocine in moderate to severe postsurgical pain [151]. Buprenorphine, 4–8 μg/kg, has been found superior to 1 mg/kg of meperidine in postoperative patients [140,143,152]. Satisfactory analgesia in chronic pain has been reported also following intramuscular injections [147] and sublingual dosing [148,153]. These studies have shown buprenorphine to have a long duration of action. Buprenorphine (0.3 mg) and morphine (10 mg) were found equianalgesic in patients with moderate to severe pain of malignant origin, although buprenorphine was found to have a significantly longer duration of action [149].

The profile of side effects observed after buprenorphine administration is similar to that observed for morphine, meperidine, and pentazocine. Nausea and vomiting were the most commonly reported side effects in a postmarketing survey of 7500 patients [154]. This study also reported a low incidence of euphoria, hallucinations, and dysphoria. In the treatment of chronic pain, buprenorphine was associated with a significantly higher incidence, greater severity, earlier onset, and longer duration of dizziness, nausea, and vomiting than morphine [149]. It is important to note that this study was conducted in cancer patients who were critically ill.

C. Other Approaches to Pain Treatment

1. Neuroleptics

A number of neuroleptics, drugs commonly used for the treatment of psychosis, have been used by themselves and in combination with narcotics for the treatment of pain. Both phenothiazines and butyrophenones have been employed in this regard.

a. Methotrimeprazine. Methotrimeprazine (Levoprome®*), a phenothiazine derivative, is a potent analgesic in patients with postoperative pain [155–157]. When administered at doses of 10–20 mg parenterally, it is equianalgesic with 10 mg of morphine. It appears to have several advantages over narcotics. Methotrimeprazine is not a narcotic since it does not bind to opiate receptors nor are its analgesic effects antagonized by naloxone [158]. No morphinelike physical dependence has been found with methotrimeprazine, although it partially suppresses morphine abstinence [159]. In clinically effective doses, it does not suppress respiration [160]. Its major disadvantages are sedation and orthostatic hypotension [161]. In fact, fainting has been reported in 70% of healthy volunteers given 10–15 mg intramuscularly during a tilt test, compared with an incidence of 20% after identical doses of morphine [162]. The high incidence of orthostatic hypotension tends to limit the clinical usefulness of methotrimeprazine.

b. Neuroleptics in combination with narcotics. The term "neuroleptanalgesia" implies the use of a butyrophenone neuroleptic in combination with a short-acting, potent analgesic as an adjunct or alternative to surgical anesthesia [163–167]. Minor surgical procedures such as insertion of eyelid sutures, nerve-blocking injections, and dressing of burns have been performed under neuroleptanalgesia. Neuroleptanalgesia combinations have also been found useful for supplementing local analgesic techniques such as in endobronchial intubation [168] and bronchoscopy procedures [169]. Neuroleptanalgesia is widely used, furthermore, as a preanesthetic medication. Of the butyrophenones available, those commonly used in neuroleptanalgesia are haloperidol and droperidol. The analgesics commonly used in neuroleptanalgesia are dextromoramide (Palfium), phenoperidine (Operidine), and fentanyl (Sublimaze) in order of increasing potency and decreasing duration of action [166].

The most common neuroleptanalgesia combination is that of fentanyl citrate and droperidol (Innovar®*). Droperidol alone produces sedation,

---

*®Trademark.

tranquilization, adrenergic blockade, and vasodilation [170,171]. The principal actions of fentanyl citrate alone are analgesia, central nervous system depression, respiratory depression, and bradycardia [172, 173]. Droperidol is reported to enhance the analgesic activity of fentanyl citrate [174]. Droperidol alone appears devoid of analgesic activity. The mechanism of the potentiation is not known, but it is doubtful that it is due to interference by droperidol with the catabolism of fentanyl citrate since the duration of analgesic action of the combination is no greater than that of fentanyl alone [174]. Some investigators, however, have found no potentiation of the analgesic effect of fentanyl by droperidol [175,176].

Fentanyl plus droperidol have been found to produce better preoperative sedation than morphine, with significantly less postoperative nausea and vomiting [177]. The concept of combining neuroleptanalgesia with light general anesthesia has been employed for a number of years. A mixture of fentanyl citrate and droperidol has been used successfully with nitrous oxide for general anesthesia in man [178]. The neuroleptics do not appear to augment the ventilatory depressant effects of the analgesics [174–176,179]. The combination, however, appears to increase the tendency of some patients to experience orthostatic hypotension [179].

2. Antidepressants

A large body of literature suggests that antidepressant agents have analgesic properties and can potentiate the analgesic activity of the narcotics both in experimental animals and man. The most widely studied agents are the serotonin-uptake inhibitors, which increase serotonin action on synaptic receptors by preventing its inactivation by reuptake from the synaptic cleft.

Fluoxetine, chlorimipramine, Org. 6582, citalopram, zimelidine, and femoxetine are all selective inhibitors of serotonin uptake which produce analgesia and potentiate morphine analgesia in rats and mice [180–185]. Norepinephrine uptake inhibitors (maprotiline, amitriptyline, and nortriptyline), on the other hand, do not appear to potentiate the analgesic effect of morphine [180].

The tricyclic antidepressants imipramine and chlorimipramine have been reported to be analgesic in man [186,187]. A reduction in pain intensity has been reported in chronic pain of malignant origin [188–190]. Imipramine was found superior to placebo in arthritic patients on antiinflammatory medication, as measured by pain relief, grip strength, and stiffness [191–193]. Zimelidine, an antidepressant that selectively inhibits serotonin uptake, produced pain relief in patients with pain syndromes of both organic and psychogenic origin [194].

The antidepressant drugs probably contribute to pain relief in three ways: (1) by improving mood, (2) by exerting a direct analgesic effect, and (3) by potentiating the effects of other analgesics. These actions are apparently secondary to the enhancement of serotonergic function provided by the inhibition of neuronal uptake of serotonin. Administration of serotonin precursors has also been reported to produce analgesia in experimental and clinical pain. Pain tolerance levels in response to tooth pulp stimulation were found to be significantly higher in subjects fed a diet supplemented with tryptophan than in those subjects given a control diet [195]. The administration of 5-hydroxytryptophan (150 mg/day) was found to lower significantly pain scores and distress levels in patients with chronic deafferentation and central pain [196].

3. Acupuncture and Brain Stimulation

This section deals briefly with two non-drug-oriented approaches for treatment of pain. These both appear to exert at least part of their effect secondary to release of endogenous opioid peptides.

In Sec. IV.B we will discuss the mechanism of action of exogenous opioids that appear to activate a descending inhibitory gate system to the spinal cord from the periqueductal grey matter via the nucleus raphe magnus. Electrical stimulation at the appropriate brain loci, such as in the periqueductal grey matter or nucleus raphe magnus, will also produce analgesia presumably by activating this same descending gate system. Evidence that endogenous opioids contribute to this stimulation-produced analgesia (SPA) is provided by the observation that naloxone blocks this phenomenon at least partially in both animals [197] and man [198,199]. Levels of endogenous opioids in cerebrospinal fluid, furthermore, are reported to increase after such stimulation [200–202]. There is much similarity between opioid-induced analgesia and SPA, but the latter will probably have more significance for the investigation of the mechanisms of pain and analgesia than it will have practical utility for the treatment of pain, except in special cases. SPA has been reviewed in more detail elsewhere [203–205].

The technique of acupuncture was developed thousands of years ago in China and has only gradually begun to be embraced in America over the last decade. The skepticism of western practitioners of medicine until very recently relegated this technique to the realm of quackery, mysticism, or even downright fraud. Developments over the last decade, however, have confirmed the efficacy of acupuncture against pain and have begun to provide a sound scientific basis for this phenomenon. Increasing numbers of controlled clinical studies are demonstrating that acupuncture is effective for alleviating pain in humans and that this effect can be at least partially antagonized by the opioid antagonist naloxone [206–211]. These same phenomena can be demonstrated also in animal models [212,213]. This modality of pain treatment has been reviewed in more detail elsewhere [214–216].

III. LIMITATIONS OF EXISTING ANALGESICS

A. General Considerations

The complete list of all adverse effects caused by analgesic drugs is extensive. Most of these are relatively rare and/or not particularly limiting to the use of these drugs. Many of these have been discussed in the previous sections. In this section we will discuss in some detail the major limiting effects associated with this class of drugs. These include respiratory depression, abuse liability (psychic and physical dependence), and psychotomimetic effects. Major efforts have been mounted over many decades to attempt separation of analgesic activity from these undesirable phenomena, but success has been limited.

The opioid agonist analgesics as a class are characterized by respiratory depression and addicting qualities as major limiting factors. The mixed agonist-antagonist analgesics as a class are characterized by reduced or altered addicting potential, but this comes at the expense of the introduction of psychotomimetic potential as a major limiting side effect. Opioid antagonists such as naloxone will reverse the respiratory depression and precipitate withdrawal in opioid-dependent subjects but generally will not alter the psychotomimetic phenomena.

The concepts and methodology for assessing abuse potential have been reviewed elsewhere for both animal models [217] and man [218]. Physical dependence or addiction liability have been generally assessed by the substitution method and the direct addiction method. In the substitution method, the ability of the compound to maintain previously established physical dependence on morphine is evaluated. This is generally measured by the ability of single doses of the test compound to suppress abstinence in morphine-dependent subjects. The human subjects used in these studies were generally dependent upon 30–240 mg morphine sulfate daily. In the direct addiction method, the ability of the compound to produce physical dependence after repeated administration over a long period is evaluated. The usual procedure in man has been to use doses of test compound equally effective to morphine and to attain maximum stabilization doses equivalent to 240 mg of morphine per day. The abstinence syndrome has been measured by the Himmelsbach point system [218].

The animal pharmacology of the opioid agonists is discussed in the reviews of these agents cited in Sec. II.A. We will concentrate here on the reports of clinical pharmacology. Some animal pharmacology will be presented, however, in the discussions of the mixed opioid agonist-antagonist analgesics to follow.

B. Discussion of Specific Analgesics

1. Morphine

Morphine depresses respiration at clinically effective doses [219–221]. The response of the brain stem respiratory centers to an increase in blood carbon dioxide tension is decreased. Morphine also reduces the excitability of the centers regulating respiratory rhythmicity [222–224]. The rate of respiration is affected more than tidal volume initially, but at higher doses periodic breathing and apnea occur [224]. Patients who are given large doses of morphine frequently become indifferent to their respiratory status, but will breathe when instructed to do so [224].

In man, physical dependence on morphine has been demonstrated following oral, subcutaneous [225], and intravenous administration [226] in as little as 18 days. Abrupt withdrawal of morphine is accompanied by the development of an abstinence syndrome which begins 8 hr after the last dose of morphine and reaches peak intensity on the second or third day of withdrawal. The intensity of this syndrome decreases slowly through a period of 4–10 weeks, while there is a secondary phase that persists for at least 6 months. The morphine withdrawal syndrome is characterized by abnormal pain, irritability, cold sweats, gooseflesh, diarrhea, nausea, and vomiting. The severity of these symptoms has been described as being uncomfortable and comparable to a severe case of flu, but these effects are not life-threatening in otherwise healthy individuals.

The intensity of the abstinence syndrome following the abrupt withdrawal of morphine was found to be directly related to the maintenance dose of morphine [227]. This abstinence syndrome can be ameliorated by the readministration of morphine in a dose-related manner [228–230].

2. Meperidine

Meperidine depresses respiration in man when given in therapeutic doses [37,221,231–236]. In equianalgesic doses, meperidine appears to produce the same degree of respiratory depression as does morphine [37]. Peak respiratory depression occurs 1 hr after dosing and lasts for approximately 2 hr, although minute volume may be depressed for as long as 4 hr [237].

Meperidine produces morphinelike subjective effects in nondependent subjects at one-seventh to one-fourth the potency of morphine [238]. In morphine-dependent subjects, meperidine substitution was found to only partially suppress the abstinence syndrome, and after 10 days of substitution its termination resulted in the occurrence of mild abstinence signs of more abrupt onset but with less subjective complaints than morphine withdrawal [228,239]. The chronic administration of meperidine in doses of 1–3 g/day in direct addiction studies produced muscular twitches and tremors, hyperactive reflexes, startle responses, seizures, and toxic psychoses [239]. Abrupt withdrawal from 2800 mg of meperidine daily resulted in an abstinence syndrome characterized by a greater degree of restlessness and muscular twitching than in morphine abstinence, but less autonomic dysfunction [240]. In studies of precipitated abstinence, 15 mg of nalorphine induced an abstinence syndrome in subjects dependent upon 1600–2800 mg of meperidine daily [240]. Meperidine seems to have an abuse potential between that of morphine and that of codeine [218].

3. Codeine

Codeine, like morphine, produces respiratory depression by reducing the responsiveness of the brain respiratory centers to carbon dioxide. In healthy subjects, 60 mg of codeine was found to be a potent respiratory depressant by both the oral and parenteral routes; this dose was less effective than 10 mg of morphine, intramuscularly, but 95.6 mg of codeine produced a similar degree of respiratory depression as 10 mg of morphine [241–243]. The administration of 120 mg of codeine subcutaneously to normal subjects affected respiration to the same extent as 10 mg of morphine [24,244]. In 125 patients with postoperative pain, 120 mg of codeine decreased respiratory minute volume to 71% of the initial value [245].

Single oral doses of 75 mg have been found to produce mild to moderate morphinelike effects in man [246]. Morphinelike subjective effects have been reported at 130–520 mg of codeine [247]. Single doses of codeine will ameliorate the morphine abstinence syndrome. In one study, subjects physically dependent upon morphine were gradually transferred to parenteral codeine and maintained on it for 2 weeks [248]. Doses of 240–600 mg of codeine were needed to substitute for 50–150 mg of morphine. When the codeine was terminated, an abstinence syndrome was observed that differed from morphine only in the delayed appearance of severe symptoms. Subcutaneous morphine has been reported to be about 15 times more potent than oral codeine in suppressing morphine abstinence [225].

Codeine has also been studied in direct addiction experiments [246,251]. The abrupt withdrawal of daily codeine after 60 days of administration resulted in an abstinence syndrome. In eight subjects with previous narcotic experience, the average daily dose of codeine obtained was approximately 1500 mg. When these subjects were challenged with nalorphine after 30–45 days of dosing, a mild to moderate abstinence syndrome was obtained.

4. Dextropropoxyphene

Dextropoxyphene does not depress respiration in therapeutic doses of 32 or 65 mg [242]. Even oral doses of 130 mg in normal subjects produced no changes in respiratory response to carbon dioxide [249], but in cases of large overdose, marked depression of respiration has been reported [74].

The effects of single oral dextropropoxyphene doses have been investigated in nonaddicted patients [229]. Minimal effects were seen with doses of 50–300 mg, but at doses of 355–650 mg patients liked the subjective effects and related them to heroin, morphine, or cocaine. Nausea, vomiting, and sedation were consistently present when the 650-mg doses of dextropropoxyphene were given.

Oral doses of dextropropoxyphene reduced the intensity of 24-hr abstinence in patients dependent upon 240–280 mg of morphine daily, but it was found less effective than codeine in this regard [229]. More recently oral dextropropoxyphene napsylate and dextropropoxyphene hydrochloride were assessed in subjects dependent upon 60 mg/day morphine [250]. It was estimated that the hydrochloride was approximately 1/24 and the napsylate approximately 1/49 as potent as morphine in suppressing abstinence.

Direct addiction experiments have been conducted also with dextropropoxyphene [229]. Five volunteers were given dextropropoxyphene for a 54-day period, with four of the subjects attaining a daily dosage of 825 mg and the remaining patient completing the study at a dose of 600 mg. During the first 2 or 3 days, all subjects liked the drug and related its effects to those of morphine, heroin, and marijuana. Their behavior resembled that of patients given an opiate. Subsequently, these patients began to complain about drowsiness, constipation, nausea, and vomiting. When the dextropropoxyphene dosing was discontinued after 54 days of treatment, all subjects complained of weakness and aching. Objective signs of abstinence were mild in nature and included yawning and rhinorrhea. The average daily Himmelsbach withdrawal scores during the first 5 days after the termination of dextropropoxyphene were 13, 14, 8, 8, and 7 points, respectively. Following withdrawl of codeine, the Himmelsbach scores were 11, 33, 30, 20, and 14 points [251].

The nalorphine-induced withdrawal syndrome from dextropropoxyphene is mild in comparison to that observed with morphine and the mixed agonist-antagonist agents. Limited morphinelike abstinence signs were observed in two of five subjects treated chronically with dextropropoxyphene at maximal doses above 600 mg daily for 54 days, followed by 10 mg of the narcotic antagonist nalorphine [229]. Patients with chronic pain given therapeutic doses of dextropropoxyphene for up to 6 months did not show significant signs of narcotic withdrawal when challenged with nalorphine [62,252].

The above studies indicate that dextropropoxyphene has a liability for physical dependence lower than that of codeine.

5. Pentazocine

Depression of respiration by pentazocine has been demonstrated in dogs [253] and rabbits [254,255]. In the rabbit, the depression of respiration did not become more severe as the total dose increased [254,255]. By either the intramuscular or the intravenous routes, pentazocine at 200 mg and morphine at 10 mg were observed to depress respiration to the same extent [93,256,257]. Pentazocine has also been reported to exert a similar degree of respiratory depression as meperidine following intramuscular [259] or intravenous administration [260,261]. Upon repeated dosing, however, ventilatory depression developed at a greater rate after meperidine than after pentazocine [262,263]. A ceiling effect for the respiratory despressant action of pentazocine occurs at about 30 mg [264,265]. The depression of respiration can be antagonized by naloxone [258].

Mice treated chronically with pentazocine do not exhibit withdrawal jumping when challenged with naloxone as do morphine-dependent mice [266]. Pentazocine does not suppress withdrawal weight loss or defecation in morphine-dependent rats [267], nor will pentazocine suppress abstinence in the morphine-dependent dog [268]. Pentazocine suppressed abstinence in monkeys dependent upon low doses of morphine but precipitated abstinence in monkeys dependent on higher morphine doses [269]. Chronically administered pentazocine produced physical dependence in monkeys, with both the precipitated and abrupt withdrawal syndromes being qualitatively different from those observed for morphine [134]. Pentazocine was found to maintain self-administration behavior in monkeys [270,271] and rats [272].

In man, pentazocine in low doses produced morphinelike subjective effects that were limited by side effects as the doses were increased [273]. Pentazocine would not substitute for morphine in subjects dependent on 240 mg of morphine per day [273]. Based upon these findings, it was concluded that pentazocine had an abuse liability lower than that of codeine. Following the introduction of pentazocine, however, reports of abuse began to appear. In a reassessment of the abuse potential of pentazocine [274], it was found that low (40 mg or less) parenteral doses of pentazocine produced morphinelike subjective effects, whereas in higher doses the effects were nalorphinelike. The abstinence symptoms in subjects dependent upon 60 mg or 240 mg/day of morphine were not suppressed by pentazocine [274]. In nonwithdrawn subjects dependent upon morphine (240 mg daily), pentazocine precipitated an abstinence syndrome.

In direct addiction studies, the abrupt withdrawal of pentazocine resulted in a mild abstinence syndrome with both morphine- and nalorphinelike features [274]. Similarly, when those subjects maintained on pentazocine were given naloxone, an abstinence syndrome of moderate severity was precipitated [274]. These results suggested that pentazocine has an abuse potential that is less than that of morphine but greater than that of nalorphine [274]. Within the past several years, pentazocine has become popular with addicts when taken in combination with the antihistamine, tripelennamine. When these drugs are combined in an intravenous injection, the result is an immediate rush similar to that obtained from heroin [275].

Psychotomimetic effects consisting of hallucinations, weird thoughts, pronounced dreaming, feelings of impending doom, anxiety, and depersonalization have been reported in patients given a wide range of intramuscular, intravenous, or oral doses of pentazocine. In the early studies on the analgesic activity of pentazocine, psychotomimetic side effects were reported only rarely. Many of the dysphoric side effects noted in these studies were thought to be a sign of pentazocine-precipitated withdrawal in patients who had previously been treated with narcotics. It has been difficult for investigators to determine whether, in patients previously treated with narcotics, dysphoric reactions after pentazocine represent borderline precipitated withdrawal, a direct psychotomimetic effect of pentazocine, or a combination of both [82]. The psychotomimetic reactions observed after pentazocine administration occur more frequently with higher doses [91,274,276–278]. All subjects given 120–140 mg in direct addiction studies experienced these reactions [274]. Psychotomimetic reactions have occurred also, however, in patients treated with intramuscular doses between 20 mg and 60 mg [80,82,91,93,279] or oral doses between 35 mg and 75 mg [51,87,280,281]. Susceptibility to these reactions varies among patients. Patients with severe chronic pain appear to be more sensitive to this side effect [82,100,101,277].

6. Nalbuphine

Nalbuphine (10 mg/kg) has been reported to produce respiratory depression approximately equal to that produced by an equal dose of morphine [282,283]. A ceiling effect for respiratory depression, however, was observed with high doses of nalbuphine given in intravenous increments. Cumulative doses of nalbuphine to 60 mg/70 kg were found not to depress respiration below the plateau established at 30 mg/70 kg [283]. A similar observation was made in a recent study in which the analgesic and respiratory effects of nalbuphine and morphine were assessed concurrently [284]. The ceiling effect of nalbuphine on respiration was paralleled by a limited analgesic effect in experimental pain.

In rats trained to discriminate between saline and two doses of morphine, nalbuphine generalized to the lower morphine dose but not the higher morphine dose [285]. In morphine-trained squirrel monkeys, on the other hand, nalbuphine did not produce morphinelike stimulus control [286]. Nalbuphine was self-administered in rats previously dependent upon morphine, but withdrawal of nalbuphine did not produce an abstinence syndrome [272].

Nalbuphine has been administered for a 1-week period at a daily dose of 40 mg to human subjects with a history of narcotic abuse [282]. Morphinelike effects were noted during the treatment period. Toward the end of the experiment, the subjects were challenged with levallorphan, which resulted in the appearance of subjective effects suggestive of a mild abstinence syndrome. After another dose, the nalbuphine was abruptly withdrawn and the subjects observed for withdrawal signs. None of the subjects exhibited any signs of withdrawal.

In another study [287], low doses nalbuphine produced morphinelike subjective effects, whereas nalorphinelike effects were observed at higher doses. In morphine-dependent patients, nalbuphine exhibited antagonist activity. Nalbuphine's ability to produce physical dependence was assessed by the administration of increasing doses of drug for a 51-day period. When naloxone was administered, it precipitated a definite abstinence syndrome. Similarly, when placebo was substituted for nalbuphine, the subjects experienced a moderate abstinence syndrome. The abstinence syndrome had both morphine- and nalorphinelike characteristics and an intensity greater than that with nalorphine or pentazocine.

Psychotomimetic reactions have been reported with nalbuphine. They appear to occur less frequently than with pentazocine [100,101, 284].

7. Butorphanol

Butorphanol was observed to depress respiration in animal studies, but there was a ceiling to this effect wherein increasing doses of butorphanol did not further increase the effect on p CO_2 and pH [106,107]. Low doses of butorphanol also depressed respiration in human volunteers. Similar to the animal studies, however, the degree of respiratory depression plateaued as the dose of butorphanol was increased [288,

289]. In patients undergoing diagnostic cardiac catheterization, butorphanol was found to produce the same degree of respiratory depression as does morphine [290]. The difference between butorphanol and morphine appears to occur only at the higher end of the dose-response curve.

Butorphanol exhibited a lower physical dependence liability than morphine, pentazocine, or dextropropoxyphene in several animal models of physical dependence. These included naloxone-precipitated mouse jumping and suppression of abstinence in morphine-dependent rodents [107,291]. Although butorphanol was self-administered in rats with a history of morphine dependence, there were no withdrawal signs upon termination of the butorphanol, which is consistent with this compound having a low liability for producing dependence [272].

During direct addiction studies in man, butorphanol produced a number of opiatelike symptoms such as constipation, nausea, and difficulty in urinating [292]. After 35 days of dosing with butorphanol, saline was substituted resulting in patient reports of typical morphine-like withdrawal symptoms. Additionally, the patients reported symptoms of the nalorphine type. A peak Himmelsbach score of 26 suggested that the withdrawal syndrome was greater than with pentazocine but less than with morphine, for which scores of 16 and 37, respectively, were reported [292].

Euphoria, dysphoria, paranoia, and hallucinations have occasionally occurred during butorphanol administration, as have feelings of floating, depersonalization, and distorted body image [100,110,111, 132,292].

8. Buprenorphine

Studies in mice, rats [133,136,137] and rabbits [293] showed that buprenorphine decreases respiratory rate. A plateau was observed in the dose-response curves, above which higher doses produced the same or less respiratory depression. The duration of respiratory depression became less as the dose of buprenorphine increased, which is in marked contrast to what is seen with morphine [136,137].

A ceiling effect to the respiratory depressant activity of buprenorphine has also been observed in human volunteers [294–296]. Several studies have indicated that at approximately equianalgesic doses morphine and buprenorphine exert about the same degree of respiratory depression [295–298]. Other investigators have reported that intravenous doses of buprenorphine produced greater depression of the respiratory response to carbon dioxide stimulation than did equianalgesic doses of morphine [299,300]. Very high doses of naloxone only partially reverse the respiratory depressant effects of buprenorphine

[295–298]. A temporary reversal of buprenorphine has been achieved by administration of the respiratory stimulant doxapram [295,296].

Buprenorphine was found not to substitute in rats undergoing morphine withdrawal [301–303] but did substitute in the chronic spinal dog [268,304]. Direct addiction experiments have been conducted in rodents [133], dogs [268], monkeys [133,134,305]. In a mouse precipitated abstinence test, buprenorphine produced less jumping than did morphine, codeine, or pentazocine [133]. In the dog, withdrawal of buprenorphine resulted in a slowly emerging withdrawal syndrome of a mild nature [286]. No signs of abstinence were observed in monkeys treated with a narcotic antagonist or abruptly withdrawn from buprenorphine treatment [133,134,305]. Monkeys self-administered buprenorphine at a rate below that for codeine but greater than for nalorphine or pentazocine [306].

Direct addiction studies have been conducted in man at a daily dose of 8 mg for up to 50 days [292,307–309]. Both observers and subjects identified buprenorphine as being morphinelike. Naloxone (4 mg) did not produce withdrawal in these subjects. Abrupt termination of drug administration resulted in a slowly emerging abstinence syndrome which at peak intensity, 13 days later, was similar to that seen for codeine, nalorphine, pentazocine, and butorphanol.

Confusion and depression have occasionally been reported following buprenorphine administration, as have euphoria and hallucinations [151]. The occurrence of mental confusion following chronic administration has been found in some subjects discontinuing treatment [153].

C. Needs and Criteria for New Analgesics

Ideally, we would like to develop a potent new analgesic agent that has good bioavailability after oral or parenteral administration, little respiratory depressant or psychotomimetic activity, and negligible abuse liability and does not introduce important new limitations such as marked hemodynamic activity. There is a place, however, for new compounds that are less than the ideal but offer significant advantages in particular circumstances.

The majority of the new introductions to the analgesic armamentarium have been mixed agonist-antagonists. They are generally effective analgesics with a relatively low abuse potential. They lack, however, the full efficacy of the pure agonists, important for anaesthetic uses and other situations involving severe pain, and their antagonistic properties complicate the use of the stronger analgesics to supplement their analgesia. Their side effects, furthermore, are similar to those of the stronger pure agonist analgesics, and they may in addition produce psychotomimetic reactions.

Far more desirable would be the development of a strong pure agonist with diminished abuse potential and without limiting respiratory depressant, psychotomimetic, or hemodynamic effects. Is this possible? The discovery of the endogenous opioid peptides raised expectations for the ideal analgesic without addicting qualities, that were shortly discouraged by reports of tolerance and physical dependence subsequent to chronic central administration of various of these opioid peptides [310,311]. The optimism and subsequent pessimism were probably both somewhat exaggerated and premature. There is still promise for improvement grounded in the development of receptor-specific ligands. The mixed agonist-antagonist analgesics presented a diminished abuse liability. This has been attributed to providing analgesia via κ-receptors in the spinal cord. Agents active on these receptors have been associated, however, with psychotomimetic activity. There is now evidence that there are δ-receptors for analgesia in the spinal cord, as well as, or rather than, the κ-receptors. Perhaps a specific δ-agonist will provide potent analgesia with greatly diminished abuse liability and without the psychotomimetic effects. The experimental tools are now available for developing such an agent.

Alternatively, there is also now evidence for nonopioid mechanisms of endogenous analgesia. Perhaps elucidation of the mechanisms of these forms of analgesia and the development of their therapeutic potential, will provide the ideal analgesic without respiratory depressant activity, abuse potential, or psychotomimetic activity.

Barring the development of the ideal analgesic, however, there are still many areas where lesser improvements would be of value. There is need for a better analgesic for general anesthesia and for postoperative care [312]. A potent but short-acting analgesic, that could be infused during short operations and had negligible psychotomimetic or hemodynamic activity, for example, could be a useful development. An effective analgesic agent, that does not cross the placental barrier could be an important contribution to obstetric analgesia.

Therapy for chronic pain is still inadequate [313,314]. This is not an insignificant problem. Nearly one-third of the population of industrialized nations have chronic pain; and in 1981 this "disease" cost the American people over 65 billion dollars for health care services, loss of work productivity, compensation, and related factors [314].

IV. MODE OF ACTION

A. Animal Models

We have already discussed the prevailing treatments for pain (analgesics) without defining pain or analgesia. This takes on more importance as we contemplate the objective measurement of experimental pain and analgesia. Pain has been defined as a more or less localized unpleasant sensation of discomfort, of varying degrees of severity, resulting from stimulation of specialized nerve endings consequent upon injury or disease or from central neuronal or emotional disorder. Analgesia has been defined more simply as the relief of pain without loss of consciousness. An analgesic is a drug that accomplishes this. This picture is complicated by the fact that the pain experience includes not only the sensations of discomfort but also the reactions to those sensations.

The development of a new technique or drug must begin with animal models. The analgesic researcher provides such models by applying an unpleasant or noxious stimulus to an animal and measuring aspects of the resulting behavioral responses that the animal makes to terminate or escape the unpleasant stimulus. This approach can provide an objective measurement but it may not be clear whether the behavioral response changes that are measured reflect changes in sensation or reaction, nor which might be the better predictor of useful analgesia in man.

The stimuli used may be mechanical, electrical, chemical, or thermal. The following is a very brief overview of several of the test systems most frequently used to assess potential new analgesics. In most laboratories engaged in the discovery of new analgesics a battery of such tests is generally utilized. There are also other methods that have been used to assess pain and analgesia and, for those who are interested, a more detailed discussion of this topic is provided in a recent review [315].

1. Mouse Writhing Test

The most common procedure for this test is to inject mice intraperitoneally with an irrritant such as phenylquinone or acetic acid and count the number of writhes induced over some subsequent time period. Both centrally and peripherally acting analgesics will reduce the number of writhes elicited. Despite the lack of specificity for centrally acting opioid analgesics and the uncertain relationship of this response to pain, this test is very useful since it is simple and fast to run and therefore serves as a convenient first screen for compounds that may have either central or peripheral analgesic activity. The use of narcotic antagonists in this test, furthermore, will differentiate central analgesics from a peripheral mechanism.

2. Tail Flick Test

This test is generally conducted with rats or mice. Radiant heat from a light source is focussed on a spot on the tail, and the time is measured until the animal flicks its tail to escape the heat stimulus. Centrally acting opioid analgesics increase this time period in a dose-dependent manner, and this effect is blocked by naloxone. This is a reflexive response mediated at the spinal level.

3. Hot Plate Test

This test is conducted most satisfactorily with mice but may be run with rats also. The most common procedure for this test is to place the test animal on a surface maintained at a noxious temperature (49–55°C, most commonly 55°C) and then measure the latency to the first incidence of hind paw licking and/or escape jumping. These responses reflect processes occurring at supraspinal levels and the two end points may distinguish perceptive versus reactive components of pain. Centrally acting opioid analgesics increase the latencies to these responses in a dose-dependent manner, and these effects are blocked by naloxone.

4. Shock Titration

This is a system for assessing pain and analgesia that is based on learned behavior and is generally conducted in rat or monkey. In this paradigm, cognitive decisions about painful stimili are made and measured because subjects are able to respond on a lever to maintain levels of potentially noxious stimuli (generally electric shock) at acceptable levels. Opioid analgesics increase acceptable levels in dose-dependent manner, and this effect can be blocked by naloxone.

5. In Vitro Assays

There are also several in vitro systems that provide surprisingly good predictions of analgesic activity. These include the isolated guinea pig ileum strip and mouse vas deferens preparations. The electrically induced contractions of these tissues are inhibited in a dose-dependent manner by opioid analgesics, and this inhibitory effect is antagonized by naloxone. The guinea pig ileum contains predominantly μ-receptors and the mouse vas deferens predominantly δ-receptors, so that the combined use of these preparations provides an assessment of the receptor type preference of active compounds. The rabbit vas deferens may contain a predominance of κ-receptors [316] and, thus, combined with the previous tissues discussed, provides a more complete assessment of receptor preference. Binding assays in brain homogenate with the appropriate labeled ligand can also provide an assesssment of the relative affinities of opioid analgesic candidates for the μ-, δ-, or κ-receptors in brain. The labeled ligands generally used to define these receptors are [^{3}H]naloxone or [^{3}H]dihydromorphine for the μ-receptors, [^{3}H]D-Ala^2-D-Leu^5-enkephalin for the δ-receptors, and [^{3}H]ethylketocyclazocine for the κ-receptors. A more detailed discussion of these in vitro assay systems is provided in several reviews [317,318].

B. Sites and Mechanism of Action

Painful stimuli are detected by peripheral receptors (nociceptors) at the site of the stimulus, and this information is transmitted via the spinal cord to various higher centers where it is perceived (at both conscious and subconscious levels), processed, and reacted to. The "reaction" consists of autonomic, somatic, and psychological components. This description is very simplistic, but the mechanisms and neuronal circuitry of this array of phenomena in response to a painful stimulus are very complex and not yet well understood. It seems to the present authors that the most desirable "analgesic" action would selectively remove the psychological suffering component of pain while leaving other components which may have some protective function, intact. Indeed, it has been suggested that this is much the way opioid analgesics might work [1], but this is not altogether clear and well established. We know very little, unfortunately, about the neurophysiological/neuroanatomical/neurochemical distinctions between these various components of reaction to painful stimuli, and very few studies of pain and analgesia, particularly in laboratories screening for new analgesic drugs, have attempted to distinguish the various components. In fact, many existing analgesics were "discovered" by their actions on a spinal reflexive response to noxious stimuli. Nevertheless, we may actually now understand the mechanisms of opioid analgesic actions better than the mechanisms of pain itself, although again at a very simplistic level.

Numerous sites in the central nervous system have been identified where opioid analgesics act to modulate perception of painful stimuli. These sites have been mapped using the technique of microinjection of opioids into stereotactically located brain regions [203,319–321]. The major supraspinal sites involved include the periaqueductal-periventricular gray, nucleus reticularis giganto-cellularis, medial thalamus, mesencephalic reticular formation, lateral hypothalamus, and raphe nuclei. The specific role of each of these sites is not yet clear, but it is generally believed that one mechanism of morphinelike analgesia is to initiate descending supraspinal inhibition of the pain input at the spinal level. Thus, opioids may induce this descending inhibition by direct action at any one or more of the sites listed. Opioids might also act to diminish the emotional-affective component of pain by some action confined to the supraspinal sites, but this has not yet been demonstrated. It has been demonstrated, however, that opioids may also act directly at the spinal level to produce analgesia [322]. All the areas noted as sites for the direct action of opioid analgesics are further characterized by being rich in endogenous opioid peptides and their receptors. These will be discussed in the next section. It seems probable that opioid analgesics produce analgesia by mimicking endogenous opioid peptides at their receptor.

The mechanism of opioid analgesia mentioned above is well illustraed by a discussion of the actions of opioids in the region of the periaqueductal gray matter (PAG). The functions of this brain region in pain and analgesia have been amply studied over the last decade [203, 204, 321]. Microinjection of opioids or electrical stimulation in this region both produce analgesia which can be antagonized at least partially by naloxone [197–199, 323–325]. Opioids are inhibitory on single neurons in the PAG [326–329] yet increase multiunit activity in this region [330], which suggests they have a disinhibitory action here resulting in an increased output of neuronal activity. There is both anatomical and electrophysiological evidence [331-334] for a direct connection from PAG to nucleus raphe magnus (NRM) and stimulation in the PAG [204] or administration of morphine, either systemically [335] or directly into the PAG [336], all excite neurons in the NRM. Excitation of either the PAG or NRM, furthermore, inhibits spinothalamic neurons and produces analgesia [337–340]. The above findings all support the hypothesis that opioids act on opioid peptide receptors in the PAG to activate a descending inhibition to the spinal cord via the nucleus raphe magnus. This scheme provides some neuroanatomical specificity to the gate control theory of Melzack and Wall [341]. A more detailed discussion of these matters is presented in several reviews [203–205]. There is evidence, furthermore, that there are both opioid and nonopioid forms of endogenous analgesic systems [342, 343] and that other neurotransmitter systems besides opioid peptidergic, such as serotonergic, function in these pathways. These other systems will be discussed further in a later section as they relate to opportunities for development of new analgesic entities.

C. Endogenous Opioids

Endogenous opioids are, for the most part, peptides, although there are reports of a nonpeptide endogenous opioid [344]. The term "endorphin" is synonymous with endogenous opioid and it is used similarly to designate the whole class of such compounds. The first identified endogenous opioids were the pentapeptides (shown in Fig. 1.3) methionine (Met)- and leucine (Leu)-enkaphalin [345]. Other larger endogenous opioid peptides, such as β-endorphin and dynorphin, have been discovered since [346–349]. β-Endorphin has potent analgesic activity if injected

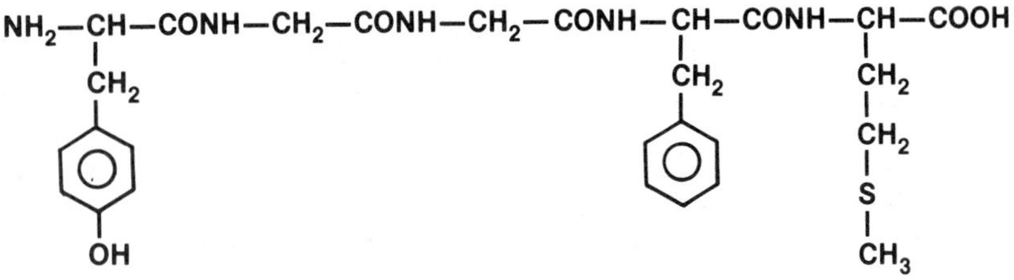

NH_2—CH—CONH—CH_2—CONH—CH_2—CONH—CH—CONH—CH—COOH

Tyr^1—Gly^2—Gly^3—Phe^4—Met^5—OH

FIG. 1.3 Structure of the endogenous opiod pentapeptide Met^5-enkephalin. The other endogenous opioid pentapeptide, Leu^5-enkephalin, has leucine in place of methionine (Met) in the 5-position. Tyr = tyrosine; Gly = glycine; Phe = phenylalanine.

directly to appropriate sites in brain [350,351], but the development of new analgesic entities has concentrated on the modification of the pentapeptide enkephalins. The present discussion will focus on these substances. The thrust of this discussion will be to provide some background on these materials and to provide evidence for a role for them in nociceptive processes.

A number of studies have made it clear that the enkephalins and β-endorphin have distinctly different distributions throughout the brain and the periphery [352–355]. Enkephalin cell bodies and terminals are broadly distributed throughout the central nervous system [356,357], and this distribution generally parallels that of the opioid receptors [358].

A large precursor protein or glycoprotein of 31 kilodaltons (proopiomelanocortin) has been identified [359] as the source of β-endorphin. There is also evidence for a distinct large common precursor for Met- and Leu-enkephalin. This precursor is referred to as either proenkephalin [360] or pre-proenkephalin [361]. This protein is composed of 263 amino acids, has a molecular weight of about 30,000, and contains four copies of metkephalin and one copy of Leu-enkephalin, each bounded by paired basic residues. The large precursor was isolated from chromaffin granules in the adrenal medulla but is suspected to exist in the brain also [362–364]. A calcium-dependent release of the enkephalins has been demonstrated from several brain regions, including globus pallidus and corpus striatum [365,366]. Among the enzymes that can digest the enkephalins are amino peptidases, carboxypeptidase A, and dipeptidylcarboxypeptidases. A specific dipeptidylcarboxypeptidase, enkephalinase A, is thought to be the means of synaptic inactivation of the enkephalins [367,368].

β-Endorphin and the enkephalins are found in blood and cerebrospinal fluid (csf). Blood levels of β-endorphin derive from the pituitary, whereas csf levels derive from the periventricular system in brain.

The source of Met-enkephalin in plasma appears to be the adrenal glands, whereas cell bodies and nerve terminals distributed throughout the brain synthesize and release enkephalins which find their way into the csf. The levels of these substances are affected by factors such as neuroendocrine disease, stress, exercise, and acupunture or brain stimulation for pain relief. Levels in blood and csf appear to be under separate control and vary differently in response to various factors or conditions. Levels of these materials in the csf may modulate pain or be a reflection of such modulation elsewhere in the brain. Plasma levels are more likely related to some different function.

Various lines of evidence support a role for the endogenous opioids in the modulation of nociceptive processes. Inhibitors of the enzymes that inactivate the enkephalins will potentiate the analgesia produced by exogenous opioid peptides and under the right conditions will by themselves produce analgesic effects that can be blocked by the opioid antagonist naloxone. Naloxone will at least partially block analgesia produced by acupunture, brain stimulation, or exposure to stress, and naloxone will, furthermore, by itself produce hyperalgesic effects. The tonic activity of these endogenous opioid systems, however, appears to be very low and must be activated to express their antinociceptive properties. The above phenomena are discussed in more detail in several recent reviews [205,369].

V. CURRENT TRENDS FOR NEW PAIN TREATMENT

A. New Synthetic Opioids

The structures of these agents are shown in Fig. 1.4.

1. Sufentanil and Alfentanil

Sufentanil, a congener of fentanyl, is an extremely potent analgesic agent; it appears to be 500–1000 times more potent than morphine [370]. It is being investigated as an i.v. anesthetic agent in man. The initial studies of sufentanil anesthesia in man indicate it to be more potent than fentanyl, with qualitatively similar effects [371].

Alfentanil, another congener of fentanyl, is a potent narcotic agonist analgesic, about one-fourth the potency of fentanyl, with an extremely short duration of action and a high margin of safety [372,373]. It is currently undergoing clinical trials as an intravenous anesthetic agent. It remains to be seen whether these new agents will provide any clinically significant advantages over fentanyl.

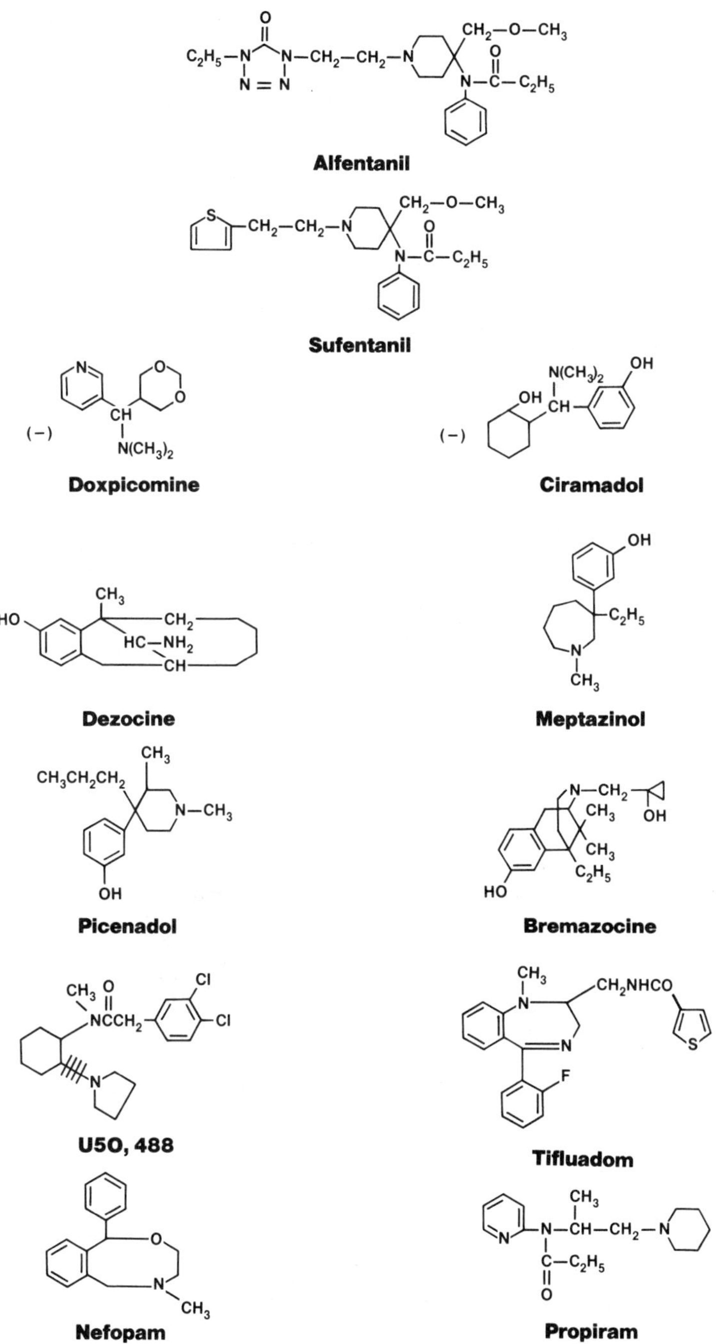

FIG. 1.4 Structures of the newer synthetic opioid analgesic candidates discussed in the text.

2. Doxpicomine

Doxpicomine is the hydrochloride salt of 1,3-[(dimethylamino)(m-dioxan-5yl)methyl]pyridine, a derivative of substituted 1,3-dioxanes [374,375]. The results of a double-blind trial indicated the analgesic activity of 400mg of intramuscular doxpicomine to be within the range of 8 mg of morphine in postoperative pain [376]. Approximately the same degree of pain relief was achieved with 400 mg of doxpicomine and 100 mg of meperidine [377]. Sedation is the most frequently reported side effect [376, 377]. There have been a few reports of a feeling of well-being after doxpicomine, but the compound appears not to produce nausea or vomiting [376].

3. Ciramadol

Ciramadol is a synthetic mixed agonist-antagonist analgesic with a benzylamine structure [378]. Oral ciramadol appears to be more potent in postoperative pain than pentazocine [379]. In patients with pain of malignant origin, ciramadol at 20 mg and 60 mg orally produced dose-related analgesia [380]. A low incidence of side effects was reported in both these studies.

4. Dezocine

Dezocine is a mixed opioid agonist-antagonist from a series of bridged aminotetralins [381,382]. In postoperative pain, dezocine (10-mg) and meperidine (50 mg) were equipotent when administered parenterally [383]. In a double-blind comparison of dezocine and morphine in postoperative pain from gynecological surgery, dezocine (10 mg) provided analgesia equivalent to morphine (10 mg) by intramuscular injection [384]. A sufficient number of studies have not been conducted to obtain a good indication of the side effect liability of this compound, but no psychotomimetic effects have yet been observed in clinical trials [383,384].

5. Meptazinol

Meptazinol, another mixed opioid agonist-antagonist, has been found effective in a number of studies for the control of moderate to severe pain in man. Analgesic efficacy has been demonstrated in pain from renal colic [385], major abdominal surgery [386–390] and arthritic pain [391]. In patients with postoperative pain, the intramuscular administration of 100 mg of meptazinol was found equianalgesic with 100 mg of meperidine with a similar frequency of side effects [392]. Meptazinol has been reported to have a low liability for producing physical dependence [267,393] and for depressing respiration at clinically effective doses [388,389], but a high incidence of nausea and vomiting has been reported [385,386,388,389].

6. Picenadol

Picenadol is an N-methyl-4-phenylpiperidine derivative, a unique structure for a narcotic with agonist-antagonist properties [394,395]. It is a racemic mixture of a D-optical isomer with potent morphinelike agonist activity and an l-optical isomer exhibiting nalorphinelike activity. Picenadol, the racemate, has a good affinity for both the μ- and the δ-opioid receptor, with the D-isomer having equal affinity for these binding sites [396]. This interesting opioid binding profile, coupled with its good rodent efficacy [396] and low abuse potential [396–398], suggested that it may have a clinical profile different from other mixed agents. It is currently under clinical investigation.

7. Bremazocine

This benzomorphan analog has been reported to be a potent long-acting analgesic in animals [399]. In preclinical studies, it appeared to be free of dependence liability and respiratory depressant action [399]. It has been suggested that it exerts its analgesic activity through the κ-opioid receptor, but it has comparable affinities for the μ- and δ-receptors [399,400].

8. U-50488

U-50488 is a chemically novel analgesic that is reported to be a pure κ-opioid receptor stimulant [401]. Its antinociceptive action in rodents appears to be mediated by a spinal mechanism [401]. Clinical efficacy has not been reported.

9. Tifluadom

Tifluadom is a 1,4-benzodiazepine that does not exhibit any affinity for the benzodiazepine binding site, but is a potent displacer of [^{3}H]bremazocine from its opioid binding site [402]. It has been characterized as a κ-opioid receptor agonist with good preclinical analgesic activity but little or no dependence potential [402]. There are no reports of its activity in clinical pain states.

10. Nefopam

Nefopam hydrochloride (Acupan*®) is a new nonnarcotic analgesic that is unrelated to any known analgesic. The analgesic properties after intramuscular administration of a 20-mg dose of nefopam have been found approximately equivalent to 12 mg of morphine [403,404], 50–100 mg of meperidine [405–407], 0.3 mg of buprenorphine [408], and 30 mg of pentazocine [408–410]. Nefopam has been reported to have a lower liability for depressing respiration than does morphine [411]. The side effects most frequently reported, such as anxiety, restlessness, and sweating appear to be associated with central nervous system stimulation [407,408,412,413]. There have also been reports of nausea [410].

11. Propiram

Propiram fumarate, N-(1-methyl-2-piperdinoethyl)-N-2-pyridyl-propionamide fumarate, is a mixed agonist-antagonist type analgesic with demonstrated efficacy in laboratory animals [414]. Clinical studies have shown that propiram is an effective analgesic in postoperative pain with an oral potency approximately one-tenth that of intramuscular morphine [415–417]. In severe postsurgical pain, 50 mg of oral propiram was found equivalent to 60 mg of oral codeine or 50 mg of oral pentazocine [418]. In postepisiotomy pain, a dose-related analgesia was seen with 50-mg and 100-mg oral doses of propiram that was greater than that seen with 60 mg of codeine [419]. The most common side effects in these studies were drowsiness, nausea, and dizziness. Propiram substituted in subjects dependent upon 60 mg of morphine per day but precipitated withdrawal, indicating antagonist activity, in subjects dependent upon 240 mg of morphine per day [420]. Propiram was also administered chronically to assesss potential for producing physical dependence. Signs of abstinence were observed upon administration of nalorphine and also after abrupt withdrawal [420]. These results suggest that propiram has an abuse potential within the range of pentazocine.

B. Peptides and Derivatives

In Sec. IV.C we briefly described the opioid peptides and the evidence suggesting their role in nociceptive processes. The endogenous opioid

---

*®Trademark.

peptides themselves have little potential utility as clinical analgesics. The enkephalins are too rapidly degraded enzymatically, and the more enzymatically stable β-endorphin does not appear to cross the blood-brain barrier readily enough. β-Endorphin produced marked and long-lasting pain relief in cancer patients with intractable pain when given intrathecally [421] but did not induce analgesia when given intravenously in experimental animals or man [422,423]. There are ways, however, to overcome these problems and develop agents with therapeutic potential. These approaches include attempts to develop inhibitors of the enzymes that inactivate the enkephalins and to develop enkephalin analogs less susceptible to anzymatic degradation than the natural peptides. Such developmental efforts are underway in several laboratories, and available information on progress in these areas will be discussed below. A brief discussion of several other peptides and derivatives with analgesic potential will also be presented.

1. Enzyme Inhibitors

As discussed earlier, there are several categories of enzymes, that will inactivate the enkephalins. The aminopeptidases are very active and effective but appear to be too ubiquitous for inhibitors of these enzymes to provide adequately selective analgesic activity. Carboxypeptidase A has not been considered a major inactiving enzyme for the enkephalins [369]. Nevertheless, D-phenylalanine, a weak inhibitor of carboxypeptidase A [424], has been reported to produce an analgesic effect in both experimental animals and in man [425–428]. It has been suggested that it produces these analgesic effects by increasing brain enkephalin levels secondary to the inhibition of carboxypeptidase [427].

Enkephalinase A (neutral metalloendopeptidase) is apparently located in the synapse [368,429], and efforts have been concentrated on developing inhibitors of its dipeptidyl carboxypeptidase activity as potential analgesic agents. An effective and relatively selective inhibitor of this enzyme, thiorphan, has been synthesized [430]. There are some similarities between enkephalinase A and angiotensin-converting enzyme (ACE), but it has now been clearly established that they are distinct encymes [431]. The structure of thiorphan is shown in Fig. 1.5. Thiorphan has been demonstrated to potentiate the analgesic activity of various enkephalin analogs in several animal models and even produced analgesia on its own under the right conditions [205,369,430].

Thiorphan itself does not appear likely to have clinical utility. Its bioavailability by systemic routes of administration does not appear adequate and the analgesic activity it exerts in the absence of an exogenous opioid peptide is too limited and dependent on conditions such

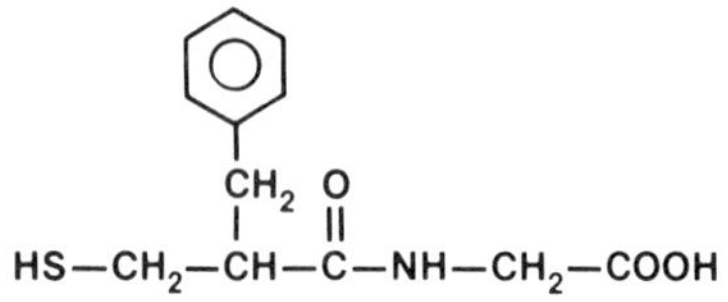

$$\begin{array}{l} \quad\quad\quad\quad\ \ C_6H_5 \\ \quad\quad\quad\quad\ \ | \\ \quad\quad\quad\quad\ CH_2\ \ O \\ \quad\quad\quad\quad\ \ |\quad\ \ \| \\ HS-CH_2-CH-C-NH-CH_2-COOH \end{array}$$

FIG. 1.5 Structure of the enkephalinase inhibitor, thiorphan (3-mercapto-2-benzylpropionyl glycine).

as the time of day, the pain model being utilized, and the state of the experimental subject. This relative lack of direct analgesic activity may be due to a very low basal activity of the enkephalinergic systems. If clinical pain were to activate these systems, however, such a compound might have very desirable clinical utility that might not be predicted by standard analgesic model systems. No such compound has yet entered clinical trial to our knowledge, but efforts are in progress in a number of laboratories to develop one.

2. Enkephalin Derivatives

Although an intact and active endogenous opioid analgesic system would be necessary to achieve the desired result with an enzyme inhibitor, this would not be a requirement for a direct-acting opioid receptor ligand. The multiple opioid receptor concept, which has been supported by the demonstation of multiple endogenous opioid ligands, provides the theoretical basis for developing receptor-selective analgesic structures devoid of physical dependence, respiratory depression, psychotomimetic effects, or other unwanted side effects. There are also other potential advantages of these new peptide-based analgesic structures and these will be discussed as we proceed with this section. Since the natural opioids are too labile to have therapeutic utility, the research challenge has been to develop analogs with desirable receptor selectivity together with sufficient bioavailability to achieve effective concentrations at the appropriate receptors in brain. Since high activity resides in the enkephalinlike pentapeptide and tetrapeptide sequences, the preparation of analogs of these or even smaller fragments is more feasible and efficient than analogs of the larger endorphins. Hundreds of such analogs have been synthesized, and considerable structure activity data have already been discussed [432,433].

Two analogs of Met-enkephalin are of particular interest because they have progressed to the clinic. These are FK 33-824 and metkephamid (LY127623) and are shown in Fig. 1.6.

FK 33-824 (Sandoz)

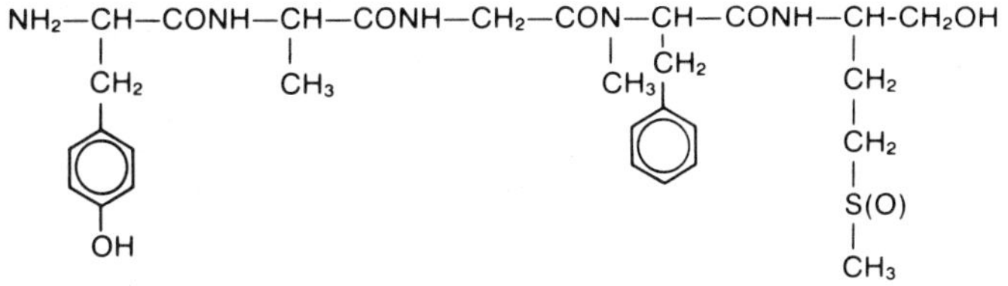

NH₂—CH—CONH—CH—CONH—CH₂—CON—CH—CONH—CH-CH₂OH

(side chains: CH₂–C₆H₄–OH; CH₃; CH₃ (on N); CH₂–C₆H₅; CH₂–CH₂–S(O)–CH₃)

LY127623 (Metkephamid, Lilly)

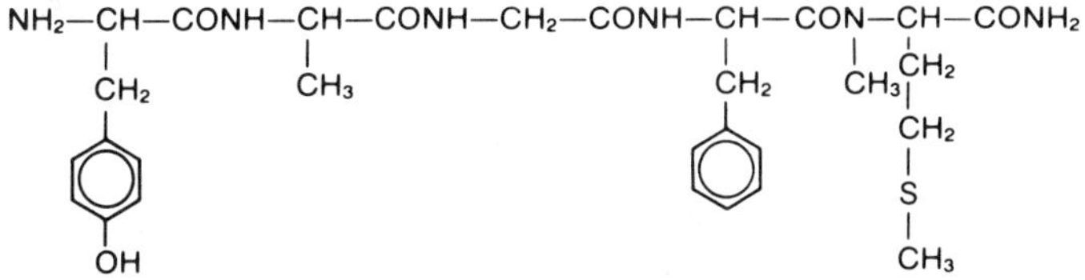

NH₂—CH—CONH—CH—CONH—CH₂—CONH—CH—CON—CH—CONH₂

(side chains: CH₂–C₆H₄–OH; CH₃; CH₂–C₆H₅; CH₃ (on N); CH₂–CH₂–S–CH₃)

FIG. 1.6 Structures of the two Met5-enkephalin analogs, FK33-824 and LY127623, which have been evaluated in clinical studies as potential analgesics.

The work with these two enkephalin analogs has confirmed the important concept that appropriate modification of the natural enkephalin structure can produce systemically active analgesic agents.

a. FK 33-824. This compound showed high activity at opioid receptors in vitro and demonstrated some slight preference for the μ-receptor compared with the δ-receptor [434]. In in vivo tests for analgesia, FK 33-824 was 100–1000 times more potent than morphine when given by the intraventricular route and was active also as an analgesic in these animal tests after systemic administration [435]. Naloxone precipitated a marked withdrawal syndrome in monkeys self-administering this compound [435].

The first report of the effects of a modified opioid peptide in man was that of Graffenried et al [436] who examined FK 33-824 in normal male volunteers. After 0.1–1.2 mg administered intramuscularly, all subjects in this study experienced a "feeling of heaviness in all the muscles of the body, often combined with a feeling of oppression in the chest or tightness in the throat which induced a certain amount of anxiety." Other symptoms noted were a marked increase in bowel sounds, redness of face, injection of the conjunctiva, chemosis, whole body flush, rhinitis vasomotorica, and a flare reaction after intradermal injection. Plasma prolactin and growth hormone were increased. Expected morphinelike effects, such as changes in emotional behavior or mental alertness, formication, and nausea, were not observed, and the unexpected signs were not blocked by opioid, histamine, serotonin, or cholinergic antagonists. The lack of blockade with nalorphine, a mixed agonist-antagonist, suggested to the authors that the effects were not mediated by opioid receptors, but a subsequent report [437] claimed that the hormonal effects and other side effects could be blocked by the pure opioid antagonist naloxone.

There have been no reports of the evaluation of intramuscularly administered FK 33-824 in pathological pain, but it was reported to have analgesic activity against experimental pain in man [438]. A single intramuscular dose of 1 mg produced a significant increase in tolerance to electrically evoked pain but caused no change in threshold to pain. Neither 0.5 mg nor 1.0 mg of FW 34-569, an [*N*-Me]Tyr^1 analog of FK 33-824, influenced pain threshold in human volunteers subjected to a hot plate analgesimeter, but both doses stimulated growth hormone and prolactin release and inhibited the release of cortisol and LH [439]. FK 33-824 did have an analgesic effect in subjects with postoperative pain after epidural administration (0.02–0.5 mg), but the effect was rated as unpredictable and dose-independent and the investigators saw no advantages over epidural morphine [440]. This compound is apparently no longer being pursued clinically as an analgesic candidate.

b. Metkephamid. Metkephamid (LY127623) is an analog of Met-enkephalin with several modifications as shown in Fig. 1.6. Like FK 33-824, it competes with labeled opioid ligands for binding in brain homogenate and produces potent naloxone-reversible depression of the electrically induced twitch of both mouse vas deferens (MVD) and guinea pig ileum (GPI), with IC_{50} values in the nanomolar range [441,442]. In the mouse vas deferens preparation, pA_2 values for naloxone versus metkephamid, normorphine and Met-enkephalin were determined to be 7.60, 8.32, and 7.54 respectively. These data suggested that metkephamid and Met-enkephalin share preference for a similar receptor, presumably the δ-receptor. This differs from normorphine, which prefers the μ-receptor. This was corroborated by the GPI:MVD ratios which were about 4.1 for metkephamid and 0.25 for morphine, suggesting a 16-fold greater δ-selectivity for metkephamid over morphine. This contrasted with the ratios for competing with [^{3}H]Nx versus [^{3}H]DADL binding in brain homogenates, which were 0.6 and 0.1, respectively, for metkephamid and morphine [442]. These latter data indicated that, although metkephamid had a sixfold greater preference for the δ-receptor than did morphine, it still had a slightly higher affinity for the μ-receptor than for the δ-receptor. This difference between the binding ratios and the ratios in the isolated muscle preparations suggests that either metkephamid has considerably greater efficacy at the δ-receptor than at the μ-receptor or that the δ-receptors in mouse deferens differ from the δ-receptors in brain. Support for the latter suggestion has been recently reported [443]. The relative analgesic potency of morphine and metkephamid after intracerebroventricular administration correlates best, however, with their relative potency on the mouse vas deferens preparation, which reflects both affinity and efficacy. Another possibility may be that metkephamid is metabolized to a product, such as the carboxyterminal acid, which has a higher preference for the δ-receptor.

In in vivo tests for analgesia, when given by the intraventricular route metkephamid was about 100-fold more potent than morphine [441, 442]. It was also analgesic by systemic routes of administration, being anywhere from one-third to 10 times as potent as morphine, depending on the test system and the route of administration.

Cross-tolerance data and differential antagonism by naloxazone (a long acting μ-antagonist) demonstrated that metkephamid could produce analgesia utilizing a different receptor, presumably the δ- receptor, than does morphine [442,443]. Metkephamid has little or no affinity for the κ-receptor [445,446].

Chronic treatment of rats with metkephamid produced little more physical dependence than did saline, unlike other drugs similarly tested such as morphine, meperidine, and pentazocine [441,442]. Metkephamid similarly produced little stimulation of locomotor activity or naloxone-precipitated withdrawal jumping in mice compared with morphine [442]. Metkephamid was also reported to have a lesser depressant effect on respiration in a rodent model than did morphine.

The ability of metkephamid to cross the placental barrier was assessed by measuring the maternal and fetal serum levels in rats and sheep at various times after intramuscular injection of metkephamid [442]. In the rat, the fetal:maternal ratio of metkephamid in blood at 1 hr after injection was about 1:60 compared with 1:1.8 for meperidine. In sheep, the fetal:maternal ratio for metkephamid was less than 1:200 compared with 1:1 or 2 reported for meperidine. This indicates a remarkable advantage of metkephamid over meperidine for use in obstetric analgesia.

In initial safety studies, metkephamid was administered to normal male volunteers in single intramuscular doses ranging from 0.5 mg to 150 mg [447,448]. No clinically relevant effects were seen by routine clinical chemistry, electrolytes, urinalysis, hemograms, EKG, blood pressure, or heart rate. At doses greater than 12.5 mg, subjects reported a mild retro-orbital burning that progressed to nasal congestion and dry mouth. A heavy sensation in the extremities, emotional detachment, and conjunctival injection were also reported, but no flushing or changes in bowel sounds were noted and a flare formation did not occur after intradermal administration. Serum prolactin was increased, but no change in serum growth hormone was observed after 75 mg.

Clinical tests in postoperative pain have demonstrated metkephamid to be efficacious as an analgesic in man [449,450]. In one controlled doubled-blind clinical trial [449], metkephamid at a single parenteral dose of 70 mg was compared with meperidine at 100 mg and placebo in 30 patients with severe postoperative pain. All measures indicated that the analgesic activity of metkephamid 70 mg was significantly greater than placebo and not less than that of meperidine 100 mg. The duration of activity was about 4 hr, and up to the 4-hr point metkephamid 70 mg appeared more efficacious than did meperidine 100 mg (Fig. 1.7). The frequency of remedication with metkephamid was also less than with meperidine or placebo. In a second controlled double-blind study [450], metkephamid at 70 mg and 140 mg intramuscularly was compared with meperidine at 100 mg and placebo in 60 postpartum women with severe pain after episiotomy. Using subjective reports as indices of response, patients rated pain intensity, pain relief, and side effects at periodic intervals for 6 hr. Metkephamid at the 140-mg dose was rated most effective, followed in order by meperidine (100 mg), metkephamid (70 mg), and placebo. Only metkephamid at 140 mg and meperidine 100 at mg showed statistically significant superiority over placebo. Both treatments took effect within 1/2 hr, peaked at 1–2 hr, and with 140 mg metkephamid, maximum analgesia was sustained for 6 hr, i.e., 2 hr longer than with meperidine.

There was a higher incidence of minor side effects with metkephamid than with the other treatments in these studies, but these effects were relatively transient and were not distressing to the patients. The side effects peculiar to metkephamid were a sensation of heavy limbs, dry mouth, eye redness, and nasal stuffiness. The spectrum of these side effects suggested that the pharmacological properties of metkephamid are different from those of standard narcotic analgesics. It has been suggested that this might be due to greater utilization of the δ-receptor than is the case with standard analgesics [450]. Metkephamid has high affinity for both the μ- and δ-receptors but little or no affinity for the κ-receptor [450,446]. This unique receptor preference of metkephamid may also contribute to its apparently lesser potential for physical dependence and respiratory depression. It is not yet clear whether more selective δ-activity or the proper combination of μ- and δ-activity is most desirable for the best analgesia versus abuse liability:respiratory depression profile. Finally, if the transfer across the placenta seen in rats and sheep proves to be the case in humans as well, metkephamid could be an important advance for obstetric analgesia.

3. Other Peptides

Evidence for analgesia deriving from agonist or antagonist action at various peptide receptors other than the opioid receptors has been generated, although no clinical candidates have yet been offered. The concept of developing a nonopioid central analgesic as an approach to

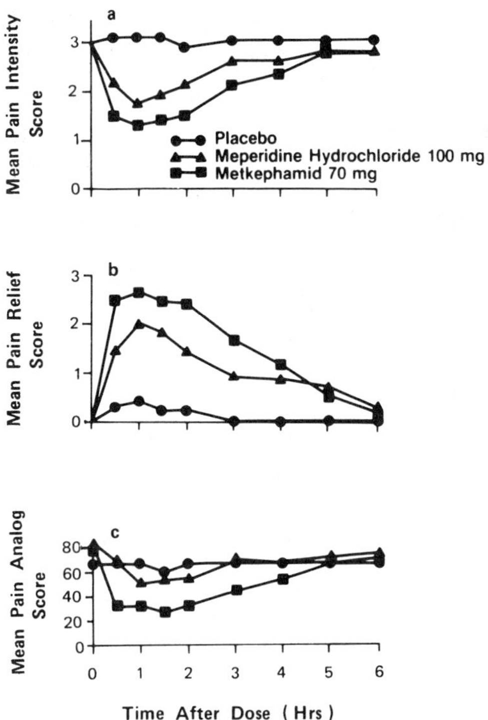

FIG. 1.7 Time-effect curves of the analgesic activity of metkephamid (70 mg, i.m.) compared with placebo and meperidine (100 mg, i.m.). Pain was assessed subjectively at each interview by: (a) a reported pain score on an ordinal scale of 0 (no pain) to 4 ("terrible" pain); (b) a reported score for pain relief compared with premedication pain level on an ordinal scale of 0 (no relief) to 4 (complete relief); and (c) an analog scale of pain consisting of a 20-cm line marked 0 ("no pain") at one end and 100 ("worst pain I have ever felt") at the other end. From these observations, the mean pain intensity scores, mean pain relief scores, and mean pain analog scores were calculated for each observation time and plotted as shown. The placebo generally had no effect on pain. By contrast, metkephamid and meperidine had begun to reduce pain by 1/2 hr, with peak analgesic effect usually at 1 hr; the analgesic effect was considerably diminished by 4 hr. Up to the 4-hr point, metkephamid (70 mg) appeared more effective than meperidine (100 mg). (Modified from Ref. 449.)

circumventing the drawbacks, discussed earlier, to existing central analgesics is appealing, and therefore we will briefly discuss the ideas and evidence behind several of these other peptides.

Convincing evidence has been reported that the endogenous undecapeptide, Substance P (SP), is a neurotransmitter for primary nociceptive afferents [451,452]. This provided a strong rationale that an antagonist of SP might be an analgesic with a very novel mechanism of action. Surprisingly, however, SP itself has been reported to produce analgesia [453–456]. This SP-induced analgesia could be antagonized by naloxone, suggesting that it was secondary to the release of endogenous opioid peptides. This action of SP was very potent but was very limited in intensity and occurred only in a narrow dose range, hyperalgesia occurring under some conditions. There is some evidence that the analgesic activity may reside in a smaller fragment of SP [457, 458]. The nature of this SP analgesia suggests that SP-related agonists would not have practical clinical utility unless the limitations are due to rapid metabolism of the active fragment. This might be circumvented by structural modifications. Two SP antagonists have been synthesized and do have analgesic properties, but these apparently are not well separated from motor effects [459,460].

The endogenous tridecapeptide, neurotensin, has been reported to produce analgesia in several species and antinociceptive test systems [461–463]. This neurotensin-induced analgesia can apparently be antagonized by thyrotropin-releasing-hormone but not by naloxone [462]. Calcitonin has also been reported to produce an analgesic action not antagonized by naloxone [464,465].

Both somatostatin [466] and the octapeptide of cholecystokinin (CCK-8) [467] have been reported to produce a naloxone-reversible analgesia. In another series of studies, to the contrary, sulfated CCK-8 was demonstrated to be an antagonist of opiate analgesia [468]. Des-tyrosine-dynorphin [469] and adrenocorticotropin (ACTH) [470] have similarly been reported to antagonize opiate analgesia.

The above-mentioned peptides are presently far from development as practical clinical analgesics, but the prospect of a unique central analgesic with a nonopioid mechanism of action is worth pursuing. In the case of the above peptides, questions concerning bioavailability and selectivity of action have not yet been considered. The topic of neuropeptides in pain and analgesia has been recently reviewed elsewhere [471].

C. Other Possible Analgesic Entities

1. Nitrous Oxide

Nitrous oxide has recently been found to have many pharmacological activities in common with morphine, suggesting that they may share some common mechanism. In experimental animals [472,473] and man

[474,475,476], nitrous oxide, like morphine, produces analgesia that is reduced by narcotic antagonists. The analgesic activity is also reduced in morphine-tolerant animals [473]. These results, in conjunction with the fact that nitrous oxide causes a displacement of [^{3}H]Nx from brain [477], have suggested that nitrous oxide may exert its analgesic activity by releasing endogenous opioids.

2. GABAergic Agents

The inhibitory neurotransmitter, γ-aminobutyric acid (GABA), has been suggested to have a role in analgesic and other opioid actions [478,479]. Antinociceptive activity, which could be antagonized by bicuculline (a GABA antagonist), has been demonstrated for GABA transaminase inhibitors, including γ-acetylenic GABA, γ-vinyl GABA, and aminooxyacetic acid [480–484]. GABA itself has been observed to produce analgesic activity when injected directly into the brain [485]. The direct-acting GABAmimetic agent, muscimol, has been reported to be active in some analgesic test systems [483,484,486], but not in others [487,488]. Kojic amine, another direct-acting GABAmimetic, is reported also to have analgesic acitivity [489]. Inhibition of GABA neuronal uptake, furthermore, by nipecotic acid ethyl ester has been observed to increase reaction time in the hot plate and tail immersion tests [489].

Baclofen, [β-(4-chlorophenyl)-γ-aminobutyric acid, Lioresal*], which is structurally related to GABA, is useful in the treatment of spasticity [490]. It suppresses pain in patients suffering this condition, but this may be secondary to muscle relaxation [491]. In animal test systems, baclofen is reported to produce analgesia at doses that do not produce ataxia, although the separation is not great [486,492–494]. Baclofen is reported not to exhibit cross-tolerance to morphine [493], but there are differing reports on antagonism by naloxone [493, 495]. There are reports, furthermore, that baclofen does not exert its pharmacological activity via the bicuculline-sensitive GABA receptor [496,497].

THIP [4,5,6,7-tetrahydroisoxazolo(5,4-c)pyridine-3-ol] is a structurally rigid analog of muscimol [498]. Analgesic activity has been observed following parenteral and oral administration in a variety of animal tests, with the exception of the mouse tail flick test [499,500]. The analgesic acitivity of THIP is not blocked by naloxone [499] nor does it appear to vary between different strains of mice in the same manner as does the analgesic activity of morphine [500]. Bicuculline does not appear to reverse its analgesic activity [499], suggesting that the bicuculline-sensitive GABA receptors are not involved in the activity of THIP. THIP has been reported to be undergoing clinical trials in Europe as an analgesic agent [501].

---

*®Trademark.

3. α-Adrenoceptor Agonists

The prototypic α-adrenoceptor agonist is the imidazoline, clonidine. Clonidine is best known for its potent antihypertensive activity which results from its stimulation of α-adrenoceptors in the central nervous system. In addition to its cardiovascular activity, clonidine produces pronounced analgesic activity in a number of animal pain models (for a complete review of the analgesic and psychopharmacological activity of clonidine, see Refs. 502–504). Clonidine has been found to exhibit antinoceptive activity in the writhing [505,506], hot-plate [507], tail-withdrawal [505,508], and Randall Sellito tests [505]. The mechanism by which clonidine exerts its analgesic activity is not known. An interaction with opioid receptors has been ruled out since it is not antagonized by naloxone [505,509] and it does not exhibit cross-tolerance to morphine [510]. It has been proposed that clonidine and other α-adrenoceptor agonists exert their analgesic activity by direct α-adrenoceptor-mediated inhibition of pain transmission [511].

VI. PROGNOSIS AND APPLICATIONS IN OTHER DISEASE AREAS

It is clear from this treatise that many treatments, both pharmacological and nonpharmacological, are available for the amelioration of pain. These treatments all have limitations that emphasize the need for improvement and provide criteria for such improvement. The limitations encompass a host of side effects that vary in seriousness, severity, and incidence. The ideal analgesic would have potency in the range of morphine, or at least meperidine, have reliable bioavailability by both the oral and parenteral routes of administration and be relatively free of tolerance, abuse potential, psychomimetic activity, respiratory depressant activity, and cardiodepressant activity. This ideal analgesic agent, which has been sought for decades, has unfortunately not yet been brought to fruition. It is important to realize, however, that there is room in our analgesic armamentarium for agents that represent significant improvement or advantage over existing therapies, even though they do not meet all the criteria for the ideal agent. Indeed, some novel compounds with unique mechanisms and advantages over existing agents are being developed.

A particularly exciting possibility is the development of nonopioid analgesics. There is evidence for many such mechanisms, some of which have been explored clinically, while others have not. The nonsteroidal antiinflammatory agents, inhibitors of prostaglandin synthesis, have progressed beyond clinical trials and have achieved a modicum of success in the market. They are found to have good utility in the treatment of mild to moderate pain states, but they do not appear to have the efficacy to treat moderate to severe pain. They have introduced, furthermore, their own set of limiting side effects such as gastrointestinal distress and renal toxicity, which may be serious or even life threatening.

Initial clinical investigation of compounds that modulate the serotonergic system have suggested that they produce analgesia and potentiate opioid analgesics. THIP, a compound that is thought to mimic the endogenous inhibitory neurotransmitter, GABA, is reported to be in clinical trial, but there are as yet no reports on its performance in these trials. None of the other nonopioid analgesic mechanisms discussed has yet reached clinical trial.

Another promising approach where there has been more progress to date is the development of receptor-selective opioids. Convincing evidence is gathering for at least four distinct opioid receptors: these are the μ-, δ-, κ-, and σ-receptors. The latter, σ-receptors, which it now seems may be identical to phencyclidine receptors, are unusual. While they are recognized by a subpopulation of opioids, they do not seem to meet the definition of opioid because their stereospecificity is opposite to that of the opioids and they are not displaced by naloxone, nor are their supposed actions antagonized by naloxone. The roles of the various receptors remain to be fully established, but some general correlations of receptor type with function can be made.

It has been generally assumed that μ-receptors mediate analgesia, and it has been suggested that κ-receptors in the spinal cord may mediate analgesia also. Analgesia produced by agents proposed to act at the latter receptors have been associated with a reduced potential of abuse. More recently, convincing evidence of δ-analgesia has been provided [442–444,512,513]. δ-Analgesia can be mediated at the spinal level [512–515], and it remains to be seen whether this occurs as well as or rather than the κ-receptor-mediated analgesia in the cord. As mentioned earlier, the σ- or PCP receptors are not opioid in nature but have been associated with the induction of psychotomimetic activity, as have the opioid κ-receptors.

Most of the new analgesic introductions have been mixed or partial agonist agents with promise of reduced abuse potential and psychotomimetic side effects. It remains to be seen whether any have real and lasting advantages over existing agents. While particular attention has not been paid to the probable receptors used by these agents, it is generally assumed they exert their activity at the μ- and/or κ-receptors.

Potential for new agents with unique mechanisms comes from development of the endogenous opioid peptides. There are as yet no inhibitors of the enkephalin degradative enzymes, enkephalinase A or aminopeptidase, in the clinic, but a number of enkephalin analogs have been examined. One of these, an analog of Met-enkephalin (metkephamid, LY127623), is still undergoing clinical trial. There is evidence that metkephamid can provide analgesia by action at δ-receptors which may be associated with less physical dependence [442,444]. If clinical data substantiate the findings in animal studies [442] of markedly reduced passage across the placental barrier in comparison to meperidine, then this new peptide-based analgesic may provide an exciting advantage for obstetric analgesia.

The dramatic proliferation of investigations inspired by the discovery of opioid receptors and their endogenous ligands has, furthermore, refocused attention on the multitude of other functions and thus other potential utilities of the opioids besides analgesia. Again, the key to realizing practical utility will probably lie in receptor-selective ligands or perhaps the correct ratio of activity at each of the subsets of receptors. There is, for example, evidence for opioid modulation and therefore possibility of opioid utility in psychotic disorders, sexual disorders, neuroendocrine disorders, depression, anxiety, obesity, hypertension, shock, epilepsy, and immune disorders [369]. For a comprehensive review of opioids in mental illness, see Refs. 516 and 517.

The specific receptor types involved in each of the proposed roles of the opioids are not yet established, but efforts are accelerating toward elucidating such correlations. Presently there is evidence that σ- and/or κ-receptors are involved in psychotomimetic activity, κ-receptors in appetite suppressant activity, and δ-receptors in the hypotensive and anticonvulsant actitivies. The development of ligands with selective agonist or antagonist activity for each subset of opioid receptors will be an exceptionally valuable endeavor. The characterization of specific receptor involvement in given disorders and the evaluation of selective agonists and antagonists in these disorders may provide major scientific and therapeutic advances.

ACKNOWLEDGMENTS

The authors gratefully acknowledge the dedicated and expert assistance of Joan Hager, Kathleen Edwards, and Georganna Irish.

REFERENCES

1. J. H. Jaffe and W. R. Martin, in *The Pharmacological Basis of Therapeutics*, 6th ed. (A. G. Gilman, L. S. Goodman, and A. Gilman, Eds.), Macmillan, New York, 1980, p. 494.
2. N. B. Eddy, *U.S. Pub. Health Repts.*, Suppl. No. 165 (1941).
3. A. Wikler, *Public Health Monograph No. 52*, U.S. Government Printing Office, Washington, D.C., 1958.
4. A. K. Reynolds and L. O. Randall, in *Morphine and Allied Drugs*, University of Toronto Press, 1957.

5. C. A. Winter, in *Analgetics Vol. 5, Medicinal Chemistry* (G. deStevens, Ed.), Academic, New York, 1965, p. 10.
6. R. K. S. Lim, in *Pain* (R. S. Knighton and P. R. Cunske, Eds.), Little, Brown and Co., Boston, 1966.
7. E. F. Domino, *Proc. Ass. Res. New Ment. Dis.*, 46:117 (1968).
8. J. W. Lewis, K. W. Bentley, and A. Cowan, *Ann. Rev. Pharmacol.*, 11:241 (1971).
9. W. R. Martin and J. W. Sloan, in *Drug Addiction 1*, (W. R. Martin, Ed.), Springer-Verlag, 1977, p. 43.
10. Merck, Sharp and Dohme Research Laboratories, Merck and Co., Inc., Medical Literature Department, *Codeine: And Certain Other Analgesic and Antitussive Agents*, Merck and Co., Inc., Rahway, NJ, 1970.
11. N. B. Eddy, H. Friebel, K. Hohn, and H. Halbach, *Codeine and Its Alternates for Pain and Cough Relief*, WHO publication, Geneva, 1970.
12. G. F. Kiplinger and R. Nickander, *J. Am. Med. Assoc.*, 216: 289 (1971).
13. R. Nickander, S. E. Smits, and M. I. Steinberg, *J. Pharmacol. Exp. Ther.*, 200:245 (1977).
14. J. D. Hardy, H. G. Wolff, and H. Goodell, *J. Clin. Invest.*, 19:649 (1940).
15. C. M. Jones and W. P. Chapman, *Arch. Int. Med.*, 73:322 (1944).
16. M. H. Seevers and C. C. Pfeiffer, *J. Pharmacol.*, 56:166 (1936).
17. H. Jackson, *Br. J. Pharmacol.*, 7:204 (1952).
18. S. Gelfand, *Can. J. Psychol.*, 18:36 (1964).
19. B. B. Wolff, T. G. Kantor, M. E. Jarvik, and E. Laska, *Clin. Pharmacol. Ther.*, 7:224 (1966).
20. B. B. Wolff, T. G. Kantor, M. E. Jarvik, and E. Laska, *Clin. Pharmacol. Ther.*, 10:217 (1969).
21. G. M. Smith, E. Lowenstein, J. H. Hubbard, and H. K. Beecher, *J. Pharmacol. Exp. Ther.*, 163:468 (1968).
22. H. K. Beecher, in *Quantitative Effects of Drugs*, Oxford University Press, New York, 1959.
23. J. E. Denton and H. K. Beecher, *J. Am. Med. Assoc.*, 141:1051 (1949).
24. L. Lasagna and H. K. Beecher, *J. Am. Med. Assoc.*, 156:230 (1954).
25. H. K. Beecher, A. S. Keats, F. Mosteller, and L. Lasagna, *J. Pharmacol.*, 109:393 (1953).
26. R. W. Houde, J. W. Bellville, and S. L. Wallenstein, *Minutes of the 23rd Meeting, Committee on Drug Addiction and Narcotics*, April 13, 1961.
27. G. M. Smith and H. K. Beecher, *J. Pharmacol.*, 126:50 (1959).

28. J. M. von Felsinger, L. Lasagna, and H. K. Beecher, *J. Am. Med. Assoc.*, 157:1113 (1955).
29. N. H. McNally, H. H. Neily, and J. Benoit, *Can. Anaesth. Soc. J.*, 9:504 (1962).
30. L. Lasagna, J. M. von Felsinger, and H. K. Beecher, *J. Am. Med. Assoc.*, 156 1006 (1955).
31. A. S. Keats and J. Telford, *J. Pharmacol. Exp. Ther.*, 143:157 (1964).
32. S. L. Wang and V. V. Gloviano, *J. Pharmacol.*, 111:329 (1954).
33. J. H. Comroe and R. D. Dripps, *Surg. Gynecol. Obstet.*, 87: 221 (1948).
34. E. M. Papper and S. E. Bradley, *J. Pharmacol. Exp. Ther.*, 74:319 (1942).
35. J. H. Drew, R. D. Dripps, and J. H. Comroe, *Anesthesiology*, 7:44 (1946).
36. E. Lowenstein, P. Hallowell, F. H. Levin, W. M. Dagget, W. G. Austen, and M. B. Laver, *New Engl. J. Med.*, 281:1389 (1969).
37. J. E. Eckenhoff and S. R. Oech, *Clin. Pharmacol. Therap.*, 1:483 (1960).
38. J. D. Crawford and B. Pinkham, *J. Pharmacol. Exp. Ther.*, 113:431 (1955).
39. O. Eisleb and O. Schaumann, *Duetsche med. Wihnschr.*, 65:967, 1939.
40. A. S. Keats, R. J. Telford and C. N. Papadopoulos, *Minutes of the 24th Meeting, Committee on Drug Addiction and Narcotics*, App. 10, 1962.
41. R. Houde and S. L. Wallenstein, *Minutes of the 19th Meeting, Committee on Drug Addiction and Narcotics*, App. D, 1958.
42. L. Lasagna, *Pharmacol. Rev.*, 16:47 (1964).
43. J. E. Eckenhoff and M. Helrich, *J. Am. Med. Assoc.*, 167:415 (1958).
44. C. M. Gruber, Jr., C. L. Miller, J. Finneran, and S. M. Chernish, *J. Pharmacol. Exp. Ther.*, 118:280 (1956).
45. C. M. Gruber, Jr., *J. Am. Med. Assoc.*, 164:966 (1957).
46. R. W. Boyle, C. E. Solomonson, and J. R. Petersen, *Ann. Intern. Med.*, 52:195 (1960).
47. W. S. Van Bergen, W. C. North, and M. Karp, *J. Am. Med. Assoc.*, 172:1372 (1960).
48. G. M. Howard, J. Levy, and J. Dougherty, *NY J. Med.*, 61: 3285 (1961).
49. N. W. Chilton, A. Lewandowski, and J. R. Cameron, *Am. J. Med. Sci.*, 242:702 (1961).
50. M. S. Sadove, M. J. Schiffrin, and S. M. Ali, *Am. J. Med. Sci.*, 241:103 (1961).
51. T. G. Kantor, A. Sunshine, E. Laska, M. Meisner, and M. Hopper, *Clin. Pharmacol. Therap.*, 7:447 (1966).

52. L. R. Orkin, S. I. Joseph, and M. Helrich, *NY J. Med.*, 57:71 (1957).
53. L. D. Prockop, J. E. Eckenhoff, and R. C. McElroy, *Obstet. Gynecol.*, 16:113 (1960).
54. R. W. Houde and S. L. Wallenstein, *Fed. Proc.*, 12:332 (1953).
55. C. M. Gruber, Jr., J. Doss, A. Baptisti, Jr., and S. M. Chernish, *Clin. Pharmacol. Therap.*, 2:429 (1961).
56. C. M. Gruber, Jr., A. Baptisti, Jr., and S. M. Chernish, *Anesth. Analg.*, 41.538 (1962).
57. J. W. Maus, W. W. Glas, and J. Silvani, *Am. J. Pharm.*, 131: 271 (1959).
58. H. G. Wolff, J. D. Hardy, and H. Goodell, *J. Clin. Invest.*, 19:657 (1940).
59. R. W. Houde, S. L. Wallenstein, and W. T. Beaver, in *Analgetics* (G. deStevens, Ed.), Academic, New York, 1965, p. 75.
60. S. L. Wallenstein, R. W. Houde, and J. W. Bellville, *Fed. Proc.*, 20:311, 1961.
61. J. S. Gravenstein, R. A. Devloo, and H. K. Beecher, *J. Appl. Physiol.*, 7:119 (1954).
62. L. J. Cass, J. T. Laing, and W. S. Frederik, *Curr. Therap. Res.*, 3:289 (1961).
63. D. A. Corgill, C. W. Ligon, and E. A. DeFelice, *Curr. Therap. Res.*, 7:263 (1965).
64. W. T. Beaver, *Am. J. Med. Sci.*, 251:576 (1966).
65. W. F. von Oettingen, in *Poisoning: A Guide to Clinical Diagnosis and Treatment*, 2nd ed., Saunders, Philadelphia, 1958, p. 309.
66. A. Pohland and H. R. Sullivan, *J. Am. Chem. Soc.*, 77:3400 (1955).
67. L. J. Cass and W. S. Frederik, *Antibiot. Med. Clin. Therap.*, 6:362 (1959).
68. R. C. Benson, *Western J. Surg. Obstet. Gynecol.*, 71:167 (1963).
69. L. E. Sunshine, J. Slafta, and E. Fleishman, *Toxicol. App. Pharmacol.*, 19:512 (1971).
70. C. M. Gruber, Jr., *J. Am. Med. Assoc.*, 237:2734 (1977).
71. R. E. S. Young, *Curr. Ther. Res.*, 24:495 (1978).
72. C. M. Gruber, Jr., A. Baptisti, Jr., and G. F. Kiplinger, *Toxicol. App. Pharmacol.*, 19:546 (1971).
73. American Medical Association Council on Drugs, *New Drugs, 1967 Ed.*, Am. Med. Assn., Chicago, 1967, p. 173.
74. A. Feinberg, *Clin. Pediat. (Phila.)*, 12:402 (1973).
75. F. S. Tennant, Jr., *Arch. Intern. Med.*, 132:191 (1973).
76. R. I. Taber, D. D. Greenhouse, and S. Irwin, *Nature*, 204: 189 (1964).
77. H. Blumberg, P. S. Wolf, and H. B. Dayton, *Proc. Soc. Exp. Biol. Med.*, 118:763 (1965).

78. W. O. Evans and D. P. Bergner, *J. New Drugs*, 4:82 (1964).
79. L. S. Harris and A. K. Pierson, *J. Pharmacol. Exp. Ther.*, 143:141 (1964).
80. R. Paddock, G. Beer, J. W. Bellville, B. J. Giliberti, W. H. Forrest, and E. V. Miller, *Clin. Pharmacol. Ther.*, 10:355 (1969).
81. J. D. Morrison, W. B. Loan, and J. W. Dundee, *Br. Med. J.*, 3:287 (1971).
82. W. T. Beaver, S. L. Wallenstein, R. W. Houde, and A. Rogers, *Clin. Pharmacol. Ther.*, 7:740 (1966).
83. B. Frankendal and D. Kjellgren, *Cancer*, 27:842 (1971).
84. I. Taylor, *J. Clin. Practice*, 25:27 (1971).
85. R. D. Wilson, L. L. Priano, and D. L. Traber, *Plas. Reconstr. Surg.*, 48:466 (1971).
86. W. T. Beaver, S. L. Wallenstein, R. W. Houde, and A. Rogers, *Clin. Pharm. Ther.*, 9:582 (1968).
87. C. G. Moertel, D. L. Ahmann, W. F. Taylor, and N. Schwartau, *New Engl. J. Med.*, 286:813 (1972).
88. R. N. Brogden, T. M. Speight, and G. S. Avery, *Drugs*, 5:6 (1973).
89. N. Guldman and K. H. Sestoft, *Clin. Trials J.*, 6:173 (1969).
90. T. Tammisto and S. Takki, *Br. J. Anaesth.*, 43:58 (1971).
91. R. C. Hamilton, J. W. Dundee, R. S. Clarke, W. B. Loan, and J. D. Morrison, *Br. J. Anaes.*, 39:647 (1967).
92. J. W. Bellville, W. H. Forrest, J. Elasihoff, and E. Laska, *Clin. Pharmacol. Ther.*, 9:303 (1968).
93. A. S. Keats and J. Telford, *J. Pharmacol. Exp. Ther.*, 143:157 (1964).
94. B. A. Berkowitz, J. H. Asling, S. M. Schnider, and E. L. Way, *Clin. Pharm. Ther.*, 10:320 (1969).
95. H. Blumberg, M. B. Dayton, and P. S. Wolf, *Pharmacologist*, 10:189 (1968).
96. W. H. Forrest, *Committee on Problems of Drug Dependence*, 1971, p. 239.
97. W. T. Beaver and G. Feise, *Clin. Pharmacol. Ther.*, 23:108 (1978).
98. G. B. Bikhazi, *Anesthesiology Rev.*, 5:34 (1978).
99. R. W. Houde, S. L. Wallenstein, and A. Rogers, *Proceedings of the 37th Annual Meeting of the Committee on Problems of Drug Dependence*, p. 162, 1975.
100. R. W. Houde, S. L. Wallenstein, A. Rogers, and R. F. Kaiko, *Proceedings of the 38th Annual Meeting of the Committee on the Problems of Drug Dependence*, p. 149, 1976.
101. R. W. Houde, *Br. J. Clin. Pharmacol.*, 7:297S (1979).
102. T. Tammisto and I. Tigerstedt, *Acta Anaesth. Scand.*, 21:390 (1977).

103. W. T. Beaver, G. A. Feise, and D. Robb, *Clin. Pharmacol. Ther.*, 29:174 (1981).
104. R. Okun, *Clin. Pharmacol. Ther.*, 32:517 (1982).
105. W. T. Beaver and G. A. Feise, *J. Pharmacol. Exp. Ther.*, 204:487 (1978).
106. A. W. Pircio, J. A. Gylys, R. L. Cavanagh, J. P. Buyniski, and M. E. Bierwagen, *Arch. int. Pharmacodyn.*, 220:231 (1976).
107. F. S. Caruso, A. W. Pircio, H. Madissoo, R. D. Smyth, and I. J. Pachter, in *Pharmacological and Biochemical Properties of Drug Substances*, vol. 2, (M. Goldberg, Ed.), Am. Pharm. Assn., Washington, D.C., 1978, p. 19.
108. A. B. Dobkin, S. Eamkaow, S. Zak, and F. S. Caruso, *Can. Anaesth. Soc. J.*, 21:600 (1974).
109. A. Del Pizzo, *Curr. Ther. Res.*, 20:221 (1976).
110. M. S. Gilbert, R. S. Forman, D. S. Moylan, and F. S. Caruso, *J. Int. Med. Res.*, 4:255 (1976).
111. M. S. Gilbert, R. M. Hanover, D. S. Moylan, and F. S. Caruso, *Clin. Pharmacol. Therap.*, 20:359 (1976).
112. M. Lippman, M. S. Mok, and S. N. Steen, *Curr. Ther. Res.*, 21:427 (1977).
113. F. L. Communale and H. S. Filtzer, *Curr. Ther. Res.*, 22:116 (1977).
114. F. M. Galloway, J. Hrdlicka, M. Losada, R. J. Noveck, and F. S. Caruso, *Can. Anaesth. Socl J.*, 24:90 (1977).
115. W. C. North and D. R. Tielens, *Clin. Pharmacol. Therap.*, 21:112 (1977).
116. I. C. Andrews, *Curr. Ther. Res.*, 22:697 (1977).
117. R. E. S. Young, *J. Int. Med. Res.*, 5:422 (1977).
118. R. E. S. Young, J. J. Quigley, W. A. J. Archambault, Jr., and L. L. Gordon, *J. Med.*, 10:239 (1979).
119. A. L. Maduska and M. Hajgkassemoli, *Can. Anaesth. Soc. J.*, 25:398 (1979).
120. R. Hodgkinson, M. Bhatt, G. Grewel, and G. Marx, *Paediatrics*, 62:294 (1978).
121. R. Hodgkinson, R. W. Huff, R. H. Hayashi, and F. J. Husain, *J. Int. Med. Res.*, 7:224 (1979).
122. A. Kliman, M. F. Lipson, and R. Warren, *Curr. Ther. Res.*, 22:105 (1977).
123. R. C. Guerreo and R. C. S. Ho, *Straub Clin. Proc.*, 44:31 (1978).
124. R. Raugel-Guerra, *J. Int. Med. Res.*, 9:120 (1981).
125. J. De La Garza, *J. Int. Med. Res.*, 9:124 (1981).
126. M. Tavakoli, G. Coresin, and F. S. Caruso, *Curr. Res.*, 55: 394 (1976).
127. L. C. Stehling and H. L. Zauser, *J. Int. Med. Res.*, 6:306 (1978).

128. R. C. Heel, R. N. Brogden, T. M. Speight, and G. S. Avery, *Drugs*, 16:473 (1978).
129. B. E. Smith and S. Walsh, *Pharmacologist*, 19:261 (1977).
130. H. M. Levin, N. P. Sanzari, M. Losada, and F. S. Caruso, *J. Int. Med. Res.*, 6:24 (1978).
131. A. B. Dobkin, S. Eamkaow, and F. S. Caruso, *Clin. Pharmacol. Therap.*, 18:547 (1975).
132. J. P. Elliott, J. W. Evans, J. O. Gordon, and L. O. Platt, *J. Urology*, 122:455 (1979).
133. J. W. Lewis and A. Cowan, *Proceedings of the 34th Annual Meeting of the Committee on the Problems of Drug Dependence*, p. 514, 1972.
134. A. Cowan, *Adv. Biochem. Psychopharmacol.*, 8:427 (1974).
135. K. Matsuki, A. Kata, H. Takei, E. Inomata, and T. Iwabuchi, *Oyo Yakuri*, 13:257 (1977).
136. A. Cowan, J. C. Doxey, and E. J. R. Harry, *Br. J. Pharmacol.*, 60:547 (1977).
137. A. Cowan, J. W. Lewis, and I. R. MacFarlane, *Br. J. Pharmacol.*, 60:537 (1977).
138. A. Cowan, *J. Pharm. Pharmacol.*, 28:177 (1976).
139. J. W. Downing, W. D. Leaky, and E. S. White, *Br. J. Anaesth.*, 49:251 (1977).
140. B. C. Hovell, *Br. J. Anaesth.*, 49:913 (1977).
141. B. C. Hovell and A. E. Ward, *J. Int. Med. Res.*, 5:417 (1977).
142. A. W. Harcus, A. E. Ward, and D. W. Smith, *Br. Med. J.*, 2:163 (1979).
143. M. M. Kamel and I. C. Geddes, *Br. J. Anaesth.*, 50:599 (1978).
144. B. Kay, *Br. J. Anaesth.*, 50:605 (1978).
145. I. Tigerstedt and T. Tammisto, *Acta Anaesth. Scand.*, 24:462 (1980).
146. M. J. Hayes, A. R. Fraser, and J. R. Hampton, *Br. Med. J.*, 2:300 (1979).
147. M. J. Ostrowski and A. W. Jackson, *Br. J. Clin. Prac.*, 33:286 (1978).
148. D. S. Robbie, *Br. J. Clin. Pharmacol.*, 7:315S (1979).
149. M. Kjaer, H. Henriksen, and J. Knudsen, *Br. J. Clin. Pharmacol.*, 13:487 (1982).
150. A. B. Dobkin, B. Esposito, and C. Philbin, *Can. Anaesth. Soc. J.*, 24:195 (1977).
151. R. C. Heel, R. N. Brogden, T. M. Speight, and G. S. Avery, *Drugs*, 17:81 (1979).
152. B. C. Hovell, *Br. J. Anaes.*, 49:913 (1977).
153. H. Andriaensen and J. Van De Walle, *Acta Anaesthesiologica Belgica*, 27:187 (1976).
154. A. H. Harcus, A. E. Ward, and D. W. Smith, *Anaesthesia*, 35:382 (1980).

155. L. Lasagna and T. J. DeKornfeld, *J. Am. Med. Assoc.*, 178: 887 (1961).
156. S. Bloomfield, S. Simard-Savoie, J. Bernier, and L. Tetreault, *Can. Med. Assoc. J.*, 90:1156 (1964).
157. E. Wallenstein, R. Dykyj, G. Onesti, and E. Cappila, *Clin. Med.*, 74:53 (1967).
158. A. B. St. John and C. K. Born, *Res. Comm. Chem. Pathol. Pharmacol.*, 26 25 (1979).
159. H. F. Fraser and D. E. Rosenberg, *Clin. Pharmacol. Ther.*, 4:596 (1963).
160. J. W. Pearson and T. J. DeKornfeld, *Anesthesiology*, 24:38 (1963).
161. P. E. Callaghan and J. S. Zelenik, *Am. J. Obstet. Gynecol.*, 95:636 (1966).
162. M. Helrich and M. I. Gold, *Anesthesiology*, 25:662 (1964).
163. J. DeCastro and P. Mundeleer, *Anesth. Analg.*, 16:1022 (1959).
164. E. Nilsson and P. Janssen, *Acta Anaesthesiol. Scand.*, 5:73 (1961).
165. P. Deligne, *Agressologie*, 2:363 (1961).
166. J. Edmonds-Seal and C. Prys-Roberts, *Br. J. Anaesth.*, 42: 207 (1970).
167. G. E. Lewis and P. B. Jennings, *Lab. Animal Sci.*, 22:430 (1972).
168. J. E. Coppen and J. W. Fox, *Anesth. Anal. Curr. Res.*, 47:70 (1968).
169. K. J. Berengi, I. Sakaya, and J. L. Snow, *Laryngoscope*, 76: 772 (1966).
170. P. A. Janssen, C. J. Niemegeers, K. H. Schellekins, F. J. Verbruggen, and J. M. Van Neuten, *Arzneimittel-Forsch.*, 13: 205 (1963).
171. J. Yelnosky, R. Katz, and E. V. Dietrick, *Toxicol. Appl. Pharmacol.*, 6:37 (1964).
172. P. A. Janssen, *Br. J. Anaesth.*, 34:260 (1962).
173. J. Gardocki and J. Yelnosky, *Toxicol. Appl. Pharmacol.*, 6:48 (1964).
174. J. Yelnosky and J. F. Gardocki, *Toxicol. Appl. Pharmacol.*, 6:37 (1964).
175. G. Corssen, E. F. Domino, and R. B. Sweet, *Anesth. An. Curr. Res.*, 43:748 (1964).
176. C. Prys-Roberts and G. R. Kelman, *Br. J. Anaesth.*, 39:139 (1967).
177. W. Norris and A. B. M. Telfer, *Br. J. Anaesth.*, 40:517 (1968).
178. M. C. Holderness, P. E. Chose, and R. D. Dreppes, *Anesthesiology*, 24:336 (1963).
179. M. H. Harper, R. F. Hickey, T. H. Cromwell, and S. Linwood, *J. Pharmacol. Exp. Ther.*, 199:464 (1976).

180. R. L. Lee and P. S. J. Spencer, *Postgrad. Med. J.*, 53 (Suppl. 4):53 (1977).
181. M. F. Sugrue, *Br. J. Pharmacol.*, 65:677 (1979).
182. R. B. Messing, L. Phebus, L. A. Fisher, and L. D. Lytle, *Psychopharmacol. Commun.*, 1:511 (1975).
183. M. F. Sugrue and I. McIndewar, *J. Pharm. Pharmacol.*, 28:447 (1976).
184. A. A. Larson and A. E. Takemori, *Life Sci.*, 21:1807 (1977).
185. M. D. Hynes and R. W. Fuller, *Drug Dev. Res.*, 2:33 (1982).
186. G. Beaumont, *J. Int. Med. Res.*, 1:435 (1973).
187. G. Beaumont, *J. Int. Med. Res.*, 4 (Suppl. 2):56 (1976).
188. R. Kocher, *Eur. Neurology*, 14:458 (1976).
189. R. Kocher, in *Advances in Brain Research and Therapy* (J. J. Bonica and D. Albe-Fessard, Eds.), vol. 1, Raven, New York, 1976, p. 579.
190. K. H. Gebhart, J. Biller, and R. Nischk, *Med. Klin.*, 64:751 (1969).
191. M. Gingras, *J. Int. Med. Res.*, 4 (Suppl. 2):41 (1976).
192. W. A. McDonald Scott, *Practitioner*, 202:802 (1969).
193. F. Hart Dudley, *J. Int. Med. Res.*, 4 (Suppl. 1):15 (1976).
194. F. Johansson and L. Von Knorring, *Pain*, 7:69 (1979).
195. S. Seltzer, R. Stock, R. Marcus, and E. Jackson, *Pain*, 13:385 (1982).
196. G. DeBenedittis, A. M. DiGiulio, K. Massie, R. Villani, and A. E. Parrerai, in *Advances in Pain Research and Therapy* J. J. Bonica and D. Albe-Fessard, Eds.), vol. 5, Raven, New York, 1983, p. 295.
197. H. Akil, D. J. Mayer, and J. C. Liebeskind, *Science*, 191:961 (1976).
198. J. E. Adams, *Pain*, 2:161 (1976).
199. Y. Hosobuchi, J. E. Adams, and R. Linchitz, *Science*, 197:183 (1977).
200. H. Akil, D. E. Richardson, J. D. Barchas, and C. H. Li, *Proc. Natl. Acad. Sci. USA*, 75:5170 (1978).
201. H. Akil, D. E. Richardson, J. Hughes, and J. D. Barchas, *Science*, 201:463 (1978).
202. Y. Hosobuchi, J. Rossier, F. E. Bloom, and R. Guillemin, *Science*, 203:279 (1979).
203. D. J. Mayer and D. D. Price, *Pain*, 2:379 (1976).
204. A. I. Basbaum and H. L. Fields, *Ann. Neurology*, 4:451 (1978).
205. R. C. A. Frederickson, in *Analgesics: Pharmacological and Clinical Perspectives* (M. Kuhar and G. W. Pasternak, Eds.), chap. 2, pp. 9-68, Raven, New York (1984).
206. B. Sjolund and M. Eriksson, *The Lancet*, 2:1085 (1976).
207. B. Sjolund and M. Eriksson, *Brain Res.*, 173:295 (1979).
208. S. A. Andersson, T. Ericson, E. Holmgren, and G. Lindqvist, *Brain Res.*, 6 :393 (1973).

209. F. Boureau, J. C. Willer, and Y. Yamaguchi, *EEG Clin. Neurol.*, 47:322 (1979).
210. R. Melzack, *Pain*: 1:357 (1975).
211. D. J. Mayer, D. D. Price and A. Rafii, *Brain Res.*, 121:368 (1977).
212. C. J. Vierck, C. G. Lineberry, P. K. Lee, and H. W. Calderwood, *Life Sci.*, 15 (7):1277 (1974).
213. B. Pomeranz and D. Chiu, *Life Sci.*, 19:1757 (1976).
214. S. J. Liao, *Yale J. Biol. Med.*, 51:55 (1978).
215. H. T. Chang, *Chin. Med. J.*, 92:7 (1979).
216. G. A. Ulett, *J. Am. Med. Assoc.*, 245:768 (1981).
217. W. R. Martin and D. R. Jasinski, in *Drug Addiction I* (W. R. Martin, Ed.), Springer-Verlag, New York, 1977, p. 159.
218. D. R. Jasinski, in *Drug Addiction I* (W. R. Martin, Ed.), Springer-Verlag, New York, 1977, p. 197.
219. R. D. Dripps and J. H. Comroe, Jr., *Anesthesiology*, 6:462 (1945).
220. A. S. Keats and H. K. Beecher, *J. Pharmacol.*, 105:210 (1952).
221. H. J. Loeschcke, A. Sweel, R. H. Kough, and C. J. Lambertsen, *J. Pharmacol.*, 108:376 (1953).
222. P. Pentiah, F. Reilly, and H. L. Boreson, *J. Pharmacol. Exp. Ther.*, 154:110, 1966.
223. J. Florez, L. D. McCarthy, and H. L. Boreson, *J. Pharmacol. Exp. Ther.*, 163:448 (1968).
224. W. B. Loan and J. D. Morrison, *Drugs*, 5:108 (1973).
225. H. F. Fraser, G. D. Van Horn, W. R. Martin, A. B. Wolbach, and H. Isbell, *J. Pharmacol. Exp. Ther.*, 133:371 (1961).
226. W. R. Martin and H. F. Fraser, *J. Pharmacol. Exp. Ther.*, 133:388 (1961).
227. H. L. Andrews and C. K. Himmelsbach, *J. Pharmacol. Exp. Ther.*, 81:288 (1944).
228. C. K. Himmelsbach and H. C. Andrews, *J. Pharmacol. Exp. Ther.*, 77:17 (1943).
229. H. F. Fraser and H. Isbell, *Bull. Narcotics*, 12:9 (1960).
230. H. F. Fraser and H. Isbell, *Bull. Narcotics*, 12:15 (1960).
231. R. I. Bodman, *Proc. Roy. Soc. Med. Sect. Anaesth.*, 46:923 (1953).
232. F. F. C. Chang, P. Sofar, and L. Lasagna, *J. Pharmacol.*, 122:370 (1958).
233. A. S. Keats, J. Telford, and Y. Kinosu, *Anesthesiology*, 18: 690 (1957).
234. C. J. Lambertsen and H. Wendel, *J. Appl. Physiol.*, 15:43 (1960).
235. L. R. Orkin, R. K. Egge, and E. A. Rovenstine, *Anesthesiology*, 16:699 (1955).
236. S. Prescott, S. G. Ranson, R. H. Throp, and A. Wilson, *Lancet*, 1:340 (1949).

237. C. J. Lambertsen, H. Wendel, and J. B. Longenhagen, *J. Pharmacol. Exp. Ther.*, 131:381 (1961).
238. D. R. Jasinski and J. G. Nutt, *Proceedings of the 35th Meeting, Committee on Problems of Drug Dependence*, p. 108, 1973.
239. C. K. Himmelsbach, *J. Pharmacol. Exp. Ther.*, 75:64 (1942).
240. H. Isbell, *Fed. Proc.*, 14:354 (1955).
241. J. W. Bellville, L. Aguto Escarragu, S. L. Wallenstein, K. C. Wang, W. S. Howland, and R. W. Houde, *J. Pharmacol. Exp. Ther.*, 136:38 (1962).
242. J. W. Bellville and J. C. Seed, *Anesthesiology*, 21:727 (1960).
243. J. W. Bellville, S. L. Wallenstein, G. H. Wald, M. D. Dowling, Jr., and R. W. Houde, *Anesthesiology*, 19:545 (1958).
244. L. Lasagna and H. K. Beecher, *J. Pharmacol. Exp. Ther.*, 112:306 (1954).
245. M. S. Sadove, A. T. Shima, and M. J. Schiffrin, *Ill. Med. J.*, 125:151 (1964).
246. H. F. Fraser, H. Isbell, and G. D. Van Horn, *J. Pharmacol. Exp. Ther.*, 129:172 (1960).
247. D. R. Jasinski, J. D. Griffith, C. B. Carr, C. W. Gorodetzky, and M. P. Kullberg, *Proceedings of the 36th Annual Meeting of the Committee on Problems of Drug Dependence*, p. 88, 1974.
248. C. K. Himmelsbach, *J. Am. Med. Assoc.*, 103:1420 (1934).
249. D. E. Burget, Jr. and N. M. Greene, *Yale J. Biol. Med.*, 35:185 (1962).
250. D. R. Jasinski, J. D. Griffith, J. S. Pevnick, and S. C. Clark, *Proceedings of the 37th Annual Meeting of the Committee on Problems of Drug Dependence*, p. 121, 1975).
251. C. K. Himmelsbach, H. L. Andres, R. H. Felix, F. W. Oberst, and L. F. Davenport, *Public Health Rep.* (*Wash.*), Suppl. 158, 1, 1940.
252. S. M. Chernish and C. M. Gruber, Jr., *Antibiot. Med. Clin. Therap.*, 7:190 (1960).
253. E. W. Ahlgren and C. R. Stephen, *Anaesth. Analges. Curr. Res.*, 45:673 (1966).
254. A. R. Hunter, *Anaesthesia*, 23:338 (1968).
255. A. R. Hunter, B. J. Plevvry, and J. M. H. Rees, *Br. J. Anaesth.*, 40:927 (1968).
256. S. Jennett, J. G. Barker, and J. B. Forrest, *Br. J. Anaesth.*, 40:864 (1968).
257. Y. Hattori, *Jpn. J. Anesth.*, 21:1319 (1972).
258. T. Kallos and T. C. Smith, *J. Am. Med. Assoc.*, 204:932 (1968).
259. I. T. Davie, G. W. Stephen, and D. B. Scott, *Br. J. Anaesth.*, 43:400 (1971).
260. V. Dysberg, P. Henningsen, and S. H. Johansen, *Acta Anaesth.*, *Scand.*, 11 77 (1967).
261. I. Davie, D. B. Scott, and G. W. Stephen, *Br. J. Anaesth.*, 42:113 (1970).

262. V. Dryberg and K. Kolliker, *Acta Anaesth. Scand.*, 15:65 (1971).
263. I. T. Davie, *Mt. Sinai J. Med., New York*, 39:146 (1972).
264. S. Engineer and S. Jennett, *Br. J. Anaesth.*, 44:795 (1972).
265. T. C. Smith, *Int. Anaesth. Clin.*, 9:125 (1971).
266. C. Kamei, K. Shimomura, and S. Ueki, *Jpn. J. Pharmacol.*, 23:421 (1973).
267. P. G. Goode, *Br. J. Pharmacol.*, 41:558 (1971).
268. W. R. Martin, C. G. Eades, J. A. Thompson, R. E. Huppler, and P. E. Gilbert, *J. Pharmacol. Exp. Ther.*, 197:517 (1976).
269. T. Yanagita, *Bull. Narcot.*, 25:57 (1973).
270. G. Deneau, T. Tamagita, and M. H. Seevers, *Psychopharmacologia (Berl,)*, 16:30 (1969).
271. F. Hoffmeister and W. Wuttke, in *Narcotic Antagonists. Advances in Biochemical Psychopharmacology* (M. C. Brande, L. S. Harris, E. L. May, J. P. Smith, and J. E. Villarreal, Eds.), Raven, New York, 1974, p. 361.
272. G. F. Steinfels, G. A. Young, and N. Khazan, *Pharmacol. Biochem. Behav.*, 16:167 (1982).
273. H. E. Fraser and D. E. Rosenberg, *J. Pharmacol. Exp. Ther.*, 143:149 (1964).
274. D. R. Jasinski, W. R. Martin, and R. D. Hoeldthe, *Clin. Pharmacol. Ther.*, 11:385 (1970).
275. C. V. Showalter, *J. Am. Med. Assoc.*, 224:1225 (1980).
276. J. W. Dundee, in *Pain: Basic Principles—Pharmacology—Therapy* (J. P. Bayne and R. A. P. Burt, Eds.), Churchill Livingstone, London, 1972, p. 346.
277. W. T. Beaver, S. L. Wallenstein, R. W. Houde, and A. Rogers, *Clin. Pharmacol. Ther.*, 9:582 (1968).
278. M. A. Yost and F. P. McKegney, *Conn. Med.*, 34:259 (1970).
279. N. DeNosaquo, *J. Am. Med. Assoc.*, 210:502 (1969).
280. G. Economou, K. Monson, and J. N. Ward-McQuaid, *Br. J. Anaesth.*, 43:486 (1971).
281. D. Levy, R. Gaillon, and M. Boron, *Presse Medicale*, 76:77 (1968).
282. H. W. Elliott, G. Nauarro, and N. Nomof, *J. Med.*, 1:74 (1970).
283. A. Ramagnoli and A. S. Keats, *Clin. Pharmacol. Ther.*, 27:478 (1980).
284. T. J. Gal, C. A. DiGazio, and J. Moscicki, *Anesthesiology*, 57:367 (1982).
285. H. E. Shannon and S. G. Holtzman, *Psychopharmacology*, 61: 239 (1979).
286. G. J. Schaefer and S. G. Holtzman, *Pharmac. Biochem. Behav.*, 14:241 (1981).
287. D. R. Jasinski and P. A. Mansky, *Clin. Pharmacol. Ther.*, 13:78 (1972).

288. H. Nagashima, A. Karamanian, R. Malovany, P. Radnay, M. Ang, S. Koerner, and F. F. Foldes, *Clin. Pharm. Ther.*, 19:738 (1976).
289. T. Kallos and F. S. Caruso, *Anaesthesia*, 34:633 (1979).
290. K. A. Popio, D. H. Jackson, A. M. Ross, B. F. Schreiner, and P. N. Yu, *Clin. Pharmacol. Ther.*, 23:281 (1978).
291. H. H. Swain, J. E. Villarreal, and M. H. Seevers, *Proceedings of the 35th Annual Meeting of the Committee on Problems of Drug Dependence, Addendum*, p. 693, 1973.
292. D. R. Jasinski, J. S. Pevnick, J. D. Griffith, C. W. Gorodetzky, and E. J. Cone, *Proceedings of the 38th Annual Meeting of the Committee on the Problems of Drug Dependence*, p. 112, 1976.
293. G. W. Stephen and L. V. Cooper, *Anesthesia*, 32:324 (1977).
294. L. Lecron, D. Levy, E. Toppet, J. Vermeulen, and L. Raynol, *Proceedings of the Sixth World Congress of Anesthesiology* (E. Hulzer, Ed.) Excerpta Medica International, Amsterdam, 1976, p. 369.
295. J. M. Orwin, *Acta Anaesthesiologica, Belgica*, 28:93 (1977).
296. J. M. Orwin, in *Pain-New Perspectives in Measurement and Management* (A. W. Harcus, R. B. Smith, B. A. Whittle, Churchill Livingstone, Edinburgh, 1977, p.141.
297. J. M. Orwin, J. Orwin, and M. Price, *Acta Anaesthesiol. Belg.*, 21:171 (1976).
298. J. M. Orwin, P. J. Robson, J. Orwin and M. Price, in *Proceedings of the Sixth World Congress of Anesthesiology* (E. Hulzer, Ed.), Excerpta Medica International, Amsterdam, p. 157, 1976.
299. T. J. Baster, J. M. Gibbs, and T. Richardson, *N. Z. Med. J.*, 84:325 (1976).
300. T. J. Baster, J. M. Gibbs, and T. Richardson, *N. Z. Med. J., and Intensive Care*, 5:128 (1977).
301. W. L. Dewey, G. A. Patrick, and L. D. Harris, *Proceedings of the 37th Annual Meeting of the Committee on Problems of Drug Dependence*, p. 64, 1975.
302. W. L. Dewey, L. S. Harris, and K. S. Ritter, *Pharmacologist*, 17:236 (1975).
303. L. S. Harris, *Ann. N.Y. Acad. Sci.*, 281:288 (1976).
304. W. R. Martin, P. E. Gilbert, C. G. Eades, J. A. Thompson, and R. E. Huppler, *Proceedings of the 37th Annual Meetings of the Committee on Problems of Drug Dependence*, p. 110, 1975.
305. H. H. Swain and M. H. Seevers, *Proceedings of the 37th Annual Meetings of the Committee on Problems of Drug Dependence*, p. 791, 1975.
306. J. H. Woods, *Proceedings of the 39th Annual Meetings of the Committee on Problems of Drug Dependence*, p. 420, 1977.

307. D. R. Jasinski, J. S. Pevnick, and J. D. Griffith, *Fed. Proc.*, 36:1025, 1977.
308. D. R. Jasinski, J. S. Pevnick, and J. D. Griffith, *Arch. Gen. Psychiatry*, 35:501 (1978).
309. J. D. P. Graham and J. W. Lewis, in *Pain—New Perspectives in Measurement and Management* (A. W. Harcus, R. B. Smith, B. A. Whittle, Eds.), Churchill Livingstone, Edinburgh, 1977, p. 84.
310. E. Wei, *J. Pharmacol. Exp. Ther.*, 216:12 (1981).
311. E. Miglecz, J. I. Szekely, and Z. Dunai-Kovacs, *Psychopharmacology*, 62:29 (1979).
312. C. C. Hug, Jr., *Sem. Anesth.*, 1:14 (1982).
313. J. M. Luce, T. L. Thompson II, C. J. Getto, and R. L. Byyny, *Hospital Practice, April*, 1979, p. 113.
314. J. J. Bonica, in *Advances in Pain Research and Therapy* (J. J. Bonica, U. Lindblom, A. Iggo, L. E. Jones and C. Benedetti, Eds.), Raven, New York, 1983, p. 1.
315. C. G. Lineberry, in *Methods of Animal Experimentation*, vol.VI (W. I. Gay, Ed.), Academic, New York, 1981, p. 237.
316. T. Oka, K. Negishi, M. Suda, T. Matsumiya, T. Inazu, and M. Ueki, *Eur. J. Pharmacol.*, 73:235 (1981).
317. H. W. Kosterlitz and A. A. Waterfield, *Annu. Rev. Pharmacol.*, 15:20 (1975).
318. R. R. Goodman and G. W. Pasternak, in *Analgesics: Pharmacological and Clinical Perspectives*, (M. Kuhar and G. W. Pasternak, Eds.), pp. 69-96, Raven, New York (1984).
319. A. Pert and T. Yaksh, *Pharmacol. Biochem. Behav.*, 3:133 (1974).
320. H. Takagi, M. Satoh, A. Akaike, T. Shibata, H. Yajima, and H. Ogawa, *Eur. J. Pharmacol.*, 49:113 (1978).
321. T. L. Yaksh and T. A. Rudy, *Pain*, 4:299 (1978).
322. T. L. Yaksh, *Pain*, 11:293 (1981).
323. Y. F. Jacquet and A. Lajtha, *Science*, 182:490 (1973).
324. D. V. Reynolds, *Science*, 164:444 (1969).
325. K. Tsou and C. S. Jang, *Sci. Sinica*, 13:1099 (1964).
326. R. C. A. Frederickson and F. H. Norris, *Science*, 194:440 (1976).
327. R. C. A. Frederickson and F. H. Norris, in *Iontophoresis and Transmitter Mechanisms in the Mammalian Central Nervous System* (R. W. Ryall and J. S. Kelly, Eds.), Elsevier, Amsterdam, 1978, p. 320.
328. J. L. Henry, *Fed. Proc.*, 34:757 (1975).
329. J. H. Wolstencroft, D. C. West, and G. P. Gent, in *Ionotophoresis and Transmitter Mechanisms in the Mammalian Central Nervous System* (R. W. Ryall and J. S. Kelly, Eds.), Elsevier, Amsterdam, 1978, p. 341.
330. G. Urca, H. Frenk, J. C. Liebeskind, and A. N. Taylor, *Science*, 197:83 (1977).

331. I. A. Abols and A. L. Basbaum, *Anat. Rec.*, 93:467 (1979).
332. D. W. Gallagher and A. Pert, *Brain Res.*, 144:257 (1978).
333. M. A. Ruda, *Anat. Rec.*, 181:468 (1975).
334. Y. Shah and J. O. Dostrovsky, *Brain Res.*, 193:534 (1980).
335. T. D. Oleson and J. C. Liebeskind, *The Physiologist*, 18:338 (1975).
336. M. M. Behbehani and S. L. Pomeroy, *Brain Res.*, 149:226 (1978).
337. G. J. Giesler, Jr., K. D. Gerhart, R. P. Yezierski, T. K. Wilcox, and W. D. Willis, *Brain Res.*, 204:184 (1981).
338. J. C. Liebeskind, G. Guilbaud, J.-M. Besson, and J.-L. Oliveras, *Brain Res.*, 50:441 (1973).
339. J.-L. Oliveras, J.-M. Besson, G. Guilbaud, and J. C. Liebeskind, *Exp. Brain Res.*, 20:32 (1974).
340. J.-L. Oliveras, F. Redjemi, G. Guilbaud, and J.-M. Besson, *Pain*, 1:139 (1975).
341. R. Melzack and P. D. Wall, *Science*, 150:971 (1965).
342. J. W. Lewis, J. T. Cannon, and J. C. Liebeskind, *Science*. 208:623 (1980).
343. G. W. Terman, J. W. Lewis, and J. C. Liebeskind, *Brain Res.*, 260:147 (1983).
344. A. R. Gintzler, A. Levy, and S. Spector, *Proc. Natl. Acad. Sci. USA*, 73:2132 (1976).
345. J. Hughes, T. W. Smith, H. W. Kosterlitz, L. A. Fothergill, B. A. Morgan, and H. R. Morris, *Nature*, 258:577 (1975).
346. C. H. Li and D. Chung, *Proc. Natl. Acad. Sci. USA*, 73:1145 (1976).
347. A. F. Bradbury, D. G. Smyth, C. R. Snell, N. J. M. Birdsall, and E. C. Hulmes, *Nature*, 260:793 (1976).
348. A. Goldstein, S. Tachibana, L. I. Lowney, M. Hunkapiller, and L. Hood, *Proc. Natl. Acad. Sci. USA*, 76:6666 (1981).
349. A. Goldstein, W. Fischli, L. I. Lowney, M. Hunkapiller, and L. Hood, *Proc. Natl. Acad. Sci. USA*, 78:7219 (1981).
350. A. Pert, in *Opiates and Endogenous Opioid Peptides* (H. W. Kosterlitz, Ed.), Elsevier, Amsterdam, 1976, p. 87.
351. W. Feldberg and D. G. Smyth, *J. Physiol.*, 260:30P (1976).
352. F. E. Bloom, E. Battenberg, J. Rossier, N. Ling, and R. Guillemin, *Proc. Natl. Acad. Sci. USA*, 75:1591 (1978).
353. A. Dupont, L. Lepine, P. Langelier, Y. Merand, D. Rouleau, H. Vaudry, C. Gras, and N. Barden, *Regulatory Peptides*, 1:43 (1980).
354. J. Rossier, T. M. Vargo, S. Minick, N. Ling, F. E. Bloom, and R. Guillemin, *Proc. Natl. Acad. Sci. USA*, 74:5162 (1977).
355. S. J. Watson, H. Akil, C. W. Richard, and J. D. Barchas, *Nature*, 275:226 (1978).
356. M. Sar, W. E. Stumpf, R. J. Miller, K.-J. Chang, and P. Cuatrecasas, *J. Comp. Neurol.*, 182:17 (1978).

357. J. C. W. Finley, J. L. Maderdrut, and P. Petrusz, *J. Comp. Neurol.*, 198:541 (1981).
358. M. J. Kuhar and G. R. Uhl, *Adv. Biochem. Psychopharmac.*, 20:53 (1979).
359. E. Herbert, *Trends Biol. Sci.*, 6:184 (1981).
360. U. Gubler, P. Seeburg, B. J. Hoffman, L. P. Gage, and S. Udenfriend, *Nature*, 295:206 (1982).
361. M. Noda, Y. Furutani, H. Takahashi, M. Toyosato, T. Hirose, S. Inayama, S. Nakanishi, and S. Numa, *Nature*, 295:202 (1982).
362. W.-Y. Huang, R. C. C. Chang, A. J. Kastin, D. H. Coy, and A. V. Schally, *Proc. Natl. Acad. Sci. USA*, 76:6177 (1979).
363. R. V. Lewis, S. Stein, L. Gerber, M. Rubenstein, and S. Udenfriend, *Proc. Natl. Acad. Sci. USA*, 75:4021 (1978).
364. A. S. Stern, R. V. Lewis, S. Kimura, J. Rossier, L. D. Gerber, L. Brink, S. Stein, and S. Udenfriend, *Proc. Natl. Acad. Sci. USA*, 76:6680 (1979).
365. J. A. Richter, D. L. Wesche, and R. C. A. Frederickson, *Eur. J. Pharmacol.*, 56:105 (1979).
366. L. L. Iversen, S. D. Iversen, F. E. Bloom, T. Vargo, and R. Guillemin, *Nature*, 271:679 (1978).
367. S. De La Baume, G. Patey, and J.-C. Schwarz, *Neuroscience*, 6:315 (1981).
368. B. Malfroy, J. P. Swerts, C. Llorens, and J. C. Schwartz, *Neurosci. Lett.*, 11:329 (1979).
369. R. C. A. Frederickson and L. E. Geary, *Prog. Neurobiol.*, 19:19 (1982).
370. C. J. E. Niemegeers, K. H. L. Schellekens, W. F. M. Van-Bever, and P. A. J. Janssen, *Arzneimettel-Forsch.*, 26:1551 (1976).
371. S. DeLange, T. H. Stanley, and M. J. Boscoe, *Anesthesiology*, 53:564 (1980).
372. C. J. E. Niemegeers and P. A. J. Janssen, *Abstracts, Seventh World Congress of Anaesthesiology*, p. 287, 1980.
373. C. J. E. Niemegeers and P. A. J. Janssen, *Drug Dev. Res.*, 1:83 (1981).
374. R. N. Booher, S. E. Smits, W. W. Turner, and A. Pohland, *J. Med. Chem.*, 20:885 (1977).
375. S. E. Smits, R. Nickander, R. N. Booher, A. Pohland, D. M. Zimmerman, D. Wong, and M. D. Hynes, in *National Institute of Drug Abuse Research Monograph* (L. S. Harris, Ed.), 34:75, 1981.
376. R. Wang and N. Robinson, *Clin. Pharmacol. Ther.*, 29:771 (1981).
377. M. S. Mok, M. Lippmann, and S. N. Steen, *Clin. Pharmacol. Ther.*, 29:266 (1981).
378. J. P. Yardley, H. Fletcher III, and P. B. Russell, *Experientia*, 34:1124 (1979).

379. F. Camu, *Eur. J. Clin. Pharmacol.*, 19:259 (1981).
380. M. J. Staquet, *Curr. Med. Res. Opin.*, 6:475 (1980).
381. M. E. Freed, J. R. Potaski, E. H. Freed, G. L. Conklin, and J. L. Malis, *J. Med. Chem.*, 16:595 (1973).
382. J. L. Malis, M. E. Rosenthale, and M. I. Gluckman, *J. Pharm. Exp. Ther.*, 194:488 (1975).
383. R. J. Fragen and N. Caldwell, *Anesth. Analg.*, 57:563 (1978).
384. J. W. Downing, J. G. Utne, A. Barclay, and I. L. Schwegmann, *Br. J. Anaesth.*, 53:59 (1981).
385. W. Oosterlinck and W. DeSy, *Curr. Med. Res. Opin.*, 3:187 (1975).
386. N. J. Paymaster, *Br. J. Anaesth.*, 46:599 (1976).
387. D. G. Mayes, M. T. Miller, and N. J. Aldridge, *S. Afr. Med. J.*, 55:865 (1979).
388. J. M. Gibbs and H. D. Johnson, *Anaesth. Intensive Care*, 8: 441 (1980).
389. R. Verschraegen, M. T. Rosseel, M. Bogaert, and G. Rolly, *Acta Anesth. Belg.*, 27:123 (1976).
390. A. Hedges, J. Rose, M. Leighton, and P. Turner, *J. Clin. Pharmacol.*, 17:125 (1977).
391. S. F. Flavell-Matts and P. J. Ward, *J. Clin. Med.*, 36:286 (1982).
392. A. Hedges, P. Turner, and J. Wadsworth, *Br. J. Anaesth.*, 52:295 (1980).
393. R. J. Stephens, J. F. Waterfield, and R. A. Franklin, *Gen. Pharmacol.*, 9:73 (1978).
394. D. M. Zimmerman, R. Nickander, J. S. Horng, and D. T. Wong, *Nature*, 275:332 (1978).
395. D. M. Zimmerman, S. E. Smits, M. D. Hynes, B. E. Cantrell, M. Reamer, and R. Nickander, in *NIDA Research Monograph* (L. S. Harris, Ed.), 41:112 (1982).
396. M. D. Hynes, S. E. Smits, B. E. Cantrell, R. Nickander, and D. M. Zimmerman, in *NIDA Research Monograph* (L. S. Harris, Ed.), 41:119 (1982).
397. M. D. Aceto, L. S. Harris, W. L. Dewey, and E. L. May, in *NIDA Research Monograph* (L. S. Harris, Ed.), 34:297 (1981).
398. J. H. Woods, F. Medzihradsky, C. B. Smith, A. M. Young, and H. H. Swain, in *NIDA Research Monograph* (L. S. Harris, Ed.), 34:327 (1981).
399. D. Romer, H. Buscher, R. C. Hill, R. Maurer, T. J. Petcher, H. B. A. Welle, H. C. C. K. Bakel, and A. M. Akkerman, *Life Sci.*, 27:971 (1980).
400. D. Romer, R. C. Hill, and R. Maurer, in *Advances in Pain Research and Therapy* (J. J. Bonica, U. Lindblom, and A. Iggo, Eds.), Raven, New York, 1983.
401. M. F. Piercey, R. A. Lahti, L. A. Schroeder, F. J. Einspahr, and C. Barsuhn, *Life Sci.*, 31:1197 (1982).

402. D. Romer, H. H. Buscher, R. C. Hill, R. Maurer, T. J. Petchek, H. Zeugner, W. Benson, E. Finner, W. Milkowski, and P. W. Thies, *Life Sci.*, 31:1217 (1982).
403. W. T. Beaver and G. A. Feise, *J. Clin. Pharmacol.*, 17:579 (1977).
404. A. Sunshine and E. Laska, *Clin. Pharmacol. Ther.*, 18:530 (1975).
405. I. Tigerstedt, J. Sipponen, T. Tammisto, and M. Turunen, *Br. J. Anaesth.*, 49:1133 (1976).
406. R. K. Furgreson and D. M. Turek, *Pharmatherapeutica*, 1:523 (1977).
407. H. Breivik and H. Siebke, *Clin. Ther.*, 2:28 (1979).
408. H. U. Gerbershagen, N. Eger, and R. Frey, *Clin. Therapeut.*, 2:22 (1979).
409. M. S. Mok, M. Lippmann, and S. N. Steen, *IRCS Med. Sci.*, 5:39 (1977).
410. L. De Thibault De Boesinghe, *Curr. Ther. Res.*, 34:646 (1978).
411. J. C. Gasser and J. W. Belville, *Clin. Pharmacol. Ther.*, 18: 175 (1975).
412. I. Tigerstedt, T. Tammisto, and P. Leander, *Acta Anaesth. Scand.*, 23:555 (1979).
413. V. M. Campas and E. L. Solis, *J. Clin. Pharmacol.*, 20:42 (1980).
414. F. Hoffmeister, G. Kroneberg, U. Schlichtung, and W. Wuttke, *Arzneim. Forsch.*, 24:600 (1974).
415. R. W. Houde, S. L. Wallenstein, and A. Rogers, in *Proceedings of the 40th Annual Meeting of the Committee on Problems of Drug Dependence*, p. 162, 1978.
416. W. H. Forrest, Jr., C. R. Brown, P. F. Shroff, and G. Tuetsch, *J. Clin. Pharmacol.*, 12:440 (1972).
417. W. H. Forrest, Jr., C. R. Brown, J. Katz, and D. C. Mahler, *J. Clin. Pharmacol.*, 16:610 (1976).
418. J. S. Finch, *J. Clin. Pharmacol.*, 20:689 (1980).
419. S. S. Bloomfield, T. P. Borden, and J. Mitchell, *Int. J. Clin. Pharmacol. Ther. Toxicol.*, 19:152 (1981).
420. D. R. Jasinski, W. R. Martin, and R. Hoeldtke, *Clin. Pharmacol. Ther.*, 12:613 (1971).
421. T. Oyama, T. Jin, R. Yamaya, N. Ling, and R. Guillemin, *Lancet*, 1:122 (1980).
422. F. E. Bloom, D. Segal, N. Ling, and R. Guillemin, *Science*, 194:630 (1976).
423. D. H. Catlin, K. K. Hui, H. H. Loh, and C. H. Li, *Commun. Psychopharmacol.*, 1:439 (1977).
424. J. A. Hartsuck and W. N. Lipscomb, in *The Enzymes* (P. Bayer, Ed.), Academic, New York, 1971, p. 1.

425. S. Ehrenpreis, R. L. Balagot, J. E. Comaty, and S. B. Myles, in *Advances in Pain Research and Therapy, Vol. 3*, (J. J. Bonica, J. C. Liebeskind, and D. G. Albe-Fessard, Eds.), Raven, New York, 1979, p. 479.
426. S. Ehrenpreis, R. L. Balagot, S. B. Myles, C. Advocate, and J. E. Comaty, in *Endogenous and Exogenous Opiate Agonist and Antagonists*, (E. Long Way, Ed.), Pergamon, New York, 1980, p. 379.
427. R. L. Balagot, S. Ehrenpreis, K. Kubota, and J. Greenberg, in *Advances in Pain Research and Therapy, Vol. 5*, (J. J. Bonica, U. Lindblom, and A. Iggo, Eds.), Raven, New York, 1983, p. 305.
428. K. Budd, in *Advances in Pain Research and Therapy, Vol. 5*, (J. J. Bonica, U. Lindblom, A. Iggo, L. E. Jones, C. Benedetti, Eds.), Raven, New York, p. 289, 1983.
429. B. Malfroy, J. P. Swerts, A. Guyon, B. P. Roques, and J. C. Schwartz, *Nature*, 276:523 (1978).
430. B. P. Roques, M. C. Fournie-Zaluski, E. Soroca, J. M. Lecomte, B. Malfroy, C. Llorens, and J.-C. Schwartz, *Nature*, 288:286 (1980).
431. J.-C. Schwartz, B. Malfroy, and S. DeLaBaume, *Life Sci.*, 29:1715 (1981).
432. R. C. A. Frederickson, *Life Sci.*, 21:23 (1977).
433. J. S. Morley, *Ann. Rev. Pharmacol. Toxicol.*, 20:81 (1980).
434. H. W. Kosterlitz, J. A. H. Lord, S. J. Paterson, and A. A. Waterfield, *Br. J. Pharmacol.*, 68:333 (1980).
435. D. Romer, H. H. Buscher, R. C. Hill, J. Pless, W. Bauer, F. Cardinaux, A. Closse, D. Hauser, and R. Huguenin, *Nature*, 268:547 (1977).
436. B. von Graffenried, E. del Pozo, J. Roubicek, E. Krebs, W. Poldinger, P. Burmeister, and L. Kerp, *Nature*, 272:729 (1978).
437. W. A. Stubbs, A. Jones, C. A. W. Edwards, D. Delitala, W. J. Jeffcoate, and S. J. Ratter, *Lancet*, 2:1225 (1978).
438. G. Stacher, P. Bauer, H. Steinringer, E. Schreiber, and G. Schmierer, *Pain*, 7:159 (1979).
439. T. Lindeburg, V. Larsen, H. Kehlet, and E. Jacobsen, *Acta Anaesth. Scand.*, 25:254 (1981).
440. H. B. Andersen, B. C. Jorgensen, and A. Engquist, *Acta Anaesth. Scand.*, 26:69 (1982).
441. R. C. A. Frederickson, E. L. Smithwick, R. Shuman, and K. G. Bemis, *Science*, 211:603 (1981).
442. R. C. A. Frederickson, C. J. Parli, G. W. DeVane, and M. D. Hynes, *NIDA Research Monograph* (L.S. Harris, Ed.), Vol. 43, pp. 150-156 (1982).
443. V. Brantl, A. Pfeiffer, A. Herz, A. Henschen, and F. Lottspeich, *Peptides*, 3:793 (1982).
444. M. D. Hynes and R. C. A. Frederickson, *Life Sci.*, 31:1201 (1982).

445. P. L. Wood, S. E. Charleson, D. Lane, and R. L. Hudgin, *Neuropharmacology* 20:1215 (1981).
446. A. Goldstein, personal communication.
447. R. C. A. Frederickson, E. L. Smithwick, and D. P. Henry, in *Neuropeptides and Neural Transmission* (C. Ajmone-Marsan and W. Z. Traczyk, Ed.), Raven, New York, 1980, p. 227.
448. Eli Lilly and Company, *LY127623. An Investigational New Drug. Clinical Investigation Manual*, 1981.
449. J. F. Calimlim, W. M. Wardell, K. Sriwatanakul, L. Lasagna, and C. Cox, *Lancet*, 1:1375 (1982).
450. S. S. Bloomfield, T. P. Barden, and J. Mitchell, *Clin. Pharmacol. Ther.*, 34:240-247 (1983).
451. M. Otsuka, S. Konishi, and T. Takahashi, *Fed. Proc.*, 34:1922 (1975).
452. R. A. Nicoll, C. Schenker, and S. E. Leeman, *Ann. Rev. Neurosci.*, 3:227 (1980).
453. J. M. Stewart, C. J. Getto, K. Neldner, E. B. Reeve, W. A. Krivoy, and E. Zimmerman, *Nature*, 262:784 (1976).
454. R. C. A. Frederickson, V. Burgis, and J. D. Edwards, *Science*, 198:756 (1977).
455. P. Oehme, H. Hilse, E. Morgenstern, and E. Gores, *Science*, 208:305 (1980).
456. J. Malick and J. Goldstein, *Life Sci.*, 23:835 (1978).
457. R. C. A. Frederickson and P. D. Gesellchen, in *Neuropeptides and Neural Transmission (IBRO Monograph No. 7)* (A. A. M. Marsan and W. Z. Traczyk, Eds.), Raven, New York, 1980, p.111.
458. J. M. Stewart, M. E. Hall, J. Harkins, R. C. A. Frederickson, L. Tenenius, T. Hokfelt, and W. A. Krivoy, *Peptides*, 3:851 (1982).
459. M. F. Piercey, L. A. Schroeder, K. Folkers, J.-C. Xu, and J. Horig, *Science*, 214:1361 (1981).
460. B. Akerman, S. Rosell, and K. Folkers, *Acta Physiol. Scan.*, 114:631 (1982).
461. B. V. Clineschmidt, J. C. McGuffin, and P. B. Bunting, *Eur. J. Pharmacol.*, 54:129 (1979).
462. A. J. Osbahr, C. B. Nemeroff, and D. Luttinger, *J. Pharmacol. Exp. Ther.*, 217:645 (1981).
463. P. W. Kalivas, G. A. Bau, C. B. Nemeroff, and A. J. Prange, Jr., *Brain Res.*, 243:279 (1982).
464. A. Pecile, S. Ferri, A. Santagostino, and V. R. Olgiati, *Experientia*, 31:332 (1975).
465. A. Fabri, C. Santoro, C. Moretti, M. Cappa, F. Fraioli, G. P. Dijulio, T. Galuzzi, and V. Lamanna, *Int. J. Clin. Pharmacol. Therap. Toxicol.*, 19:509 (1981).
466. M. Rezek, V. Havlicek, L. Leybin, F. S. Labella, and H. Friesen, *Can. J. Physiol. Pharmacol.*, 56:227 (1978).

467. G. Zetler, *Neuropharmacology*, 19:415 (1980).
468. P. L. Faris, B. R. Komisaruk, L. R. Watkins, and D. J. Mayer, *Science*, 219:310 (1983).
469. J. M. Walker, D. E. Tucker, D. H. Coy, B. B. Walker, and H. Akil, *Eur. J. Pharmacol.*, 85:121 (1982).
470. G. Belcher, T. Smock, and H. L. Fields, *Brain Res.*, 247:373 (1982).
471. G. M. Abrams and L. Recht, *Int. J. Acupuncture Electrother.*, 7:105 (1982).
472. B. A. Berkowitz, S. H. Ngai, and A. D. Finck, *Science*, 194: 967 (1976).
473. B. A. Berkowitz, A. D. Finck, M. D. Hynes, and S. H. Ngai, *Anesthesiology*, 51:309 (1979).
474. W. C. Clark and J. C. Yang, *Pain Abstracts, 2nd World Congress on Pain*, 1:14, 1978.
475. C. R. Chapman and C. Benedetti, *Anesthesiology*, 51:135 (1979).
476. J. C. Yang, W. C. Clark, and S.-H. Ngai, *Anesthesiology*, 52:414 (1980).
477. M. D. Hynes and B. A. Berkowitz, *J. Pharmacol. Exp. Ther.*, 220:499 (1982).
478. W. R. Buckett, *Rev. Pure Appl. Pharmacol. Sci.*, 2:115 (1981).
479. F. V. DeFeudis, *Drug Dev. Res.*, 3:1 (1983).
480. W. R. Buckett, *Br. J. Pharmacol.*, 68:129 (1980).
481. W. R. Buckett, *Neuropharmacology*, 19:715 (1980).
482. W. R. Buckett, *Eur. J. Pharmacol.*, 69:281 (1981).
483. T. C. Spaulding, J. Little, K. McCormack, and S. Fielding, *Brain Res. Bull.*, 4:711 (1980).
484. J. Sawynok and F. S. LaBella, *Neuropharmacology*, 21:397 (1982).
485. E. I. Danilova, V. N. Grafova, and G. N. Kryzhanovsky, *Byul. Eksp. Biol. Med.*, 87:525 (1979).
486. J. M. Liebman and G. Pastor, *Neurosci. Abst.*, 4:461 (1978).
487. D. Biggio, D. Della Bella, V. Frigeni, and A. Guidotti, *Neuropharmacology*, 16:149 (1977).
488. P. Mantegazza, R. Tammisto, L. Vincentini, F. Zambotti, and N. Zonta, *Br. J. Pharmacol.*, 67:103 (1979).
489. D. A. Kendall, M. Browner, and S. J. Enna, *Soc. Neurosci. Abstr.*, 7:335 (1981).
490. E. Pedersen, P. Arlien-Soborg, and J. Mai, *Acta Neurol. Scand.*, 50:665, 1974.
491. O. de S. Pinto, M. Polikar, and G. Debono, *Postgrad. Med. J.*, 48:18 (1972).
492. D. A. Cutting and C. C. Jordan, *Br. J. Pharmacol.*, 54:171 (1975).
493. R. A. Levy and H. K. Proudfit, *J. Pharmacol. Exp. Ther.*, 202:445 (1977).

494. R. A. Levy and H. K. Proudfit, *Eur. J. Pharmacol.*, 57:43 (1979).
495. R. C. A. Frederickson, V. Burgis, and J. D. Edwards, *Fed. Proc.*, 36:965 (1977).
496. D. R. Curtis, C. J. A. Game, G. A. R. Johnston, and R. M. McCulloch, *Brain Res.*, 70:493 (1974).
497. S. R. Naik, A. Guidotti, and E. Costa, *Neuropharmacology*, 15:479 (1976).
498. P. Krogsgaard-Larsen, G. A. R. Johnston, D. Lodge, and D. R. Curtis, *Nature*, 268:53 (1977).
499. R. C. Hill, R. Maurer, H.-H. Buscher, and D. Romer, *Eur. J. Pharmacol.*, 69:221 (1981).
500. A. Grognet, F. Hertz, and F. V. DeFeudis, *Drug Alcohol Depend.*, 9:269 (1982).
501. *Chemical and Engineering News*, 59:5, 1981.
502. S. Fielding and H. Lal, *Med. Res. Rev.*, 1:97 (1980).
503. H. Lal and G. T. Shearman, *Prog. Clin. Biol. Res.*, 77:99 (1981).
504. G. T. Shearman and H. Lal, in *Neuropharmacology: Clinical Applications* (W. Essman and L. Valzelli, Eds.), Spectrum, New York, 1982, p. 221.
505. S. Fielding, J. Wilker, M. Hynes, M. Szewczak, W. Novick, and H. Lal, *J. Pharmacol. Exp. Ther.*, 207:899 (1978).
506. G. A. Bentley, I. W. Copeland, and J. Starr, *J. Clin. Exp. Pharmacol. Physiol.*, 4:405 (1977).
507. H. Schmitt, J. C. LeDouarec, and N. Petillot, *Neuropharmacology*, 13:289 (1974).
508. R. D. E. Sewell and P. S. J. Spencer, *Br. J. Pharmacol.*, 54:256 (1975).
509. G. Paalzow and C. Paalzow, *Naunyn-Schmiedeberg's Arch. Pharmacol.*, 292:119 (1976).
510. T. C. Spaulding, F. Fielding, J. J. Venafro, and H. Lal, *Eur. J. Pharmacol.*, 58:19 (1979).
511. S. V. R. Reddy, J. L. Maderdrut, and T. L. Yaksh, *J. Pharmacol. Exp. Ther.*, 213:525 (1980).
512. A. S. Tung and T. L. Yaksh, *Brain Res.*, 247:75 (1982).
513. L.-F. Tseng, *Life Sci.*, 31:987 (1982).
514. J. L. K. Hylden and G. L. Wilcox, *Eur. J. Pharmacol.*, 86:95 (1983).
515. G. F. S. Ling and G. W. Pasternak, *Brain Res.* (in press).
516. K. Verebey (Ed.), *Opioids in Mental Illness: Theories, Clinical Observations and Treatment Possibilities*, The New York Academy of Sciences, New York, 1982.
517. N. S. Shah and A. G. Donald (Eds.), *Endorphins and Opiate Antagonists in Psychiatric Research: Clinical Implications*, Plenum, New York, 1982.

2
Antidepressants

DAVID C. HORWELL *Parke-Davis Research Unit, Addenbrookes Hospital Site, Cambridge, England*

I. INTRODUCTION

Among the disorders of the central nervous system, it is depression, which is both a normal and an abnormal phenomenon, that most reflects the human condition. It would indeed be regarded as abnormal if depression did not follow a traumatic experience such as bereavement or redundancy, and it may follow a great personal success, such as passing an examination or giving birth. Such depression can be controlled by the passing of time or by various activities such as counseling with family, friends, priest, or doctor, or by taking up new interests and relationships. However, depression can become so disabling that it leads to the inability to communicate, or to the thought or even the act of suicide. Such abnormal depression certainly warrants treatment by drugs or hospitalization.

Human beings have treated themselves for centuries with concoctions prepared from natural herbs and substances to unburden their minds of melancholic thoughts. Usually these preparations have provided relief of a transient and euphoric nature, such as that experienced with marijuana, cocaine, alcohol, morphine, or the hallucinogens like mescaline, psylocibin, and khat. More recently in this century, we have seen the advent of electroconvulsive therapy (ECT) as an effective treatment for depression. In addition, a useful armory of drugs has been developed since the 1950s. The first major class of drugs to receive widespread acclaim was the so-called monoamine oxidase (MAO) inhibitors. These drugs, which were first introduced into the clinic for the treatment of tuberculosis, were found to have a marked stimulant effect in some of the patients. Reinvestigation of these drugs as a treatment for depression quickly testified to their efficacy in this condition. The MAO inhibitors are particularly effective in the treatment of reactive (or secondary) depression, but it repeatedly has been emphasized that care must be exercised in their use, as these drugs can precipitate a hypertensive crisis when ingested with certain other drugs and a wide variety of common foods that contain sympathomimetic amines, such as tyramine and phenylethylamine. These include cheese, red wine, marmite, and pickled herrings.

The most widely prescribed drugs for the treatment of depression are the tricyclic antidepressants, so called because of the three fused rings that characterize their chemical structure. The prototype of this class of compound is imipramine which was first investigated as a treatment for schizophrenia, but without success. However, reinvestigation of the drug by Kuhn in Switzerland in 1957 showed it to be effective in the treatment of many types of depression.

During the 1970s we have seen the development of a "second generation" of antidepressants that appear to have less pronounced cardiovascular and anticholinergic side effects than the tricyclics. It appears that the sedative tricyclics amitriptyline and doxepin, as well as the newer drugs nomifensine, mianserin, and trazodone, have anxiolytic properties in addition to their antidepressant effects.

It is intended in this chapter to review the properties of the major classes of drugs currently used in the treatment of depression and to refer the reader to more detailed articles on the clinical, psychiatric, diagnostic, and social aspects of the disease itself. A brief survey of the epidemiology, classification, and etiology of depression is followed by a description of the major classes of antidepressants: the tricyclics, the MAO inhibitors, second-generation drugs, lithium, ECT, and amphetamine and related compounds. The concluding discussion focuses on the areas of research that may offer scope for the development of truly novel third-generation drugs for the 1980s; emphasis in recent research has centered on the role of biogenic amines, electrolyte imbalance, and neuroendocrine mechanisms in depression.

II. EPIDEMIOLOGY OF DEPRESSION

Depression is now the most common mental illness diagnosed by psychiatrists [1,2]. However, the full extent of depressive illness is not easy to estimate, and it depends on the criteria used to assess symptoms that are very subjective in nature. The presenting symptoms that general practitioners are faced with may cover the whole continuum between neuroses and psychoses. Unless the history of the patient's illness is known, it is often difficult to identify the underlying syndrome of depression. Patients who remain under the care of a general practitioner are invariably at some time treated with antianxiety agents, and to a lesser extent, by neuroleptics or even placebos. However, those patients who are subsequently referred to a psychiatrist and who may ultimately require hospital treatment may represent a separate subclass. The cases actually treated as depression may be considerably less than the total number that require antidepressant therapy [3,4]. There are several yardsticks for measuring the epidemiology of depression. In 1976 the National Institute of Mental Health, and other sources, estimated that up to 15% of the adult population of the United States suffered from a serious depressive disorder in any given year [5–7]. In the same year in the United States, 400,000 cases were treated for depression and 20,000–26,000 suicides were attributed to acute mental depression [5,5]. This places depression as ranking number 10 in the diseases that cause death. Other surveys show the range of depression that is severe enough to impair normal mental function as high as 23% of the population [6]. In the United Kingdom, it has been estimated that approximately 5% of the general practitioner's workload and 2% of the total bill of the National Health Service are directed toward treatment of depression [8]. The world market of antidepressant drugs in 1977 has been estimated as being worth $520 million, compared with $700 million for antianxiety, and $300 million for neuroleptic drugs [9]. It is widely believed that women suffer from depression more than men in a ratio of approximately 2:1 [6,8], although this ratio varies widely on age and subclass of depression [10].

III. CLASSIFICATION OF DEPRESSION

It is convenient to classify mental illness into two groups, neurosis and psychosis [11]. The former usually manifests itself as anxiety and is invariably treated with the antianxiety agents such as the benzodiazepines. Psychosis may include schizophrenia, depression, and mania. It is important to bear in mind that neurosis and psychosis are part of a spectrum of syndromes that may show very similar symptoms. Indeed, classification is often difficult even if the history of the illness has been long established. The diagnosis of depression on the basis of acute symptoms may lead to the choice of the wrong drug or other therapeutic regimen for chronic maintenance of the condition. Depression is now often diagnosed as either the neurotic or psychotic type. Neurotic depression often appears as anxiety, coupled with some somatic complaints and behavioral disturbances. Psychotic depression is less common, with signs of mental agitation or retardation, morbid outlook, delusions, and even hallucinations. "Masked depression" is a useful term where depression is suspected but where the symptoms appear to be those of anxiety or phobia. The term schizo-affective disorder also has a role in describing the interface condition between the psychoses

1. Feelings of sadness, hopelessness, gloom
2. Inability to experience pleasure
3. Loss of appetite with associated weight loss
4. Insomnia
5. Fatigue, lethargy
6. Retardation
7. Agitation
8. Anxiety, tension
9. Decrease in libido
10. Feelings of guilt
11. Loss of interest in usual activities such as work
12. Loss of ability in rational though
13. Thoughts of suicide
14. Bodily complaints

Rating Scales

a. Global Assessment, involve scales of improvement, graded as moderate-some-none-worse
b. Clinical Interview, e.g., Hamilton Rating Scale
c. Self-Reports, mainly used by outpatients, e.g., Zung, Beck
d. Ratings by Nursing Staff, mainly used for day or inpatients, e.g., N.O.S.I.E.

FIG. 2.1 Some symptoms of depression and rating scales. (From Ref. 15.)

of schizophrenia and depression. Several excellent new books on the description of masked depression [12], the psychology of depression [13], and somatic manifestations of depressive disorders [14] offer an insight into these types of disorders and the problems of classification.

Psychotic depression may be further classified as either reactive (secondary) or endogenous (primary): Reactive depression is more prevalent in the younger age groups, endogenous depression more so in the elderly. Reactive depression is alleged to account for about 60% of treated cases, as this diagnosis is common where doctors believe they know the cause of a patient's depression. Therefore, this depression is perceived as being reactive to, or secondary after, a traumatic primary event such as bereavement, loss of job, or break up of a loving relationship. Endogenous depression accounts for about 30% of treated cases, the diagnosis of which occurs where the doctor is unable to determine the cause. Thus, the disease is perceived as being intrinsic in nature, or the primary cause of the symptoms. Although depression presents itself as a spectrum of anxiety or psychotic symptoms, several well characterized swings of mood, or behavioral polarized states, have been described. Endogenous depression has often been described as being of the unipolar (depressive) or bipolar (manic-depressive) type. The former is characterized by recurring bouts of deep melancholy and feelings of guilt that may vary in their duration, intervals, and severity; the latter is characterized by periods of overactivity, sometimes of a violent nature, followed by periods of deep depression. However, the manic and depressive phases do not necessarily alternate, nor are they of equal severity or duration. Mania is sometimes classified as a separate syndrome and is characterized by recurring episodes of overactivity, often of an extremely disturbing intensity. The diagnostic scales are based on necessarily subjective assessment of the symptoms of depression. Fig. 2.1 lists some of these symptoms together with some of the more commonly used rating scales, the details of which are described elsewhere [4,6,15–17].

IV. ETIOLOGY OF DEPRESSION

There are many causative factors in the development of depression in human beings, including genetic factors, stress induced by toxic substances, or environmental conditions. Akitstal and McKinney have surveyed the evidence for this multietiological input into depression [18]. Their conclusions are summarized in Fig. 2.2. These etiologies appear to manifest themselves in three main areas, both centrally and peripherally:

1. As biochemical changes of biogenic amine levels and turnover rates both in the central nervous system and peripherally
2. As changes in electrolyte balance (Na^+/K^+) with concomitant changes in stimulated ATPase
3. As changes in endocrine function.

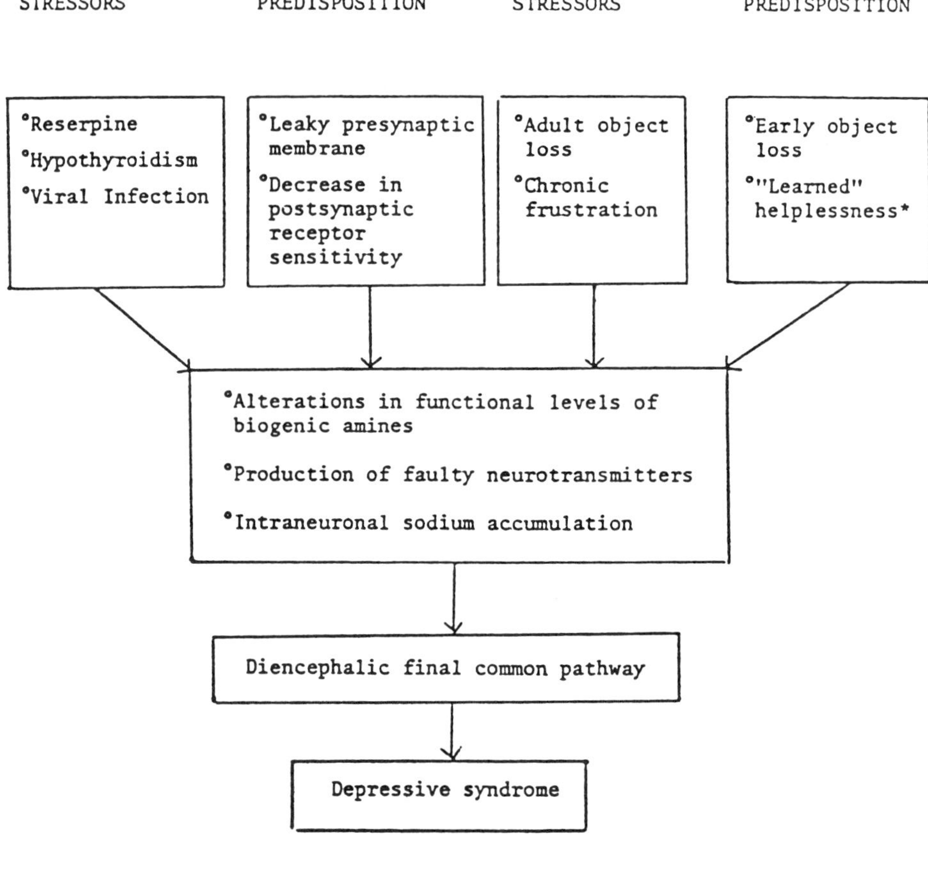

* NOTE : See ref. 13

FIG. 2.2 Multetiological input to the depressive syndrome.

V. THE MAJOR CLASSES OF ANTIDEPRESSENT DRUGS

The major classes of drugs used in general practice for the treatment of depression in the United Kingdom are given in Table 1.1 together with their approximate percentage use in both acute (first week) and chronic maintenance therapy [9, see also Ref. 193]. Clearly, the tricyclics dominate this therapeutic area, with the antianxiety agents being important in maintenance therapy.

TABLE 2.1 The Major Classes of Antidepressant Drugs and Their Approximate Percentage of Use

Drug class	Acute therapy (first week) (= %)	Chronic maintenance therapy (= %)
Tricyclics	84	53
MAO inhibitors	1	2
Antianxiety agents	7	34
Antipsychotics (neuroleptics)	1	6
Others (e.g., stimulants, β-Blockers, etc.)	7	5

Note: Noncompliance indicates approximately 60% of patients who were still depressed after 6 weeks no longer took medication.

A. The Tricyclic Antidepressants

1. Efficacy

There are 20–30 of this class of drugs currently available for the treatment of depression. The most widely prescribed and studied members of this group are listed in Fig. 2.3, together with their recommended daily doses [1,7,19]. These are the drugs of choice for the treatment of psychotic depression, and clinical evidence is increasing for their effectiveness in neurotic depression [20,21]. Estimates of their efficacy vary widely. Surveys, as assessed on a variety of rating scales (see Fig. 2.1), have shown that the tricyclics are effective in 70% of treated patients as compared with 20–40% on placebo during the same period [22]. However, other surveys indicate that the tricyclics are "only just better than placebo" [Ref. 5, p. 87]. The tricyclics appear to be a relatively homogenous group, the most widely prescribed being various commercial brands of imipramine and amitriptyline either alone or in combination particularly with antianxiety agents [23]. In depressed patients, the antidepressant activity does not usually appear until 14–21 days of multiple daily dosing, although the major side effects appear within a few days. This may, in part, account for the high percentage of noncompliance with these drugs. The most troublesome side effects are those associated with the anticholinergic properties of the drug (e.g., dry mouth, sedation, blurred vision, constipation) and the cardiovascular effects, particularly hypotension. Cardiotoxicity has proved fatal in the elderly and in patients with heart disease [24].

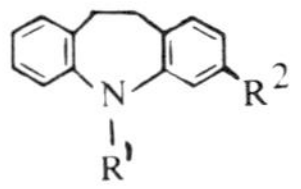

$R^1 = (CH_2)_3N(CH_3)_2$: $R^2 = H$, imipramine (Tofranil, Presamine) (75-300)

$R^1 = (CH_2)_3NHCH_3$; $R^2 = H$ desipramine (Pertofran (e), Norpramin) (75-200)

$R^1 = (CH_2)_3N(CH_3)_2$; $R^2 = Cl$, clomipramine (Anafranil) (50-150)

$R^1 = CH_2CH(CH_3)CH_2N(CH_3)_2$ trimipramine (Surmontil) (50-100)

$R^1 = (CH_2)_3N$⟨ ⟩N-CH_2-CH_2OH, (with bridgehead double bond)

Opipramol (Insidon, Ensidon), (100-150)

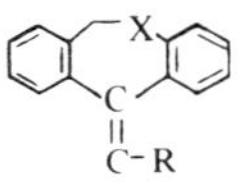

X = CH_2; R = $(CH_2)_2N(CH_3)_2$, amitriptyline (Tryptizol, Elavil, Lentizol) (75-300)

X = S, R = $(CH_2)_2N(CH_3)_2$, dothiepin (Prothiaden) (75-150)

X = O, R = $(CH_2)_2N(CH_3)_2$ doxepin (Sinequan, Adapin) (75-300)

X = CH_2, R = $(CH_2)_2NHCH_3$ nortriptyline (Aventyl) (Allegron) (75-100)

X = CH_2, R = $CH(CH_3)N(CH_3)_2$ butriptyline (Evadyne) (75-100)

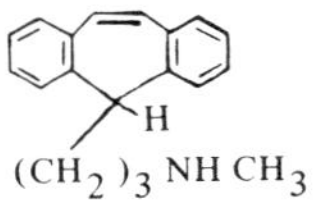

protriptyline (Concordin, Triptil, Vivactil) (15-60)

Notes: Also used in combination with other drugs, e.g., amitriptyline + perphenazine (Triavil, Etrafon). Recommended daily dose ranges (m.g., orally) are given in parenthese after the names. (From Refs. 17,19).

FIG. 2.3 Some tricyclic antidepressant drugs.

2. Metabolism and Pharmacokinetics

The metabolism of imipramine has been studied in detail in many animal species; considerably less work has been directed toward the other tricyclics. There have been 24 metabolites of imipramine identified, of which the 6 major ones are shown in Fig. 2.4 [25–27]. The most important metabolite is desmethylimipramine (DMI) which also has potent pharmacological actions and is a drug in its own right known as desipramine (see Fig. 2.3). The *N*-oxide of imipramine has been shown to be reconverted to the parent compound on second pass and may therefore be an important circulating prodrug. Indeed, amitriptyline *N*-oxide has been recently introduced into the clinic as a tricyclic that is claimed to have less cardiovascular toxicity [Ref. 24, p. 203].

There is a species difference in the metabolic profile of imipramine. In man, rats, mice, rabbits, and guinea pigs demethylation to DMI is the major primary metabolic process, whereas pigs produce mainly the *N*-oxide [28–31]. The formation of a high proportion of inactive metabolites in some members of the population may account for the approximate 30% failure rate in the clinic. The central pharmacological effects of the tricyclics are now believed to be due to a combination of the properties of both the tertiary and secondary amines.

Virtually all the tertiary amine tricyclics give the corresponding desmethyl metabolites which are also active antidepressants. The dibenzocycloheptadienes, amitriptyline and nortriptyline, give the bridgehead 10-hydroxy derivative as a major metabolite, which quickly forms a glucoronide [32]. In contrast, the dibenzapines like imipramine and chlorimipramine, show no evidence for bridgehead hydroxylation. The drugs with a 10,11-double bond, such as protriptyline and opipramol, give a 10,11-dihydroxy metabolite, possibly derived from the 10,11-epoxide. The epoxide has been observed in up to 40% of the total metabolites present in rat urine with protriptyline, but only in small amounts for opipramol [33,34].

The tricyclics are well absorbed on oral dosing. However, they are notoriously difficult to assay accurately in blood, as they are rapidly metabolized, and a high percentage is bound to plasma protein with only 10% actually circulating as free drug. Thus, these drugs have a low and variable bioavailability and estimates therefore vary widely as to the effective minimum blood levels [35–39].

Of a single dose of imipramine in humans, 30–50% is excreted in the urine within 24 hr. Bilary excretion is of secondary importance, but the drug is removed by both routes mainly as glucoronide conjugates [40,41].

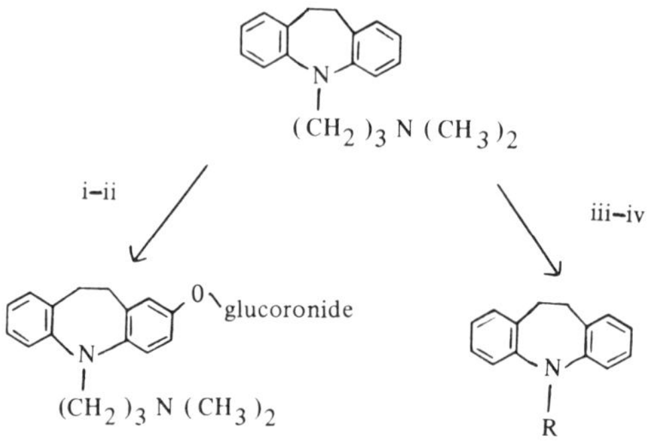

i. Hydroxylation

ii. Glucoronidation

iii. Demethylation, R = $(CH_2)_3NHCH_3$ (desipramine, active metabolite)

iv. Di-demethylation, R = $(CH_2)_3NH_2$

v. *N*-oxidation, R = $(CH_2)_3N(CH_3)_2$ (with ↓ O on N)

vi. Complete loss of side chain, R = H

FIG. 2.4 Major metabolites of imipramine.

3. Side Effects

The major side effects of the tricyclics are related to their anticholinergic and cardiovascular properties. The latter are complicated by the diverse activities of these drugs on the heart and vascular tissue, which include both α- and β-adrenergic effects, anticholinergic effects, and modification of atrio- and intraventricular conduction [42]. The effects on the cardiovascular system are not solely related to, nor correlated with, their potency on the noradrenaline (NA) responses.

The typical anticholinergic effects such as dry mouth (perhaps the most bothersome to patients), blurred vision, constipation, and sedation are apparent in clinical use almost immediately, although some degree of tolerance is achieved after a few days. A major compliance problem encountered in the clinic is that the patient is asked to take medication that will make him feel worse during the first few days before the antidepressant properties appear. However, some degree of sedation is often considered beneficial for patients who have had a history of insomnia and show symptoms of anxiety. There is a good correlation between peripheral and central anticholinergic effects, as measured by acetylcholine-induced guinea pig ileum contraction, and competitive binding experiments in synaptosomes prepared from whole rat brain using [^{3}H]propyl benzilyl choline mustard, respectively (see Table 2.2, entry 8).

The direct effects of the tricyclics on the heart have proved fatal in some cases and great care must be exercised in administration of these drugs to the elderly and those with a history of heart disease. It is advised that a pretreatment electrocardiogram (ECG) be run in suspect patients. A typical ECG produced on dosing tricyclics, such as imipramine, amitriptyline, nortriptyline, protriptyline, and doxepin, has similarities in both man and animals. Studies in rabbits indicate these drugs induce broadening of S waves, ST changes, and extremely deformed QRS complexes, which appear to be greatest with amitriptyline and doxepin [43—45]. Depressed patients treated with tricyclics often show prolongation of the P-R interval and broadening of QRS complexes, which may lead to a complete partial heart block in some cases. Increase in pulse rate is invariably associated with administration of the tricyclics, though hypotension is the most troublesome of the cardiovascular side effects seen in general practice. It has been indicated that approximately 20% of patients experience a considerable reduction in systolic blood pressure [46,47]. Unlike the anticholinergic effects, there appears to be no tolerance developed to hypotension, which manifests itself as dizziness and ataxia, with the inevitable result of falling and bone fractures, to which the elderly are particularly prone.

4. Mode of Action

In healthy man and animals, the tricylics induce sedation and mild depression. They are able to block the mouse-killing (muricidal) action of rats [48] and reduce spontaneous exploratory behavior in rats in open field studies [49]. The tricyclics antagonize the effects of the natural product reserpine, and several other synthetic depressants such as tetrabenazine. They also markedly potentiate the effects of the biogenic and sympathomimetic amines, particularly those due to NA, dopamine (DA), and serotonin, also known as 5-hydroxytrptamine (5-HT). A sample of these effects is shown for the most widely studied tricyclics in Tables 2.2 [50—52] and 2.3 [53].

a. Antagonism of the effects of reserpine. The naturally occuring rauwolfia alkaloid reserpine was introduced into clinical practice in the western world in 1954 as a treatment for arterial hypertension and was found to induce symptoms of similar character to depression in up to 15% of the patients [5,10]. The condition was found to be so severe in some cases that electroconvulsive therapy (ECT) was required. Animal studies both in vivo and in vitro have shown that reserpine decreases the functional levels of the brain neurotransmitter amines

Table 2.2 Some Biochemical and Pharmacological Effects of Selected Tricyclic Antidepressants

	1	2	3	4
Tricyclic antidepressant	Reserpine ptosis [ED_{50} (mg/kg)]	Apomorphine gnawing [ED_{50} (mg/kg)]	Antagonism of 6-OHDA of heart NA (ED_{50} mg/kg i.p.)	Antagonism of PCA depletion of of brain 5-HT (ED_{50} mg/kg i.p.)
Imipramine	3.5	3.7	3.4	No effect
Desipramine	0.8	6.9	0.25	No effect
Amitriptyline	13	3.6	5.4	No effect
Nortriptyline	5	4.9	1.2	>32
Protriptyline	0.4	7.9	0.12	≅30
Chlorimipramine	3.5	5.0	6.0	10
Opipramol	>40	62.6	—	—
Trimiprimine	20	22.8	—	—
Doxepin	42	4.0	4.7	No effect

Entries 1,2,5,6,8 adapted from Ref. 50; and from 3,4 Ref. 52; and 7 from Refs. 50 and 51.

NA, DA, and 5-HT. Reserpine induces this effect mainly through a mechanism where the presynaptic storage granules of these amines are made leaky, probably by membrane destabilization.

Most tricyclics antagonize reserpine-induced ptosis (Table 2.2, entry 1), catalepsy, and hypothermia (Table 2.3) in animal models, and this test has been widely used as a primary screen for antidepressants in laboratory animals. Reserpine-induced ptosis is believed to be mainly a peripheral response to antagonism of NA transmission, whereas catalepsy is mainly attributed to antagonism of DA transmission. The hypothermia is believed to be due to antagonism of NA effects in the whole animal. Imipramine, desipramine, and nortriptyline potentiate the initial hyperthermic phase and inhibit the subsequent hypothermic phase when dosed to animals before the reserpine. Imipramine, desipramine, amitriptyline, and nortriptyline dosed *after* reserpine induce

5	6	7			8	
Potentiation of NA pressor response in pitched rat (ED_{50} mg/kg i.v.)	Potentiation of 5-HT effects (ED_{50} mg/kg)	Inhibition of uptake in rat brain synaptosomes (IC_{50} μm) prepared from			Anticholinergic effects (IC_{50} μm)	
		Hypo-thalamus	Corpus striatum		peripheral	central
		NA	DA	5-HT	(G.P. ileum)	$[^3H]$-PrBCM binding
0.35	20	0.066	20	0.81	0.43	0.48
0.07	>20	0.0056	21	3.4	1.5	3.4
4.0	21	0.13	13	1.2	0.12	0.047
2.1	>20	0.025	11	1.7	0.45	0.48
0.025	>20	0.018	12	2.6	0.45	0.12
3.5	8.8	0.11	8.1	0.099	0.69	0.31
>4.0	>40	4.8	3.0	42	5.0	—
	>20	7.7	6.6	26	0.42	—
	54	0.12	24	2.9	0.52	0.54

a marked increase in body temperature above the control level [54]. Table 2.3 summarizes the effects of pretreatment (i.p.) with some tricyclics on reserpine hypothermia in mice. Body temperature is increased in a dose-related manner for drugs that are clinically effective antidepressants (e.g., imipramine, DMI, amitriptyline, and doxepin) as well as the MAO-inhibitors (e.g., isocarboxazide) and some stimulants (e.g., amphetamine). However, compounds that are not clinically effective antidepressants can also be very active in this test, including some hallucinogens, neuroleptics (e.g., CPZ), anthistamines (e.g., tripelennamine), and anticholinergics (e.g., atropine)[55]. Furthermore, several of the second-generation clinically effective antidepressants e.g., mianserin, iprindole, and trazodone, have little or no activity in these tests. Thus, reversal of reserpine effects is not a specific test for antidepressants, but needs to be used in conjunction with other tests.

TABLE 2.3 Temperature Change of Mice Pretreated in 1 Hr before Reserpine (5 mg/kg i.v.)

Compound	Dose (mg/kg i.p.)	Mean % change in body temperature
Imipramine	5	+40 (dose related $<$40 mg/kg)
Desipramine	1	+54 (dose related $<$5 mg/kg)
Amitriptyline	10	+62 (dose related $<$40 mg/kg)
Nortriptyline	5	+64 (dose related $<$20 mg/kg)
Trimipramine	5	+5 (not dose related)
Doxepin	10	+23 (dose related $<$20 mg/kg)
Isocarboxazide	5	+4 (dose related $<$20 mg/kg)
Amphetamine	1.25	+24 (dose related $<$10 mg/kg)
Chlorpromazine	5	+16 (not dose related)
Chlordiazepoxide	2.5	-22 (dose related $<$20 mg/kg)
Atropine	5	+29 (dose related $<$20 mg/kg)
Tripelennamine	5	+16 (dose related $<$40 mg/kg)

Source: Adapted from Ref. 53.

b. Potentiation of the effects of biogenic and sympathomimetic amines. The tricyclics that stimulate DA and NA intensify the gnawing syndrome elicited by apomorphine [56] (Table 2.2, entry 2), and potentiate the gnawing induced in mice by DOPA, the biosynthetic precursor of both DA and NA, combined with the peripheral decarboxylase inhibitor Ro-4-4602 [57]. Potentiation of the peripheral responses to NA has been demonstrated in both the pithed rat preparation [58] (Table 2.2, entry 5) and the cat nictitating membrane [59]. The tricyclics also potentiate the effect of 5-HTP, the biosynthetic precursor of 5-HT, with the tertiary amine chlorimipramine being particularly effective in this regard [10,60] (Table 2.2, entry 6).

The considerations discussed above are evidence for the indirect involvement of the biogenic amines NA, DA, and 5-HT in the mode of action of antidepressants. The potent peripheral activity of the tricyclics on NA and 5-HT function led Sigg [61] to speculate that their antidepressant properties may be due to a similar stimulation of central noradrenergic neurons. Much evidence is now available to support this hypothesis. Indeed, it has been shown that although both the tricyclics and the neuroleptic CPZ inhibit peripheral NA uptake [62], only the tricyclics are active in brain tissue [63]. Thus, the tricyclics inhibit NA uptake in both mouse brain cortical slices [64] and hypothalamic synaptosomal preparations [65], both areas being rich in NA-containing neurons. Imipramine and DMI are potent in this regard, consistent with the whole animal data described above. The tricyclics also inhibit uptake of 5-HT from synaptosomes prepared from the hypothalamic area. Chlorimipramine is the most potent against 5-HT uptake, being much greater than imipramine in this regard [10,66,67; Table 2.2, entry 7]. Many of the tricyclics have only weak activity against DA uptake, but the newer clinically effective antidepressant, nomifensine is potent in this regard (see Table 2.5). The inhibition of uptake of ^{14}C-labeled NA in synaptosomes prepared from rat brain hypothalamus, and ^{14}C-labeled DA and 5-HT in synaptosomes prepared from rat brain corpus striatum, has recently been studied for many tricyclics, which confirms the earlier findings discussed above (Table 2.2, entry 7).

In many animal models, including monkey but not man [10], the compounds α-methylparatyrosine (α-MPT, a tyrosine hydroxylase inhibitor which blocks biosynthesis of both NA and DA [68]), and ρ-chlorophenylalanine (PCPA, an inhibitor of 5-HT biosynthesis) both induce apathy and withdrawal similar to that seen in depression. The tricyclics antagonize these effects [10]. Similarly, the compound 6-hydroxydopamine (6-OHDA) depletes NA and DA, and PCPA depletes 5-HT, and these have been used as in vivo methods for evaluating potential antidepressant activity [52] (Table 2.2, entries 3,4).

c. Studies on biogenic amine metabolism in depressed man.

1. 5-HT. It has been shown that 5-hydroxyindole acetic acid (5-HIAA, a major metabolite of 5-HT) is lower in some depressed patients than in controls in both urine and cerebrospinal fluid (csf). In more limited studies, autopsied brains of diagnosed depressed patients who had committed suicide contained less 5-HT and 5-HIAA than controls [10]. Tryptophan, the biosynthetic precursor to 5-HT, has been reported as being effective in the treatment of depression both alone and in combination with MAO inhibitors.

2. NA. The metabolism of NA is complex [69]. However, approximately 50% of the major metabolite, 3-methoxy-4-hydroxy-phenylglycol (MHPG) that is found in urine is believed to be derived from NA metabolism in the brain. This metabolite has been shown to have a lower concentration in urine of depressed patients than controls, indicating a lower turnover of NA in these patients. However, later work has not supported these findings [70]. Thus, the value of measuring levels of amine metabolites in urine or CSF as an indicator of depression or, *vide infra*, as a measure of the antidepressant activity of drugs may be limited.

d. Biogenic amine involvement in the mode of action of antidepressants. The information above may be summarized by stating that in depression both the amines NA and 5-HT have decreased functionality in the central nervous system, and that antidepressants are drugs that increase the levels of functional amines at their central receptor sites [71]. There is much evidence to support this hypothesis [72]. It should be borne in mind that although these specific biochemical events are often implicated in the mode of action of all the antidepressant therapies, both their efficacy and side effects may be due to a combination of these and other factors. It has been suggested that there is a correlation between the inhibition of 5-HT uptake with the clinically observed "elevation of mood," and the inhibition of NA uptake with the "increase in drive" seen on administration of these drugs to depressed patients. Amitriptyline and doxepin also have some direct NA receptor-blocking action which has been correlated with their clinically observed antianxiety properties [73–76]. Several objections may be raised to such correlations: first, there is little dramatic difference in the clinical experience with the drugs and, indeed, they represent a remarkably homogeneous group. Second, the picture is complicated by the fact that the tertiary amines (e.g., imipramine) are metabolized in vivo to the secondary amines, the latter often being more potent against NA uptake than 5-HT (see Table 2.2, entry 7). Third, and perhaps most importantly, the blockade of uptake can be demonstrated both in vitro and in vivo to occur very quickly on single dosing, whereas the antidepressant activity in the clinic only appears after 14–21 days of multiple daily dosing. Recent ideas that attempt to rationalize this problem are discussed later in Sec. VI.

However, despite such limitation, the investigations of the role of biogenic amines has proved an extremely useful approach to our understanding of the etiology of depression and an attractive explanation of the mode of action of the major types of antidepressant drugs. Therefore, it is instructive to consider the simplified model of a central noradrenergic synapse (Fig. 2.5). A similar discussion would apply to events at a 5-HT synapse. The hypothesis now widely supported is that in depression there is not sufficient functional NA available at the postsynaptic receptor on the effector cell and that the antidepressants increase this functional NA at the postsynaptic receptor sites by different mechanisms and to a varying degree:

1. Tricyclics (e.g., imipramine, amitriptyline) inhibit uptake of NA, hence maintaining a high concentration of NA at the postsynaptic receptor. Tricyclics also inhibit MAO, affect endocrine function and electrolyte balance, as well as facilitate presynaptic release.

2. MAO inhibitors (e.g., phenelzine, tranylcypromine) inhibit the monoamine oxidases, hence decrease the formation of deaminated metabolites. This increases the amount of NA that is transferred to functional pools, and hence transmitted to postsynaptic receptors.

3. Stimulants (e.g., amphetamine) facilitate the release of NA from functional pools, hence increasing the amount of NA available to enter the synaptic cleft.

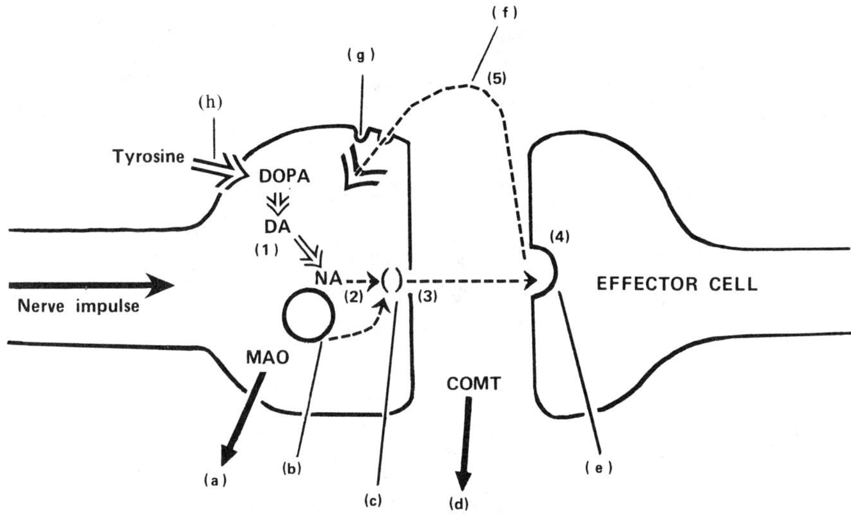

(----) Movement of NA; (⇨) biosynthesis of NA; (➡) metabolism of NA; (NA) noradrenaline; (DA) dopamine; (MAO) monoamineoxidase enzyme; (COMT) catechol-*O*-methyltransferase enzyme; (NMN) normetanephrine; (MHPG) 3-methoxy-4-hydroxyphenylglycol; (α-MPT) α-methylparatyrosine.

Notes:

1. NA biosynthesized from extracellular tyrosine. Dopamine converted to NA cellularly.
2. NA transferred to functional pool.
3. Nerve impulse (action potential) activates release of NA from functional pool into synaptic cleft.
4. Transmission of impulse to effector cell by activation of postsynaptic receptor.
5. NA taken up again for further use.
   (a) Deaminated metabolites; formation inhibited by MAO inhibitors.
   (b) Deep-pool storage granules; depleted by reserpine
   (c) Release of NA from functional pool; increased by amphetamine.
   (d) Methoxylated metabolites (NMN, MHPG).
   (e) Postsynaptic receptor; stimulated by functional NA; becomes subsensitive after chronic stimulation.
   (f) Uptake of NA; blocked by tricyclics.
   (g) Inhibitory presynaptic or autoreceptors.
   (h) NA biosynthesis; blocked by α-MPT.

FIG. 2.5 A simplified noradrenergic synapse.

4. Sympathomimetic amines mimic the stimulatory effects of NA at the receptor sites.

5. ECT may increase the rate of biosynthesis of NA by stimulating the enzymes involved in its formation from tyrosine. It also induces degranulation of storage granules, which increases the availability of NA, and induces a subsensitivity of presynaptic α- or postsynaptic β-adrenergic receptors (see Sec. VI). However, the stimulation of 5-HT biosynthesis is considered the more dominant factor.

5. Summary

The tricyclic antidepressants appear to be a homogeneous class of clinically effective drugs which are the major prescribed treatment for depression. Amitriptyline and imipramine are still the most popular drugs, administered mainly alone but also in combination with neuroleptics and antianxiety agents. Chlorimipramine, protriptyline, nortriptyline, and doxepin are also popular. Amitriptyline and especially doxepin are indicated as useful in the treatment of depression with an accompanying anxiety component. However, the apparent relief of anxiety may be attributed to the sedative effects of these particular tricyclics. A consensus has emerged that these drugs exert their antidepressant activity by virtue of their ability to potentiate the central effects of NA and 5-HT, mainly through their potent inhibitory properties on uptake of these amines in central neurons. However, changes in endocrine function and electrolyte balance may augment these effects in a poorly defined manner. The major side effects are well characterized and have been related to their anticholinergic and cardiovascular properties. A further limitation is that their antidepressant action does not appear until at least 14 days after multiple daily dosing, and overdosage can easily prove fatal. However, depression is a condition that needs to be treated promptly, as suicide is a risk. These drugs, on the whole, do offer a good benefit-to-risk ratio.

B. The Monoamine Oxidase Inhibitors

In recent years, several informative reviews on the pharmacology [77–79], selectivity [80–81], and side effects [24] of the MAO inhibitors have appeared in the literature.

1. Introduction and History

The enzyme monoamine oxidase (MAO) is widely distributed in animal organs, tissue, and blood platelets. Together with the enzyme catechol-O-methyl-transferase (COMT), these enzymes are responsible for the detoxification of extraneous primary amines. Both NA and DA are substrates for MAO and COMT, whereas 5-HT is almost exclusively oxidized by MAO. Intracellular amines mainly are oxidized by MAO whereas COMT primarily detoxifies circulating amines.

The MAO inhibitors are classified by their chemical structures, either as the group that contain a hydrazine, hydrazide, or amine moiety, or the more recently characterized acetylenic compounds (Fig. 2.6). Phenelzine is the most widely prescribed of these drugs today, whereas iproniazid, isoniazid, and pargyline are receiving less popularity. Pargyline is mainly prescribed to treat hypertension.

Isoniazid was first introduced into the clinic in 1951 for the treatment of tuberculosis. It soon became apparent that this compound, and its isopropyl derivative iproniazid, caused a marked central nervous system and motor stimulation in hospitalized tuberculosis patients. The MAO-inhibiting property of iproniazid was demonstrated by Zeller in 1953 and later, in 1957, Kline introduced this compound into the treatment of depressed patients with positive results. Kline described the compound as a "psychic energizer," and later work, both in Europe and the United States, confirmed its antidepressant properties.

2. Side Effects and Efficacy

The hydrazide compounds have often been shown to cause hepatotoxicity and orthostatic hypotension. Indeed, pargyline is mainly used to treat hypertension. Overdose of the drugs leads, during a 24-hr period, to symptoms of headache, agitation, tremor, variations in blood pressure, hyperreflexia, hyperpyrexia, and, rarely, hallucinations and convulsions [24]. However, the side effect that has been the cause of most concern has been the precipitation of a hypertensive crisis when these drugs are taken with a wide variety of common foods such as cheese, red wine, chocolate, pickled herrings, and marmite. These foods often have a high content of primary amines which are known to elicit pressor responses. The major monoamine in cheese is tyramine, and the so-called "cheese syndrome" has led to fatalities in the early use of these drugs, although the incidence is not as great as commonly believed. The occurrence of the side effects is often unpredictable because of:

1. Variability of distribution and activity of MAO from patient to patient
2. Variability of monoamine content in foods, for example, different batches of the same cheese can contain 100-fold difference in tyramine concentration
3. Poor patient compliance to a controlled diet during, and for a time, after treatment

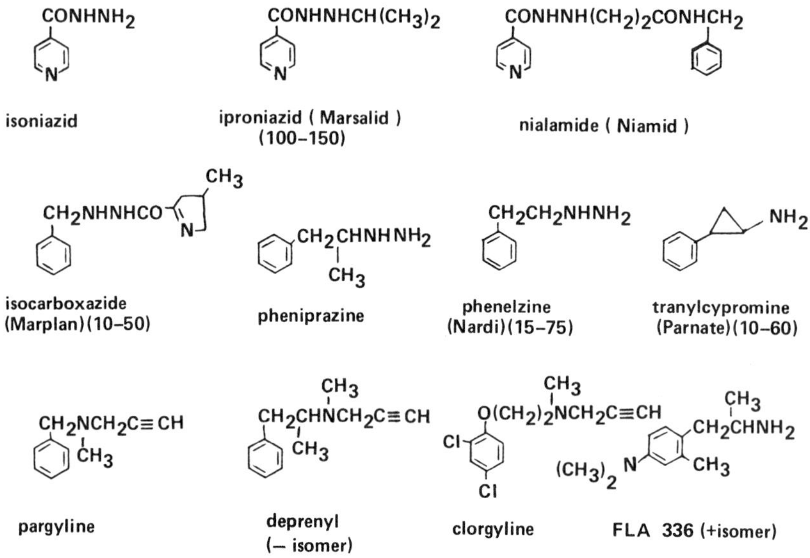
CONHNH2
isoniazid
CONHNHCH(CH3)2
iproniazid (Marsalid)
(100–150)
CONHNH(CH2)2CONHCH2
nialamide (Niamid)
CH3
CH2NHNHCO
isocarboxazide
(Marplan)(10–50)
CH2CHNHNH2
CH3
pheniprazine
CH2CH2NHNH2
phenelzine
(Nardi)(15–75)
NH2
tranylcypromine
(Parnate)(10–60)
CH2NCH2C≡CH
CH3
pargyline
CH3
CH2CHNCH2C≡CH
CH3
deprenyl
(– isomer)
CH3
O(CH2)2NCH2C≡CH
Cl
Cl
clorgyline
CH3
CH2CHNH2
(CH3)2
CH3
FLA 336 (+isomer)

FIG. 2.6 Some monoamine oxidase inhibitors. (From Refs. 7 and 19.)

4. The cross-reaction with a variety of other drugs such as the narcotic analgesics, tricyclic antidepressants, and insulin, as well as many over-the-counter decongestants that contain sympathomimetic amines or anticholinergics.

These effects, coupled with the rise in popularity of the tricyclics during the 1960s, have led to a steady decrease in the use of MAO inhibitors in the therapy of depression. Although phenelzine, in common with most of the hydrazine derivatives, produces some incidence of hepatotoxicity, there appears to be a resurgence in its use, as it is believed to produce the least incidence of hypertensive effects. This drug has FDA approval in the Unites States as an effective antidepressant. Multiple trials indicate the efficacy of phenelzine is mainly in depressive outpatients with associated phobic-anxiety states, but it is not considered so effective in hospitalized retarded patients as compared with the tricyclics [82,83). In common with the tricyclics, antidepressant effects do not appear until after several weeks of multiple daily dosing. Human platelets are rich in MAO type B (see Sec. 5.B. 3, below) and offer a convenient source of assay for inhibiting activity [84]. The delay in clinical efficacy correlated reasonably well with the blood platelet assay, where phenelzine, dosed at 60 mg/day shows maximal inhibition of 80% of MAO activity after 2 weeks [85].

3. Multiple Forms and Selective Inhibitors of Types A and B

There appear to be multiple forms of MAO present in most animal tissue, including brain. There may in fact be only one enzyme that occurs in different forms and environment. Two major forms are designated as types A and B: type A is selective in oxidizing NA and 5-HT, whereas type B, the major enzyme form in brain, is selective towards benzylamine and phenylethylamine. Tyramine and DA appear to be substrates for both forms of the enzyme [7,80,81,86–90] (see Table 2.4). A drug that selectively inhibits MAO-A should, therefore, not induce a pressor response precipitated by ingestion of foods containing phenylethylamine (e.g., chocolate). These compounds should increase 5-HT and NA levels in the brain, which should therefore be antidepressants in accord with the biogenic amine hypothesis (see Sec. A.4.d and Fig. 2.5). A selective MAO-B inhibitor should not potentiate cardiac problems associated with stimulation of NA. Thus, there may be a role for both selective type-A and -B inhibitors in antidepressant therapy. The early MAO inhibitors show little selectivity, but several new agents have been developed that appear to be selective against both types A and B. A body of opinion is now emerging that a selective, reversible type-A inhibitor would be clinically useful [80,91]. Clorgyline has been shown to be a selective inhibitor of type A and deprenyl is selective against type B [81]. These acetylenic compounds appear to inhibit MAO by irreversibly forming a covalent bond with the flavin cofactor of the enzyme [81]. The nonacetylenic compound (+)-FLA-33 appears to be both a selective and reversible inhibitor of brain MAO-A and raises brain 5-HT levels at low doses and NA levels at higher doses, with minimal elevation of tyramine. The compound has been shown to be a competitive inhibitor of 5-HT in vitro in rat brain hypothalamic mitochondria. The major metabolite, the desmethyl compound (+)-FLA-788, also selectively inhibits MAO-A [80].

Limited metabolic studies have shown that deprenyl is metabolized to amphetamine and methamphetamine, which may complicate the in vivo pharmacology and apparent MAO selectivity based on extrapolation from the in vitro data. Clorgyline is the only acetylenic compound that has so far been shown to be a clinically useful antidepressant [80]. Deprenyl appears to be devoid of the pressor potentiation of tyramine and has, so far, found limited clinical use in the treatment of the akinetic effects of L-dopa therapy in patients suffering from Parkinson's disease [80]. The development of selective MAO inhibitors should be treated with caution as the sensitivity and selectivity of the enzyme varies in different peripheral and central nervous system locations [86].

TABLE 2.4 Selectivity of Monoamine Oxidase Substrates and Inhibitors

	Common substrates		
	Type A	(A and B)	Type B
Selectivity for natural substrates	5-HT,NA, normetanephrine	DA, tyramine, tryptamine	Benzylamine, phenyethylamine
Selectivity of inhibitors	Chlorgyline, Lilly-51641, cimoxatone, MD-780515, FLA-336, FKA-788, Moclobemide (Ro-11-1163), Toloxatone (weakly selective) [Ref. 124b]	Pargyline, isocarboxazid, phenelzine, iproniazid, nialamide, pheniprazine, α-ethyltryptamine, tranylcypromine	Deprenyl (selegiline), caroxazone (weakly selective)

4. Summary

The popularity of the MAO inhibitors has diminished in recent years due to their unpredictable efficacy and notorious side effects, and to the advent of the more reliable tricyclics. The occurrence of a hypertensive crisis on ingestion of these drugs with a wide variety of common foods and other commonly prescribed drugs is overexaggerated, but still gives cause for concern. The identification of subclasses of MAO-A and MAO-B has stimulated interest in findings selective inhibitors. Sufficient clinical data are not yet available to predict the role for such drugs in the therapy of depression. However, a body of opinion is emerging that a selective, reversible inhibitor of MAO-A, with potent activity in the brain and minimal peripheral effects, would be a useful antidepressant.

C. The Second-Generation Drugs

1. Introduction

Evidence for an antidepressant-antianxiety broad-spectrum profile has been cited for the second-generation drugs nomifensine, mianserin, and trazodone. However, more extensive clinical data will probably need to be generated before a consensus of opinion is available on these claims.

In general, the many newer antidepressants that have been developed since the tricyclics have either:

1. No better efficacy or any less side-effects than the tricyclics
2. An increased antianxiety component in their clinical evaluation
3. A decreased incidence or severity of side effects, particularly those found most troublesome with the tricyclics, such as the cardiovascular and anticholinergic effects. The side effects that are specific to the newer drugs will undoubtedly appear on their more extensive usage, and in many cases have yet to be determined [92].

A list of some of the more recently developed antidepressants is given in Table 2.5, which indicates some of the features of these compounds that have been highlighted in the literature. Leading references are given to their biological and clinical data where applicable. There is a large number of new antidepressants under investigation. In the year June 1980–1981 alone, there have been 7 new products introduced onto the market, 28 in phases I–III clinical trials, and 46 under laboratory investigation with published animal data available.

TABLE 2.5 Some Second-Generation Antidepressant Drugs

Generic name (Brand name) (Company)	Comments: General animal data (Clinical Status, September 1981)	References (General/ clinical)
Amoxapine (Lederle)	Tricyclic; desmethyl derivative of the antipsychotic, loxapine; sleep patterns resemble amitriptyline; selective inhibitor of NA uptake	[93]
	Clinically effective against both psychotic and nonpsychotic depression; similar efficacy with imipramine; Anticholinergic (AC) side effects common	[94,95]
Amineptine (Sevier)	Tricyclic; DA agonist, less AC than imipramine; stimulant	–
	Clinically similar to DMI, but less AC effects; popular in France	[96a]
Maprotiline (Ludiomil) (Ciba-Geigy)	Rigid analog of DMI; more potent inhibitor of NA than 5-HT uptake	See text
	Clinically useful in agitated depression; sedative; similar profile to classical tricyclics	[97]
Oxaprotiline (Geigy)	Analog of maprotiline; inibitor of NA uptake	–
	Useful in psychotic depression	[98]
Nomifensine (Merital) (Hoechst)	Tetrahydroisoquinoline derivative; potent inhibitor of both DA and NA uptake; stimulant; No AC effects	See text [99,100]
	Clinically effective in psychotic depression; sleep disturbance and motor restlessness in some patients; nonsedative; safer in overdose than tricyclics	[101,102]
Moxefensine (Diclofensine) (Roche)	Structurally related to nomifensine; potent inhibitor of DA uptake; stimulant	–
	Clinically effective (phase III)	[103,104]

TABLE 2.5 (Continued)

Generic name (Brand name) (Company)	Comments: General animal data (Clinical Status, September 1981)	References (General/ clinical)
Bupropion (Wellbatrin) (Wellcome)	Selective inhibitor of DA uptake; pharmacological profile intermediate between tricyclics and amphetaminelike stimulants	[105]
	Antidepressant effects seen within 8 days in a phase-III double-blind placebo controlled trial; less AC and cardiovascular (CV) effects than tricyclics	[106]
FS-32 (Chugai)	Potent inhibitor of DA uptake; also inhibits NA and 5-HT uptake; major metabolite (FS-37) long acting; weak central but no peripheral AC activity;	[107a,b,c]
	Profile similar to imipramine in animals	–
HRP-197 (Hoechst)	Very potent inhibitor of both NA (IC_{50} = 0.2 μm) and DA (IC_{50} = 0.5 μm) uptake; potentiates effects of 5-HTP; inhibits tetrabenazine ptosis	[108]
LR-5182 (Lilly)	Bicyclooctylamine derivative	–
	Potent inhibitor of both NA and DA (very potent) uptake; stimulant; under laboratory investigation	[109, 110a,b]
Tandamine (Ayerst)	More potent inhibitor of NA than 5-HT uptake; similar to DMI against reserpine syndrome	[111a]
	Clinically effective antidepressant, but with marked AC and CV effects	[111b]
Pirandamine (Ayerst)	More potent inhibitor of 5-HT uptake than Tandamine	[111a]

TABLE 2.5 (Continued)

Generic name (Brand name) (Company)	Comments: General animal data (Clinical Status, September 1981)	References (General/ clinical)
Fluoxetine (Lilly)	First selective inhibitor of 5-HT uptake; minimal CV or AC effects; long-acting desmethyl metabolite	[112,113]
	Highly effective in preliminary clinical trials	[114]
Zimelidine (Zelmid)	Selective inhibitor of 5-HT uptake, 10× more potent than chlorimipramine; the long-acting desmethyl metabolite 10× more potent than zimeldine against 5-HT uptake	See text [115]
	Clinically effective; some AC effects, but less than amitriptyline; desmethyl metabolite also under clinical investigation [nor-zimelidine (nomelidine)]	[116,117]
Fluvoxamine (Solvay)	Selective inhibitor of 5-HT uptake	[118,119]
	Initial clinical trials indicate effective and well tolerated in 12 depressed hospitalized patients	[120,111b]
	Later studies show adverse ECG and gastrointestinal disturbance in some patients	[194]
FG-4963 Femoxitine (Ferrosan)	Selective inhibitor of 5-HT uptake	–
	Less effective than amitriptyline clinically; some headache and sleep disturbance; low bioavailability due to extensive first-pass metabolism	[121,122]
Toloxatone (Delande)	Potentiates tryptamine and 5-HTP effects; antagonizes reserpine-induced ptosis and hypothermia, and PGO spikes in EEG; selective MAO-type A inhibitor; no AC effects	[123, 124a,b]

TABLE 2.5 (Continued)

Generic name (Brand name) (Company)	Comments: General animal data (Clinical Status, September 1981)	References (General/ clinical)
Nitalapram, Citalopram (Lundbeck)	Long-acting selective 5-HT uptake inhibitor, 4–10× activity of chlorimipramine; no MAO-inhibiting properties	[125,126]
Indalpine (Pharmuka)	Selective inhibitor of 5-HT uptake, 6–7× activity of fluoxetine	[127]
	Clinically effective (phase III); brain steady-state reached after 7 days compared with 14 days for imipramine; no AC effects	[128]
Org-6582 (Organon)	Potent selective inhibitor of 5-HT uptake; more potent and longer activity than fluoxetine	[129,130] –
Etoperidone (Angelini)	Selective inhibitor of 5-HT uptake, but less potent than chlorimipramine; structurally related to trazodone and similary lacks AC and CV effects	[131]
	Antidepressant effects in man	[131]
Trazodone (Molipaxin, Desyrel) (Roussel)	Both a potent central 5-HT uptake inhibitor at high doses, and 5-HT antagonist at lower doses; no AC or CV effects; no effects on reserpine syndrome or potentiation of effects of catecholamines or L-Dopa	See text
	Well-tolerated clinically effective antidepressant, with antianxiety properties; minimal AC and CV effects; some sedation	[132,133]
Mianserin (Bolvidon) (Organon)	5-HT antagonist; introduced as an antidepressant as EEG patterns similar to amitriptyline in human volunteers	[134,135]
	Clinically as effective as tricyclics, but with minimal CV and AC effects; both antidepressant and antianxiety properties	[136–139]

TABLE 2.5 (Continued)

Generic name (Brand name) (Company)	Comments: General animal data (Clinical Status, September 1981)	References (General/ clinical)
	have been demonstrated; safer in overdose than tricyclics; sedative	
Org-2305 (Organon)	Analog of mianserin; EEG similar to mianserin	[140]
	Antidepressant-anxiolytic profile similar to mianserin (phase II)	[140]
Org-3770 (Organon)	Anlog of mianserin; EEG profile indicates 3× activity of mianserin	[140]
	Phase-II clinical trial	[140]
Binodaline (Siegfried)	Antagonizes the effects of tetrabenazine; more active against muricidal activity than imipramine; devoid of atropinelike effects	[141]
Pirlindole (Pirazol) USSR source (Cassella, Hoechst)	No AC, CV, or sedative effects	[142]
	Clinically similar to tricyclics, but better tolerated	[143]
Caroxazone (Timostenil) (Montedisan, Farmitalia)	Similar profile to amitriptyline in animal studies, but less AC effects; slightly selective but weak MAO-B-inhibiting activity	[144, see text]
	Double-blind phase-III clinical trials show a similar efficacy with amitriptyline and well tolerated	[145,146]
Pridefine (Robins)	No AC effects, profile otherwise similar to imipramine	–
	Clinically similar to imipramine in unipolar depression; less side effects and well tolerated	[147,148]
Ciclazindol, WY-23409 (Wyeth)	Structurally similar to the anorectic agent Mazindol; no AC effects; peripheral α-blocker; selective inhibitor of NA uptake	[149,150]

TABLE 2.5 (Continued)

Generic name (Brand name) (Company)	Comments: General animal data (Clinical Status, September 1981)	References (General/ clinical)
Ciclazindol, WY-23409 (Continued)	Clinically as effective as amitriptyline, but incidences of headache, tiredness, dizziness, and anorexia; minimal AC effects	[151]
HRP-459 (Hoechst)	Potent inhibitor of NA uptake (IC_{50} = 0.021 μm)	[152]
	Potent memory-enhancing properties in animal models.	–
Indeloxazine (Yamanouchi)	Antidepressant and memory-enhancing properties	[153–156]
	Similar EEG-theta wave changes to Hydergine; structurally related to viloxane, but pharmacology resembles amitriptyline	–
Metraindole (Incazan)	Similar properties to imipramine, but stimulant rather than sedative; hence contraindicated in patients with anxiety syndromes	[157] –
Viloxazine (Vivalan) (I.C.I.)	Amphetaminelike stimulant in animals; selective but weak inhibitor of NA uptake	See text [153]
	Clinical efficacy comparable with imipramine; no AC or CV effects; stimulant rather than sedative; some nausea and vomiting; toxic effects in overdose	[159,160]
Iprindol	Investigative drug; clinically effective antidepressant but does not block uptake of NA or 5-HT	[161]
RX-77368 (Reckitt & Colman)	Peptide TRH analog, with dimethyl group on proline residue in 3-position; more potent than either amitriptyline, mianserin, or TRH in learned immobility test	[162]

TABLE 2.5 (Continued)

Generic name (Brand name) (Company)	Comments: General animal data (Clinical Status, September 1981)	References (General/ clinical)
RX-77368 (Continued)	Clinically appears to be a stimulant rather than antidepressant	–
DN-1417 (Takeda)	Peptide TRH analog	[163]
Selective MAO-inhibitors		See Table 3

The list in Table 2.5 is not exhaustive, but it does indicate the drugs that are representative of recent trends. The compounds are grouped together as much as possible in terms of their major points of interest.

The great majority of the drugs has been selected for clinical trial on the basis of animal data generated by the pharmaceutical companies. Biochemical profiles of these drugs have been extensively studied due to the precedence that the tricyclics show central uptake-inhibiting effects of both NA and 5-HT. Much attention has been focused on developing a selective inhibitor of 5-HT uptake. A compound with this property hopefully would clarify the question concerning the importance of 5-HT over NA uptake in antidepressant therapy and perhaps produce none of the cardiovascular effects characteristic of the tricyclics. The first of the selective 5-HT uptake inhibitors to be developed was fluoxetine; this drug has been followed by zimelidine, nor-zimelidine, citalopram, fluvoxamine, pirandamine, indalpine, Org. 6582, etoperidone, and napactadine, among others. The natural biochemical precursor to 5-HT, L-tryptophan, has recently received more attention as a potential antidepressant, although clinical efficacy and safety have not been adequately demonstrated [192].

Several drugs have been developed that inhibit the uptake of both NA and DA such as nomifensine, moxefensine, butriptyline, FS-37, HRP-197, and bupropion (a selective but weak DA uptake inhibitor). Some of these compounds, such as nomifensine, viloxazine, bupropion, and the investigative drug LR-5182, elicit a distinct central nervous system amphetaminelike stimulation in rats, probably related to their DA properties. These drugs are expected to be more useful in psychotic rather than neurotic depression.

Selective MAO-A and MAO-B inhibitors have also been developed, with the possibility of less incidence of the "cheese syndrome" and cardiovascular toxicity, as described in Sec. B.3. Computer-analyzed electroencephalography (EEG) is emerging as having an important role in both the discovery and clinical evaluation of new antidepressants. Mianserin is one of the most interesting of the new drugs that was shown to have antidepressant activity after comparison of its EEG spectrum with that of the tricyclics in healthy patients [134,139].

The antidepressant and central nervous system-stimulant effects of several hormones and peptides such as ACTH, TRH, and substance P have not received much attention, but several recently synthesized analog of TRH are now under clinical investigation (e.g., RX-773681 and DN 1417).

Some of the compounds (Fig.2.7) that have received most interest in the recent literature, or represent novelty, are discussed below.

2. Mianserin [134–139]

Mianserin was originally shown in animal models to be both an antihistamine and 5-HT antagonist. Therefore, the drug was introduced into clinical trial as an antiallergy agent and for the treatment of migraine. The computer-analyzed EEG profile in both healthy volunteers and depressed patients showed similarities with imipramine and particular with amitriptyline. The common characteristics of the EEG are a decrease in α-activity and an increase in slow waves, with an increase of superimposed fast β-activity [164,165]. The compound was shown to be sedative, but to have little central or peripheral anticholinergic activity as compared with amitriptyline. Sedation is probably due to the antihistamine activity. The drug was reevaluated as an antidepressant agent and shown to be clinically effective in the usual dose range of 40–80 mg/day [138,139]. Mianserin has no apparent effects on NA uptake, and lacks the cardiodepressant and negative ionotropic effects of the tricyclics [166] as compared with amitriptyline [139]. Some incidences of convulsions in overdose have been reported [167] but none proved fatal [168]. The drug has been shown to reverse the weight gain caused by amitriptyline therapy in a small group of patients [169]. Mianserin is well absorbed, peak plasma concentrations being measured at 2–3 hr after oral dosing. Mean elimination half-life is estimated at 10–17 hr. The minimal effects on the heart and cardiovascular system allow the drug to be well tolerated in the elderly and those with heart disease [139]. Comparison with diazepam has indicated mianserin to have the superior antianxiety properties when administered in divided daily doses [137], but its role in neurotic depression has yet to be established.

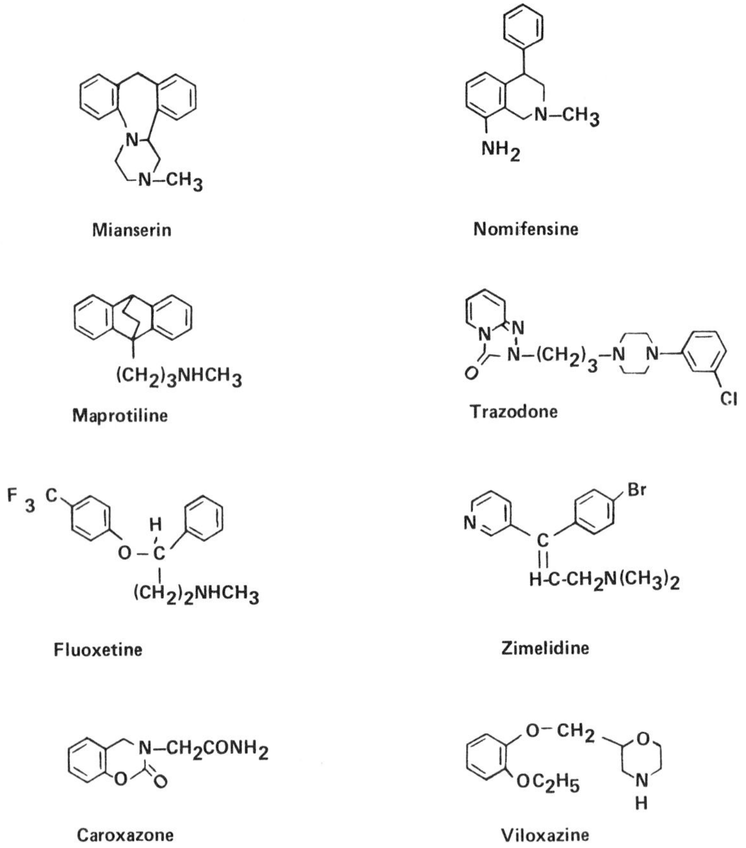

Mianserin

Nomifensine

Maprotiline

Trazodone

Fluoxetine

Zimelidine

Caroxazone

Viloxazine

FIG. 2.7 Chemical structures of the second-generation antidepressants discussed in the text.

3. Nomifensine [99–102]

Nomifensine, being a stimulant rather than a sedative, has a distinctly different profile of activity than mianserin [102]. The compound has a novel chemical structure as a tetrahydroisoquinoline derivative. Mainly outpatient-controlled and open clinical trials indicate the drug to have antidepressant activity in the range 50–150 mg daily. A more rapid onset of activity than with the tricyclics has been reported, but this may be due to the lack of sedation and mild stimulation that occurs on administration of this drug. There appears to be minimal anticholinergic activity and effects on the heart, as compared with the tricyclics. The major side effects appear to be related to the stimulant properties of the drug, as approximately 10% of patients have shown sleep disturbance and signs of motor restlessness [101].

Nomifensine was discovered by animal screening and showed to reverse reserpine and tetrabenazine effects. In particular, the compound is a potent inhibitor of uptake of DA as well as NA, but has little effect on 5-HT. The DA and NA effects are in common with those of amphetamine; each drug shares the chemical structural feature of phenylethylamine, and both cause a dose-related increase in stereotyped behavior in rats. However, comparison with diazepam in the clinic has indicated some antianxiety component in the action of nomifensine [102].

4. Viloxazine [160]

The chemical structure of viloxazine has similarities with the β-blockers, but the compound has a distinctly different pharmacological profile. Antidepressant antivity has been demonstrated to be comparable with imipramine in controlled clinical trials in both hospitalized and outpatients. The dose range is 100–300 mg/day. The drug is rapidly absorbed, extensively metabolized, and more rapidly excreted than either imipramine or amitriptyline. In contrast to impramine, viloxazine has little anticholinergic or adrenergic effects in man, but has a central stimulant activity similar to amphetamine. This latter property may be related to the claims of a faster onset of activity of antidepressant effects than the tricyclics. Clinical trials give contradictory data on this point. The main side effects appear to be nausea (18.8%) and vomiting (4.7%), accrued from data on 771 patients in 29 clinical trials [170]. In a limited study, these gastrointestinal disturbances are reduced when the drug is given as enterically coated tablets [171].

5. Maprotiline [197]

This compound is an analog of the tricyclic antidepressant DMI, where the central tricyclic ring is made rigid by an ethane bridge, thus forming a tetracyclic structure. Like DMI, maprotiline is a more potent inhibitor of uptake of NA than 5-HT. Maprotiline is effective in the treatment of both psychotic and neurotic depression, perhaps being more useful in the latter subgroup. This may correlate with the more potent activity against NA uptake. The drug is usually effective repeated daily oral dosing in the range 75–150 mg, often given as a single dose at night due to its sedative properties. Clinical experience has shown maprotiline to have no discernible advantages over the tricyclics imipramine and amitriptyline, showing a similar profile of sedative, anticholinergic, and cardiovascular effects. In addition, there appears to be a higher incidence of convulsions (42% of all antidepressant) [167,172] and, on 14 days chronic treatment, a 3% incidence of skin rashes [173].

6. Zimelidine [115–117,174]

Fluoxetine was the first selective 5-HT uptake inhibitor to be identified from animal screening and it has been shown to be a clinically effective antidepressant. However, to date zimelidine has more published clinical data available. The major active metabolite, the desmethyl derivative nor-zimelidine, is even more potent against 5-HT uptake, and has itself been introduced into the clinic as an antidepressant agent. In healthy volunteers, the elimination half-lives have been shown to be 5.1 hr for zimelidine and 15.1 hr for nor-zimelidine after i.v. infusion, and 5.4 hr and 21.1 hr on oral dosing, respectively. Zimelidine dosed at 100 mg/day over 7 days produced some evidence of decreased heart rate and prolong Q–T interval, but no effect on systolic time intervals in contrast to amitriptyline [166]. Limited clinical studies indicate no sedative properties, slight weight loss, and few untoward cardiac effects with this compound [174]. Zimelidine does have some anticholinergic properties which cause dry mouth and constipation. The drug also appears to cause insomnia to which tolerance develops during the first 7 days of therapy [116]. Longer-term clinical studies will be necessary to establish the role of this drug and the other selective 5-HT uptake inhibitors in antidepressent therapy.*

7. Trazodone [132,133]

Trazodone has emerged as an effective, broad-spectrum antidepressant that is well tolerated and has minimal tricycliclike side effects. Clinical trials show it to be equally efficacious with amitriptyline, DMI, doxepine, and dothiepin on well-known and widely accepted rating scales, such as the Hamilton Depression Rating Scale. Furthermore, trazodone, when compared with diazepam, chlorodiazepoxide, and lorazepam has been shown to have a good antianxiety profile. However, the latter findings have yet to be widely accepted. Thus, the drug appears to be particularly promising in the treatment of depression mixed with an anxiety component, perhaps the major class of depression treated in general practice. Trazodone appears to have no anticholinergic or cardiovascular effects at the usual dose of 150–600 mg/day. Some sedation does occur, but this is minimised by dosing at bedtime.

---

*Note added in proof: Zimelidine has now been withdrawn due to unexplained fatalities.

Trazodone has a novel chemical structure where a triazolopyridine ring is joined to a *m*-chlorophenylpiperidine ring by a propane bridge. The compound has structural features in common with both the antidepressant, antianxiety, and neuroleptic agents. Trazodone was developed primarily on the basis of animal behavioral models of depression which involve schedules that monitor responses to unpleasant and noxious stimuli, rather than the classical screens related to the amine hypothesis of depression. Biochemical studies have revealed that the compound is a 5-HT uptake inhibitor at high doses, but a potent peripheral and central 5-HT antagonist at lower doses. The drug will compete with [^{3}H]spiperone for 5-HT binding sites in mouse brain frontal cortex, an activity in common with doxepin and mianserin [175,176].

It may appear paradoxical that trazodone is a 5-HT antagonist and yet a clinically effective antidepressant. The compound also has α-adrenergic blocking effects. According to the biogenic amine hypothesis, antidepressants should be either a direct or indirect postsynaptic agonist of NA or 5-HT. One explanation is that 5-HT acts as an inhibitory transmitter in many parts of the brain and that the 5-HT antagonistic effects of trazodone may counteract the inhibition. Thus, the drug indirectly stimulates the activity of other neurotransmitters such as NA and DA in selective areas of the brain. It has been pointed out that trazodone contains an *m*-chlorophenylpiperidine moiety in its chemical structure, this latter compound being a well-known 5-HT agonist. However, trazodone is well absorbed and the major metabolite in man is oxotriazolepyridine propionic acid. There is no evidence at present for the formation of *m*-chlorophenyl piperidine in man, but it has been found in rats [175]. The mode of action of trazodone has, therefore, still to be determined conclusively [177].

8. Caroxazone [144–146]

Caroxazone is a benzoxazine-acetamide derivative that has been shown by screening to reverse the effect of reserpine in mice, rats, cats, and monkeys. The drug has a novel chemical structure for an antidepressant and was selected for further progression as a clinical candidate on the basis of its classical pharmacological profile. Biochemical studies showed the compound to be selective towards inhibiting the uptake of 5-HT rather than NA in rat brain slices. The compound appears to have no anticholinergic or antihistaminic activity [178].

Double-blind studies have indicated caroxazone to be better than placebo and equiactive with imipramine and amitriptyline after 7–21 days daily dosing, as assessed by the Hamilton Depression Rating Scale. The compound appears to be particularly useful in neurotic depressed patients [146].

Caroxazone appears to elicit a disinhibiting effect, which may be accounted for by the more recent discovery that the compound is also a reversible MAO inhibitor [179]. No classical MAO inhibitor side effects, such as a hypertensive crisis or postural hypotension, have yet been reported [146].

9. Summary

The extensive research programs throughout the world to look for new antidepressant agents in the era 1960–1980 have involved a wide range of animal testing involving behavioral, biochemical, endocrinological, and EEG studies. A vast collection of clinical data now testify, to the efficacy and limiting side effects of the tricyclics, MAO inhibitors, and other antidepressant therapies, such as ECT. This work has led to the development of a large number of antidepressant candidate drugs, some representative examples of which are listed in Table 2.5. Many of the new drugs have not sufficient published clinical data available to warrant definitive comment. Several compounds appear to offer no advantage over the classical drugs but, as with most psychotropic agents, individual patients may tolerate one drug better than a closely related compound. Progress does appear to have been made in reducing the major side effects of the tricyclics and MAO inhibitors, particularly the anticholinergic and cardiovascular effects, and toxicity in overdose, such as convulsions. Thus, these drugs should be better tolerated in the elderly and in those patients with a history of heart disease. Claims that an antianxiety component may offer a broader-spectrum antidepressant are still regarded with some scepticism. At the time of writing, trazodone, mianserin, and perhaps nomifensine appear to be the safest, best tolerated, and have the broadest spectrum of the newer drugs. No indications have yet appeared to suggest that any of these drugs cure or directly affect the pathology of the condition of depression.

D. Miscellaneous Treatments of Depressive Illness

1. Lithium [180–185]

The major role of lithium is in the therapeutic treatment of mania and the prophylactic management of manic-depression (bipolar depression), for which it is now the treatment of choice. Lithium has little value in the management of unipolar depression.

The use of lithium in the treatment of mental illness has a long and checkered history. Earlier in this century, lithium bromide was used as an anticonvulsant; the chloride salt gained notoriety in the 1940s when it was used as a salt substitute in cardiac and hypertensive patients, as it was the cause of several fatalities and was quickly withdrawn from therapy. Cade, working in Australia in 1949, showed lithium to be extremely effective in the treatment of mania [186]. This important discovery went virtually unheralded in the 1950s, when the newly discovered neuroleptics, antihistamines, and antidepressants were all being investigated in mania. Extensive reinvestigation of lithium in the 1960s in North America and Europe confirmed both the therapeutic use of lithium in the treatment of mania, and later its prophylactic use in the management of manic-depression [183]. The drug is now most often used as the water-soluble carbonate salt, given orally in the range 600–2500 mg in divided daily doses for the control of acute mania but which may be reduced to 300–1500 mg/day for prophylactic use. Lithium carbonate is quickly absorbed, peak plasma concentrations being achieved after 0.5–2 hr, with a plateau lasting for 12–24 hr [180]. The lithium ion is virtually completely excreted in the urine, with an elimination half-life of about 24 hr. The drug does not appear to be effective in controlling the paranoid symptoms of schizophrenia, which often have phases of similar behavioral characteristics, perhaps indicating a fundamentally different etiology in these conditions. The therapeutic index for lithium is low, the effective maintenance blood levels being in the range 0.4–1.4 μm/ml; levels of 1.6 μm/ml often lead to toxicity and 2.0 μm/ml nearly always so [180]. The symptoms of lithium intoxication gradually develop over months or even years; these include apathy, muscular rigidity, ataxia, and later, irregular tremor leading if not remedied, to coma and death. Fortunately, the lithium ion is readily and accurately estimated in blood by a flame photometric assay, hence blood levels can easily be monitored. The chronic use of lithium is now recognized to cause renal impairment, which often raises the blood levels to dangerously high levels. Blood levels may be reduced in such cases by ingestion of sodium chloride solution or just plain water, but acute lithium intoxication is best treated by hemodialysis or peritoneal dialysis, when the ion is quickly removed. The progress of renal impairment may be accelerated by the patient allowing himself to become dehydrated. From the start of treatment, it has been recommended that patients should drink at least 2–3 liters of fluid a day to minimize lithium accumulation in the kidneys [183].

The mode of action of lithium is still uncertain, and hypotheses favor effects on electrolyte imbalance and a consequent decrease in action potential that decreases the firing rate of the (*vide infra*, overactive) dopaminergic neurons.

2. Electroconvulsive Therapy (ECT) [187,188]

Although this chapter is concerned with the drug treatment of depression, ECT has stood the test of time and is still considered the most effective treatment for retarded depression. It is often used in patients who have failed to respond to other therapies.

ECT is one of several shock therapies introduced in the 1930s for the treatment of depression; it was found to be effective long before lithium, MAO inhibitors, and the tricyclics were used. ECT was first introduced as a treatment for schizophrenia, when it was erroneously believed that schizophrenia and epilepsy never occurred in the same patient. It was therefore believed that the induction of an epileptic-like seizure, either electrically with ECT or chemically with a large dose of insulin, would produce a state of the brain that was incompatible with schizophrenia. ECT has little value in the treatment of schizophrenia, but was quickly shown to be extremely useful in the treatment of retarded depression. The treatment appears to be of little value in the milder neurotic depressions. Perhaps because of the emotive use of the phrase "shock therapy," ECT has become regarded by some as a last-resort therapy. In patients refractory to other treatments, particularly the tricyclics, ECT is firmly established as the most effective therapy. The application of ECT has been dramatically improved by:

1. Using muscle relaxants to prevent skeletal damage
2. Using rubber guards in the mouth to prevent jaw and tongue damage
3. Using the minimum voltage necessary to effect a seizure, which is ensured to have occurred by monitoring with EEG
4. Using unilateral electrode placement over the nondominant hemisphere (right hemisphere for right-handed persons) which appears to minimize memory loss.

The major side effect of ECT therapy is loss of memory, which is most intense for short-term memory and may last for several hours or even days. Thus, outpatient treatment should require a protocol involving a recovery period in the hospital. Therapy is often most effective after six to seven daily sessions. Evidence has been obtained to show that maintenance on tricyclics after ECT does not appear to further improve the antidepressant effects, but does reduce the incidence of relapse.

In common with other antidepressant therapies, ECT appears to work only after multiple dosing after 2–3 weeks. Suggestions regarding its mode of action range from increase in NA and 5-HT by electrical activation of the enzymes involved in their biosynthesis, to Sulser's ideas on subsensitive receptors (see Fig. 2.5 and Sec. VI).

3. Amphetamine and Related Compounds [180,190,192]

Amphetamine is one of the most widely studied drugs in both animals and man. This compound has been used in the treatment of such diverse disorders as obesity, narcolepsy, minimal brain dysfunction (MBD) or the hyperkinetic syndrome in children, and depression. In common with other well-known stimulants, amphetamine has been abused, and the liability to addiction is of major concern [189].

In the treatment of depression, amphetamine is given in daily doses ranging from 5 mg to 30 mg. Amphetamine is well absorbed and extensively metabolized; in man 90% of the drug is excreted in the urine over 3–4 days, with a biological half-life estimated as approximately 12 hr [190].

Amphetamine has a wide spectrum of biological activity, the major stimulant effects most often being related to a sharp increase in the release of the neurotransmitters NA and DA from presynaptic storage vesicles. The NA and DA synthesis inhibitor, α-methylparatyrosine, given before amphetamine, greatly reduces the stimulant and euphoric effects of amphetamine in man [191].

Stimulants were, in fact, used in the treatment of depression before the tricyclics and MAO inhibitors were available, but their use still appears to be controversial and there is a paucity of well-controlled clinical data that testify to their therapeutic efficacy. Some authors discourage the use of stimulants in depression, in that their effects are not antidepressant at all, but are only transient and euphoric in nature, with withdrawal symptoms that often lead to a more severe depression than that originally being treated [190,192]. Amphetamine may have a role in the treatment of mildly depressive neurosis, but not in agitated depression where the stimulant properties may potentiate the symptoms of the illness.

Hypertension appears to be the side effect of amphetamine of most concern to clinicians. However, it has been pointed out that fatalities with amphetamine treatment are rare and, perhaps, of less concern than those that occurred with the use of the tricyclics [2]. The most common complaint from patients taking amphetamine is insomnia. Chronic administration can lead to tolerance, but the dependence is regarded as being psychological rather than physical. Stimulants may also precipitate an acute syndrome with symptoms similar to schizophrenia. In fact, schizophrenics themselves are particularly susceptible to this syndrome.

The use of stimulants in the treatment of depression remains controversial. However, they may have value where acute management of the condition is considered advantageous, for example, in acute mild neurosis, as the tricyclics or MAO inhibitors take 2–3 weeks for their antidepressant effects to develop. Cross-reaction of the stimulants with antidepressants and other drugs should also be considered.

Perhaps the clinically effective newer antidepressants nomifensine, bupropion, and viloxazine, with amphetaminelike stimulant properties will supersede the use of "pure" stimulants in the treatment of depression.

VI. DISCUSSION OF SOME CURRENT TRENDS IN RESEARCH INTO DEPRESSION

The development of the next generation of antidepressant drugs will be supported by an ever increasing background of clinical experience, basic animal pharmacological, and biochemical data. There is a need for a reliable internationally acceptable method for classification of the disease based on a sound scientific rationale, so that real progress can be made in the development of a truly novel drug. This process is complicated by what may be different subclasses of depression treated by general practice and by hospital psychiatry [Ref. 193, p. 455].

The desire for a unifying concept has led to much interest in the role of biogenic amines in depression. Although uptake blockade of NA and 5-HT caused by a single dose of antidepressants can be readily demonstrated in vitro and in vivo on both peripheral and central neurons, their andtidepressant effects do not appear until multiple daily dosing for at least 14 days. Furthermore, the clinically effective antidepressants mianserin and iprindole have little inhibiting effects on uptake of NA or 5-HT, whereas the non-antidepressant cocaine is a very potent uptake inhibitor. Therefore, the uptake-blocking properties may be of little importance in the therapeutic efficacy of antidepressant drugs.

Alternative correlations between effects of a antidepressants on the biogenic amines have been sought. In animal studies, chronic treatment with fluoxetine [194] and zimelidine [195] leads to a reduction in postsynaptic 5-HT receptor sensitivity during 14 days. Sulser has explored the effects of chronic dosing with other antidepressants on NA and 5-HT receptors [177,196,197]. Several tricyclics, MAO inhibitors, ECT, and mianserin induce a subsensitivity of brain presynaptic α_2- or postsynaptic β-receptors [198,199] on multiple dosing. Furthermore, antidepressants can induce low-affinity sites in cortex and hypothalamus and can reduce the number of high-affinity binding sites in the hypothalamus and frontal cortex for 5-HT [194,200].

These changes do correlate with the onset of antidepressant effects, but whether they are responsible for the antidepressant activity of these drugs remains to be verified. A corollary has been proposed that antidepressant therapy represents a method of adaptation to stress in which the treatments mimic the down-regulation, or subsensitising, actions of stress at central NA and 5-HT receptors [201]. The regulation of impulse-mediated release of NA has also been suggested [202].

Interest has also focused on the influence of the brain amines on the hypothalamus-pituitary-adrenocortical axis. The amines histamine, acetylcholine, NA, DA, and 5-HT, functioning in the limbic area of the brain, have all been shown to influence peptide transduction mechanisms in the hypothalamus that regulate the secretion of hormones from the pituitary gland. Peptidal analogs of the neurosecretory hormone

TRH have been synthesized as potential antidepressants (see Table 2.5), and ACTH, substance P, and pineal melatonin have all been implicated in depression. A finding of great potential is that patients suffering from endogenous depression appear to lack circadian variation in circulating cortisol levels. These levels are not affected by the suppression of the hypothalamus-pituitary-adrenocortical axis induced by dexamethasone in these patients. The dexamethasone suppression test is now recommended as a routine diagnostic for endogenous depression. Dexamethasone (1 mg) is administered orally at night and cortisol blood levels measured at intervals during the next 24 hr. Cortisol levels of greater than 0.05 μg/ml are regarded as abnormal and have a good correlation with the incidence of endogenous depression [203].

Several new behavioral models of depression in animals have been recently developed, including Irwin's swimming rat test, muricidal rats, and infant monkey deprivation. However, difficulties have been encountered in differentiating antidepressant from stimulant activity in these models [204]. The phenomenon of "learned helplessness" is regarded as a response to the stress caused by our modern complex and hierarchal society, which can manifest itself as symptoms of depression (see Figs. 2.1 and 2.2 and Ref. 13). A behavioral model in animals that attempts to mimic this phenomenon [205] has given a useful test in which imipramine has been shown to be effective [206]. The procedure involves exposing one animal to an electric shock that can be avoided (the "executive"), and another where the shock cannot be avoided (the "yoked") as it is controlled by the executive animal. A control animal is also used. Correlation of these behavioral effects with changes in brain 5-HT activity are under investigation [207].

Alternative drug therapies currently under exploration include treatment with vitamins, β-blockers such as propranolol, and combinations such as lithium with 5-HTP and chlorimipramine with tryptophan [193].

Alternatives to drug therapy that have been, or are being, investigated include jogging, sleep deprivation (paradoxical, as sleep disturbance is a symptom of depression), counselling in private and discussion groups, and even psychosurgery [208].

VII. SUMMARY

This chapter has outlined the epidemiology, classification, and etiology of depression and has traced the development of the major classes of antidepressant therapies. The large number of terms used in attempted classifications testify to the complexity of this syndrome and its etiology. A consensus is developing that depression may be classified as neurotic or psychotic, the latter being either unipolar or bipolar.

Since the discovery of ECT as an effective treatment of psychotic depression, many drug therapies have been developed. The amphetaminelike stimulants are now regarded as not truly antidepressant. Lithium has emerged as the major prophylactic treatment of mania, but careful monitoring of blood levels is recommended to minimize the incidence of intoxication. Treatment of depression with the MAO inhibitors such as phenelzine has been largely superseded by the use of the tricyclic antidepressants. Selective MAO inhibitors may have a role to play in the treatment of neurotic depression, but the distribution and activity of MAO-A and MAO-B may be too variable to allow the selective activity to be of therapeutic value.

The tricyclic antidepressants, such as imipramine, amitriptyline, and doxepine, are currently the major class of drugs used in the treatment of depression. Mianserin, trazodone, and nomifensine have emerged as second-generation drugs of equal clinical efficacy with the tricyclics, but appear to have a broader-spectrum antidepressant-antianxiety profile and minimal anticholinergic and cardiovascular toxicity. Therefore, these drugs may be better tolerated, particularly in the elderly, and less dangerous in overdose. The selective 5-HT uptake inhibitors fluoxetine and zimelidine hold great promise as effective antidepressants devoid of NA properties at the therapeutic doses. However, on further evaluation, the selective 5-HT uptake inhibitor fluvoxamine has been shown to cause cardiotoxic and gastrointestinal disturbance [209], and zimelidine has been withdrawn due to unexplained fatalities.

More recent modifications to the biogenic amine hypothesis of depression indicate that the central blockade of uptake of the neurotransmitters NA and 5-HT may only be partly responsible for antidepressant activity. Down-regulation or subsensitivity of both β-NA or 5-HT receptors has been demonstrated with all the major antidepressant therapies, and this correlates better with the clinical observation that their antidepressant effects develop only after 2–3 weeks of daily dosing.

Many of the newer drugs need more extensive clinical data to be generated before their role in antidepressant therapy can be evaluated. There is no evidence that the currently available therapy alters the pathology of depression. The next generation of antidepressants will be developed with support from an even wider background of clinical and basic biological data. Biochemical data at present appear to offer the best chance of correlation with clinical observations and thus a scientific basis for classification and treatment. The analysis of behavioral and EEG data from animals has been considerably improved, but correlation with the complex human condition of depression is still regarded by many as unachievable. However, such data has been extremely valuable in the development of the newer drugs that are being shown as clinically effective antidepressants.

REFERENCES

1. G. D. Burrows, *Drugs*, 11:209 (1976).
2. C. Brewer, *World Medicine*, March 24th, 1976, p. 37.
3. G. S. Dykes, *J. Int. Med. Res.*, 3 (Suppl. 1):1 (1975).
4. R. L. McGhie, H. O'Hara, J. O'Hara, N. H. Brodie, H. G. Dunckly, and A. A. Schiff, *J. Int. Med. Res.*, 5:354 (1977).
5. L. E. Hollister, *Clinical Use of Psychotherapeutic Drugs*, Charles C. Thomas, Springfield, Illinois, 1973, chap. 4.
6. J. H. Greist and T. H. Greist, in *Antidepressant Treatment—The Essentials*, Williams and Wilkins, Baltimore, 1979, p. 10.
7. L. E. Hollister, *Current Antidepressant Drugs: Their Clinical Use, Drugs*, 22:129 (1981).
8. D. G. Taylor, *J. Int. Med. Res.*, 3 (Suppl. 1):22 (1975).
9. Eli Lilly Market Survey, 1977, private communication.
10. W. Linford-Rees, *J. Int. Med. Res.*, 3, (Suppl. 1):12 (1975).
11. C. Duncan, *Mims Magazine*, August 15th, 1981, p. 44.
12. S. Lesse, (Ed.), *Masked Depression*, Aronson, New York, 1974.
13. R. J. Friedman and M. Katz (Eds.), *The Psychology of Depres-*
13. *sion*, Winston, Washington D.C., and Halsted (Wiley), New York, 1974.
14. A. Kiev (Ed.), *Somatic Manifestations of Depressive Disorders*, Excerpta Medica, Elsevier, Amsterdam and New York, 1974.
15. F. D. A. Guidelines for Psychotropic Drugs, *Psychopharmaocol. Bull.*, 19:70 (1974).
16. R. C. B. Aitken, *J. Int. Med. Res.*, 3 (Suppl. 1):18 (1975).
17. M. Metcalfe, A. L. Johnson, and A. Coppen, *Br. J. Psychiatry*, 126:41 (1975).
18. H. G. Akiskal and W. T. McKinney, *Arch. Gen. Psychiatry*, 32:285 (1975).
19. R. M. Cain and N. N. Cain, *Drug Ther.*, 105, (1975).
20. L. Covi, R. S. Lipman, R. Derogatis, J. E. Smith, and J. H. Pattison, *Am. J. Psychiatry*, 131:191 (1974).
21. S. S. Friedman, *Arch. Gen. Psychiatry*, 32:619 (1975).
22. L. L. Simpson (Ed.), *Drug Treatment of Mental Disorder*, Raven, New York, 1976, chap. 9.
23. *The Medicinal Letter*, 18:90 (1976).
24. B. Blackwell, *Drugs*, 21:201 (1981).
25. M. H. Bickel, *Prog. Drug. Res.*, 11:121 (1968).
26. L. F. Gram, *Dan. Med. Bull.*, 21:218 (1974).
27. C. I. Judd and R. C. Ursillo, in *Antidepressants*, (S. Fielding and H. Lal, Eds.), p. 231, Futura, New York, 1975.
28. J. V. Dingell, F. Sulser, and J. R. Gillette, *J. Pharmacol. Exp. Ther.*, 143:14 (1964).

29. P. L. Gigon and M. H. Bickel, *Biochem. Pharmacol*, 20:1921 (1971).
30. M. H. Bickel, *Xenobiotica*, 1:313 (1971).
31. G. P. Quinn, M. J. Hurwick, and J. H. Perel, in *Psychotherapeutic Drugs* (E. Usdin and I. S. Forrest, Eds.), Marcel Dekker, New York, 1976, p. 605.
32. H. B. Hucker, A. J. Balletto, J. Demetriades, B. H. Arison, and A. G. Zacchei, *Drug. Metab. Dispos.*, 5:132 (1977).
33. H. B. Hucker, A. J. Balletto, J. Demetriades, B. H. Arison, and A. G. Zacchei, *Drug. Metab. Dispos.*, 3:80 (1975).
34. A. Frigero and C. Pantarotto, *J. Pharm. Pharmacol.*, 28:665 (1976).
35. C. J. S. Walter, *Proc. Royal Soc. Med.*, 64:282 (1971).
36. A. Nagy and L. Treiber, *J. Pharm. Pharmacol.*, 25:599 (1973).
37. R. A. Braithwaite, R. Goulding, G. Theano, J. Bailey, and A. Coppen, *Lancet*, 1:1297 (1972).
38. D. G. Spiker, A. N. Weiss, and S. S. Chang, *Clin. Pharmacol. Ther.*, 18:539 (1975).
39. J. M. Petit, D. G. Spiker, and J. F. Ruwitch, *Clin. Pharmacol. Ther.*, 21:47 (1977).
40. J. L. Crammer, B. Scott, and B. Rolfe, *Psychopharmacologia*, 15:207 (1969).
41. M. H. Bickel and H. J. Weder, *Arch. Int. Pharmacodyn. Ther.*, 173:433 (1968).
42. E. Bachmann and G. Zbinden, *20th Congress of the European Society of Toxicology*, West Berlin, June 25th–28th, 1978.
43. E. Elonen, M. J. Mattila, and L. Saarnivaara, *Eur. J. Pharmacol.*, 28:178 (1974).
44. E. Elonen, *Med. Biol.*, 53:231 (1975).
45. E. Elonen and M. J. Mattila, *Med. Biol.*, 53:238 (1975).
46. J. R. Hayes, G. F. Born, and A. H. Rosebaum, *Mayo Clinic Proceedings*, 52:509 (1977).
47. S. J. Kantor, A. H. Glassman, J. T. Bigger, J. M. Perel, and E. V. Giardina, *Am. J. Psychiatry*, 135:534 (1978).
48. Z. P. Horovitz, J. J. Piala, J. P. High, J. C. Burke, and R. C. Leaf, *Int. J. Neuropharmacol.*, 5:405 (1966).
49. W. J. Kinnard, H. Barry, N. Watzmann, and J. P. Buckely, in *Proceedings of the First International Symposium on Antidepressant Drugs*, S. Garattini (Ed.), Excerpta Medica Foundation, Amsterdam, 1967, p. 89.
50. M. Nielsen, Psychotropic Agents in *Experimental Pharmacology* (F. Hoffmeister and G. Stille, Eds.), vol. 55/1, Springer-Verlag, New York, 1980, chap. 18, p. 401, 403, 475.
51. F. Sulser and P. L. Mobley, Psychotropic Agents, in *Handbook Experimental Pharmacology* (F. Hoffmeister and G. Stille, Eds.), vol. 55/1, Springer-Verlag, New York, 1980, chap. 21a, p. 475.

52. R. W. Fuller, H. D. Snoddy, and B. B. Molloy, *Psychopharmacol. Commun.*, 1:455 (1975).
53. H. van Riezen and A. Delver, *Arzneim. Forsch.*, 21:1562 (1971).
54. S. Garratini and A. Jori, in *Proceedings of the First International Symposium on Antidepressant Drugs* (S. Garratini, Ed.), Excerpta Medica Foundation, Amsterdam, 1967, p. 179.
55. B. Benz and P. G. Waser, *Arzneim. Forsch.*, 21:654 (1971).
56. V. Pederson, *Acta. Pharmacol. Toxicol.*, 25:63 (1967).
57. L. Molander and A. Randrup, *Psychopharmacology*, 45:261 (1976).
58. I. Møller Nielsen, M. Nymark, W. Hougs, and V. Pedersen, *Arzneim.-Forsch.*, 16:135 (1966).
59. K. D. Carincross, M. W. McCulloch, and F. Michelson, *J. Pharmacol. Exp. Ther.*, 149:365 (1965).
60. A. Delini-Stula, E. Radeke, and A. Vassout, *J. Int. Med. Res.*, 6:421 (1978).
61. E. B. Sigg, *Can. Psychiatr. Assoc. J.*, 4:S75 (1959).
62. J. Axelrod, L. G. Whitby, and G. Hertting, *Science*, 133:383 (1961).
63. J. Glowinski and J. Axelrod, *Nature*, 204:1318 (1964).
64. S. B. Ross and A. L. Renyi, *Eur. J. Pharmacol.*, 2:181 (1967).
65. S. B. Ross and A. L. Renyi, *Acta. Pharmacol. Toxicol.*, 36:382 (1975).
66. A. S. Horn and R. C. A. M. Trace, *Br. J. Pharmacol.*, 51:399 (1974).
67. A. S. Horn, *Postgrad. Med. J.*, 52:25 (1976).
68. O. Eränko, *Ann. Rev. Pharmacol.*, 7:203 (1967).
69. J. Axelrod, *Pharmacol. Rev.*, 18:95 (1966).
70. W. E. Bunney, *Psychopharmacol. Commun.*, 1:599 (1975).
71. G. W. Aschcroft, D. Eccleston, L. G. Murray, A. I. M. Glen, T. B. B. Crawford, I. A. Pullar, P. J. Shields, D. S. Walter, I. M. Blackburn, J. Connechan, and M. Lonergran, *Lancet*, 573 (1972).
72. H. M. Van Praag, *Depression and Schizophrenia: A Contribution to Their Chemical Pathologies*, Spectrum, New York, 1977.
73. A. Carlsson, H. Corrodi, K. Fuxe, and T. Hökfeld, *Eur. J. Pharmacol.*, 5:357 (1969).
74. A. Carlsson, H. Corrodi, K. Fuxe, and T. Hökfeld, *Eur. J. Pharmacol.*, 5:367 (1969).
75. O. Benesová and K. Náhunek, *Psycholpharmacologia*, 20:337 (1971).
76. N. E. Andén, A. Carlsson, and J. Haggendal, *Ann. Rev. Pharmacol.*, 9:119 (1969).
77. *Neuropyschopharmacology of monoamines and their regulatory enzymes. Advances in biochemical psychopharmacology* (E. Usdin, Ed.), vol. 12, Raven, New York, 1974.

78. P. A. Berger and J. D. Barchas, *Monoamine oxidase inhibitors* in *Psychotherapeutic Drugs* (E. Usdin and I. Forrest, Eds.), Marcel Dekker, New York, 1977.
79. R. J. Baldessarini, Mood Drugs in *Disease-a-Month* (H. F. Dowling, Ed.), vol. 24, 2, Year Book Medical Publishers, Chicago, 1977.
80. *Monoamine Oxidase Inhibitors—The State of the Art*, (M. B. H. Youdim and E. S. Paykel, Eds.), Wiley, New York, 1981.
81. C. J. Fowler, L. Oreland, and B. Callingham, *J. Pharm. Pharmacol.*, 33:341 (1981).
82. E. S. Paykel, R. R. Parker, R. Penrose, and E. Rassaby, *Neuropharmacology*, 17:1055 (1979).
83. E. S. Paykel, in *Psychopharmacology of Affective Disorders* (E. S. Paykel and A. Coppen, Eds.), Oxford University Press, Oxford, 1979.
84. D. S. Robinson, A. Nies, C. L. Ravaris, J. O. Ives, and D. Bartlett, Clinical psychopharmacology of phenelzine: MAO activity and clinical response in *Psychopharmacology: A Generation of Progress* (M. A. Lipton, A. DiMascio, and K. F. Killam, Eds.), Raven, New York, 1978.
85. *Arch. Gen. Psychiatry*, 35:629 (1978).
86. D. D. Schoepp and A. J. Azzaro, *J. Neurochem.*, 36:2025 (1981).
87. J. P. Johnston, *Biochem. Pharmacol.*, 17:1285 (1968).
88. R. W. Fuller, *Adv. Biochem. Psychopharmacol.*, 5:339 (1972).
89. M. B. Youdim, *Br. Med. Bull.*, 29:120 (1973).
90. H. Y. T. Yang and N. H. Neff, *J. Pharmacol. Exp. Ther.*, 187:365 (1973).
91. R. W. Fuller, *Prog. Neuropsychopharmacol.*, 2:303 (1978).
92. B. Blackwell, *Drugs*, 21:273 (1981).
93. D. R. Brebbia, M. H. Branchey, E. Pyne, J. Watson, A. F. Brebbia, and G. F. Simpson, *Psychopharmacol.*, 45:1 (1975).
94. D. M. Gallant, *Curr. Ther. Res.*, 15:56 (1973).
95. V. N. Bagadia, L. P. Shati, P. V. Pradhari, and M. T. Gada, *Curr. Ther. Res.*, 26:417 (1979).
96. *Therapie*, 35:733 (1980).
97. R. M. Pinder, R. N. Brogden, T. M. Speight, and G. S. Avery, *Drugs*, 13:321 (1977).
98. *Curr. Ther. Res.*, 29:363 (1981).
99. I. Hoffman, *Arzneim. Forsch.*, 23:45 (1973).
100. C. Braestrup and J. Scheel-Krüger, *Eur. J. Pharmacol.*, 38:305 (1976).
101. K. Tauber, *Symposia. Medica. Hoechst.* 10:51 (1974).
102. R. N. Brogden, R. C. Heel, T. M. Speight, and G. S. Avery, *Drugs*, 18:1 (1979).
103. *Curr. Ther. Res.*, 28:837 (1980).
104. *Curr. Ther. Res.*, 29:567 (1981).

105. W. C. Stern, J. Rogers, V. Fang, and H. Meltzer, *Life Sci.*, 25:1717 (1979).
106. L. Fabre and D. M. McLendon, *Curr. Ther. Res.*, 23:393 (1978); and also see A. W. Peck, C. E. Bye, M. Clubley, T. Henson, and C. Riddington, *Br. J. Clin. Pharmacol.*, 7:469 (1979).
107a. T. Koide and K. Uyemura, *Eur. J. Pharmacol.*, 62:147 (1980).
107b. *Neuropharmacology*, 19:349 (1980).
107c. Y. Ikeda, N. Takano, H. Matsushita, Y. Shiraki, T. Koide, R. Nagashima, Y. Fujimura, M. Shindo, S. Suzuki, and T. Iwasaki, *Arzneim-Forsch.*, 29:511 (1979).
108. *Fed. Proc.*, 39:404 (1980).
109. C. H. Cashin, J. Fairhurst, D. C. Horwell, I. A. Pullar, S. Sutton, G. H. Timms, E. Wildsmith, and F. Wright, *Eur. J. Med. Chem.*, 13:495 (1978).
110a. D. T. Wong and F. P. Bymaster, *Life Sci.*, 23, 1041 (1978).
110b. R. Fuller, K. W. Perry, and A. Snoddy, *Neuropharmacology*, 18:197 (1979).
111a. T. Pugsley and W. Lippman, *Psychopharmacology*, 47:33 (1976).
111b. Also see H. Schanda and B. Saletu, *Pharmakopsychiatrie*, 12: 338 (1979).
112. D. T. Wong, *Fed. Proc.* 40:249 (1981).
113. R. W. Fuller, K. W. Perry, and B. B. Molloy, *Life Sci.*, 15: 1161 (1974).
114. H. M. Rowe, R. H. Carmichael, and S. Oldham, *Science*, 199: 436 (1978).
115. A. Coppen, V. A. Rama Rao, C. Swade, and K. Wood, *Psychopharmacology*, 63:125, 199 (1979).
116. R. J. Simpson, *Br. Med. J.*, 1:1133 (1980).
117. *Proc. Br. Pharmacol. Soc.*, (Aberdeen), C. 81 (1980).
118. V. Claasen, J. E. Davies, G. Hertting, and P. Placheta, *Br. J. Pharmacol.*, 60:505 (1977).
119. D. P. Droogen, *Neuropharmacology*, 19:1215 (1980).
120. J. H. Wright and H. C. B. Denber, *Curr. Ther. Res.*, 23:83 (1978).
121. K. Ghose, R. Gupta, A. Coppen, and J. Lund, *Eur. J. Pharmacol.*, 42:31 (1977).
122. C. Borup, I. M. Petersen, P. le Fevre Honore, and L. Wetterberg, *Psychopharmacology*, 63:241 (1979).
123. G. Raynaud, C. Gouret, M. J. Bourniol, M. Mazadier, and G. Anton, *Eur. J. Med. Chem.*, 11:75 (1976).
124a. C. Gouret, *Therapie*, 28:1197 (1973).
124b. See also P. E. Keane, J. P. Kan, N. Sontag, and N. Strolin-Benedetti, *J. Pharm. Pharmacol.*, 31:752 (1979).
125. A. J. Bigler, K. P. Bogeso, A. Toft, and V. Hansen, *Eur. J. Med. Chem.*, 12:289 (1977).

126a. J. Hyttel, *Psychopharmacol.*, 51:225 (1977).
126b. See also K. F. Overton, *Eur. J. Clin. Pharmacol.*, 14:69 (1978).
127. G. Le Fur, M. Kabouche, and A. Uzan, *Life Sci.*, 19:1959 (1979).
128. *Eur. J. Drug. Metab. Pharmacokinet.*, 1:9 (1979).
129. M. F. Sugrue, I. Goodlet, and S. E. Mireylees, *Eur. J. Pharmacol.*, 40:121 (1976).
130. S. E. Mireylees, I. Goodlet, and M. F. Sugrue, *Biochem. Pharmacol.*, 27:1023 (1978).
131. M. Ramacci, O. Ghirardi, F. Maccari, L. Pacifici, and P. Sale, *Arzneim-Forsch.*, 29:294 (1979).
132. M. M. Al-Yassiri, S. I. Ankier, and P. K. Bridges, *Life Sci.*, 28:2449 (1981).
133. R. N. Brogden, R. C. Heel, T. M. Speight, and G. S. Avery, *Drugs*, 2:1, 401 (1981).
134. M. Fink, *Psychopharmacol. Bull.*, 15:27 (1979).
135. M. Raiteri, F. Angelini, and A. Bertollini, *J. Pharm. Pharmacol.*, 28:483 (1976).
136. W. L. Shaw, *Curr. Med. Res. Opin.*, 6 (Suppl. 7):44 (1980).
137. L. Conti and R. M. Pinder, *J. Int. Med. Res.*, 7:285 (1979).
138. R. V. Magnus, *Br. J. Clin. Pract.*, 33:251 (1979).
139. R. N. Brogden, R. C. Heel, T. M. Speight, and G. S. Avery, *Drugs*, 16:273 (1978).
140. *Pharmaprojects*, July, 1981.
141. F. Schatz, U. Jahn, T. W. Jaaregg, L. Zirngibl, and K. Thiele, *Arzneim. Forsch.*, 30:919 (1980).
142. P. A. Martorana and R. E. Nitz, *Arzneim. Forsch.*, 29:946 (1979).
143. M. D. Mashkovsky and N. I. Andrejeva, *Arzneim. Forsch.*, 31:75 (1981).
144. *7th Int. Cong. Pharmacol.* (Paris), Abs. 625, 1978.
145. *Curr. Ther. Res.*, 27:458 (1980).
146. S. Cecchini, P. Petri, R. Ardito, S. R. Bareggi, and A. Torriti, *J. Int. Med. Res.*, 6:388 (1978).
147. *Curr. Ther. Res.*, 24:734 (1978).
148. *Psychopharmacol. Bull.*, 15 (1979).
149. V. M. Soh, R. S. B. Ehsanullah, M. Leighton, and M. J. Kirby, *Psychopharmacol.*, 60:177 (1979).
150. K. Ghose, *Psychopharmacology.*, 57:109 (1978).
151. S. Levine, *J. Int. Med. Res.*, 7:1 (1979).
152. *8th Int. Cong. Pharmacol.*, (Tokyo), Abs. P527, 1981.
153. *Jpn. J. Pharmacol.*, 29 (S):31p (1979).
154. *8th Int. Cong. Pharmacol.*, (Tokyo), Abs. p. 854 (1981).
155. M. Harada and H. Maeno, *Biochem. Pharmacol.*, 28:2645 (1979).
156. S. Tachikawa, M. Harada, and H. Maeno, *Arch. Int. Pharmacodyn.*, 238:81 (1979).

157. U. K. Patent No. 1409935, and U.S. No. 3959470.
158. T. A. Ban, *Psychopharmacol. Bull.*, 15:22 (1979).
159. J. F. Chevalier, *Ann. Med.-Psychol.* 133:363 (1979).
160. R. M. Pinder, R. N. Brogden, T. M. Speight, and G. S. Avery, *Drugs*, 13:401 (1977).
161. A. P. Zis and F. K. Goodwin, *Arch. Gen. Psychiat.*, 36:1097 (1979).
162. *Proc. Br. Pharmacol. Soc.* (London), p. 14 (1980).
163. *Pharmaprojects*, June, 1981.
164. T. M. Itil, *Dis. Nerv. Syst.*, 33:557 (1972).
165. T. M. Itil, in *Psychopharmacology, Sexual Disorders and Drug Abuse* (T. A. Ban, J. R. Boissier, G. J. Gessa, H. Heimann, L. Hollister, H. E. Lehmann, I. Munkvad, N. Steinberg, F. Sulser, A. Sandwell, and O. Vinar, Eds.), Amsterdam, London, North Holland, 1973, p. 13.
166. C. D. Burgess, S. Montgomery, J. Wadsworth, and P. Turner, *Postgrad. Med. J.*, 55:704 (1979).
167. J. G. Edwards, *Lancet*, 2:1368 (1979).
168. W. L. Shaw, *Curr. Med. Res. Opinion*, 6 (Suppl. 7):44 (1980).
169. W. Williams, *Med. J. Austr.*, 1:132 (1980).
170. J. E. Murphy, *J. Int. Med. Res.*, 3 (Suppl. 3):47 (1975).
171. I. Ichimaru, *Jpn. J. Int. Med. Res.*, 3 (Suppl. 3):97 (1975).
172. P. Crome and B. Newman, *J. R. Soc. Med.*, 72:649 (1979).
173. W. A. Forrest, *J. Int. Med. Res.*, 5 (Suppl. 4):112 (1977).
174. A. Aberg and G. Holmberg, *Acta. Psychiat. Scand.*, 59:45 (1979).
175. J. Maj, W. Palider, and A. Rawlow, *J. Neur. Transm.*, 44:237 (1979).
176. S. Clements-Jewery, P. A. Robson, and L. J. Chidley, *Neuropharmacology*, 19:1165 (1980).
177. J. Maj, *T.I.P.S.*, 80 (March 1981).
178. G. K. Suchowsky and L. Pegrassi, *Arzneim. Forsch.*, 19:643 (1969).
179. A. Moretti and C. Caccia, *Communication at 6th International Meeting of the International Society for Neurochemistry*, Copenhagen, 1977.
180. L. F. Hollister, *Clinical Use of Psychotherapeutic Drugs*, Charles C. Thomas, Springfield, Illinois, 1977, chap. 3.
181. J. H. Greist and T. H. Greist, in *Antidepressant Treatment—The Essentials*, Williams and Wilkins, Baltimore, 3.8, 1979, p. 177.
182. *Drug Treatment of Mental Disorders* (L. L. Simpson, Ed.), Raven, New York, 1976, chap. 12 and 13.
183. H. E. Hansen, *Drugs*, 22:461 (1981).
184. M. Schou, Psychotropic Agents in *Handbook Experimental Pharmacology* (F. Hoffmeister and F. Stille, Eds.), vol. 55/1, Springer-Verlag, New York, 1980, chap. 25.

185a. Also see 19 papers on lithium, *Arch. Gen. Psychiat.*, 20:833 (1979).
185b. L. E. Eleshefsky, A. M. Gilderman, and C. M. Jewett, *Drug. Intel. Clin. Pharm.*, 13:403, 492 (1979).
185c. F. N. Johnson, *Neurosci. Biobehav. Rev.*, 3:15 (1979).
185d. M. Schou, *Neuropsychobiol.*, 5:241 (1979; 6:1 (1980).
186. J. F. J. Cade, *Med. J. Austr.*, 36:349 (1949).
187. T. J. Crow, *Psychol. Med.*, 9:401 (1979).
188. J. H. Greist and T. H. Greist, in *Antidepressants—The Essentials*, Williams and Wilkins, Baltimore, 3:12, 1979, p. 199.
189. Drug Addiction II, Amphetamine, Psychotogen and Marijuana Dependence, in *Handbook of Experimental Pharmacology*, vol. 45, (G. V. R. Born, O. Eichler, A. Farah, H. Herken, and A. D. Welch, Eds.), Springer-Verlag, New York, 1977.
190. *Drug Treatment of Mental Disorders* (L. L. Simpson, Ed.), Raven, New York, 1976, chap. 11.
191. L. E. Jonsson, E. Anggard, and L. M. Gunne, *Clin. Pharmacol. Ther.*, 12:889 (1971).
192. J. H. Greist and T. H. Greist, in *Antidepressant Treatment—The Essentials*, Williams and Wilkins, Baltimore, 3.10, 1979, p. 192.
193. Proceedings of an International Symposium, *Acta. Psych. Scand.*, 63 (Suppl. 290), Munksgaard, Copenhagen, 1981.
194. D. T. Wong, *Fed. Proc.*, 40:Abst. 73 (1981).
195. S. Ögren, K. Fuxe, L. F. Agnati, J. A. Gustafsson, G. Jonsson, and A. C. Holm, *J. Neurol. Transm.*, 46:85 (1979).
196. J. Vetulani and F. Sulser, *Nature*, 257:195 (1975).
197. F. Sulser, in *Towards Understanding Receptors*, (J. W. Lamble, Ed.), Elsevier, 1981, p. 99.
198. S. P. Banerjee, L. S. Kung, S. J. Riggi, and S. K. Chanda, *Nature*, 268:455 (1977).
199. B. McMillen, W. Warnack, D. G. German, and P. A. Shore, *Eur. J. Pharmacol.*, 61:239 (1980).
200. K. Fuxe, S. O. Ögren, and L. P. Agnati, *Neurosci. Lett.*, 13:307 (1979).
201. E. Stone, *Res. Commun. Psychol. Psychiat. Behav.*, 4:241 (1979).
202. T. C. Westfell, *Physiol. Rev.*, 57:659 (1977).
203. B. J. Carroll, M. Feinberg, and J. F. Greden, *III World Congress, Biological Psychiatry*, S.50, Stockholm, 1981.
204. N. C. Tye, Lilly Research cCentre, Windlesham, Surrey, U. K., personal communication.
205. M. E. P. Seligman and S. F. Maier, *J. Exp. Psychol.*, 74:1 (1967).
206. F. Petty and A. D. Sherman, *Commun. Psychopharmacol.*, 3: 371 (1980).

207. F. Petty and A. D. Sherman, *Drug. Dev. Res.*, 2:43 (1982).
208. J. H. Greist and T. H. Greist, in *Antidepressants—The Essentials*, Williams and Wilkins, Baltimore, 3:15–19 (1979).
209. M. Schachter and J. D. Parkes, *J. Neurol. Neurosurg. Psychiatry*, 43:171 (1980).

3
Benzodiazepines and Barbiturates: Drugs for the Treatment of Anxiety, Insomnia, and Seizure Disorders

KELVIN W. GEE and HENRY I. YAMAMURA *Department of Pharmacology, University of Arizona Health Sciences Center, Tucson, Arizona*

I. INTRODUCTION

The clinical indications for the barbiturates and benzodiazepines are very similar. Prior to the introduction of the benzodiazepines, barbiturates were widely used as antianxiety and sedative-hypnotic agents. The prevalent use of barbiturates was also associated with drug abuse, drug dependency, and overdose fatalities. Currently, the major clinical applications of the barbiturates are limited to the treatment of certain epilepsies and as an intravenous anesthetic. The use of the barbiturates as antianxiety agents and as sedative-hypnotics has been eclipsed by the advent of the safer benzodiazepines, just as the barbiturates made the use of the bromides, paraldehyde, and chloral hydrate obsolete. The latter compounds of the prebarbiturate era are now only of historical interest. Thus, the following discussion of the drugs useful in the treatment of anxiety, insomnia, and certain convulsive disorders will be confined to the benzodiazepines. The barbiturates will be covered in a limited manner, since they now have a more confined therapeutic application than the benzodiazepines.

This chapter is divided into two major sections. The benzodiazepines are discussed first and then the barbiturates are considered in the second section. The basic pharmacology of these compounds is presented along with the general principles underlying their current clinical application in the treatment of specific central nervous system (CNS) disorders. Particular emphasis is placed upon the discussion of the possible mechanisms of action of these compounds and how they relate to the possible biological basis of the disorders treated by these compounds. The advantages and limitations of the current drug therapies are also discussed. Finally, some insights into the future directions of drug research aimed at the development of compounds with improved specificity for CNS disorders currently amenable to therapeutic intervention by the benzodiazepines and the barbiturates are included.

II. BENZODIAZEPINES

A. Historical Perspective

The discovery of the therapeutically useful benzodiazepines in the late 1950s is attributed to the systematic search for an orally active muscle relaxant [1,2]. The benzodiazepines are derivatives of the 4,5-benzohept-1,2,6-oxodiazines first described in the 1930s. The pharmacological screening of these compounds by Randall and co-workers resulted in an observation that the benzodiazepines produced a "taming" effect on various test animals including primates [2]. Since the "taming" effect on animals occurred at doses less than those producing ataxia or sedation, the clinical application of these compounds as antianxiety agents was suggested. Benzodiazepines became commercially available in the early 1960s with the introduction of chlordiazepoxide (Librium*®) as an antianxiety agent. Since the introduction of the benzodiazepines, this class of compound has become one of the most commonly prescribed drugs. In the United States alone, over 8000 tons of benzodiazepines were consumed by an estimated 51 million people in 1977 [3]. The widespread use of the benzodiazepines is, in part, attributable to the effectiveness of these compounds in the symptomatic treatment of nonpsychotic anxiety and to the relative safety of these drugs.

B. Chemistry, Biotransformation, and Pharmacokinetics

The general structure of the 1,4-benzodiazepines is depicted in Table 1. Over 2000 of these compounds have been synthesized but only the currently marketed compounds are included in Table 3.1. The structure-activity relationships have been extensively reviewed by Sternbach [4]. Briefly, substitutions in positions 7,1 and ring C are all-important in modifying the potency of these compounds (Table 3.1). Recently the introduction of the triazolo-1,4-benzodiazepine analogs have yielded a

*® Trademark.

TABLE 3.1 Names and Structures of Various Benzodiazepines Available for Clinical Use

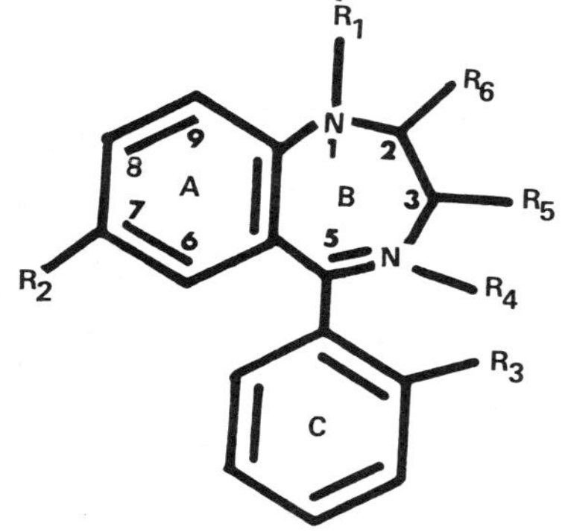

Name	R_1	R_2	R_3	R_4	R_5	R_6
Chlordiazepoxide (Librium*®)	H	Cl	Cl	O	H	$—NHCH_3$
Clorazepate (Tranxene*®)	H	Cl	H	–	—COOH	=O
Clonazepam (Clonopin*®)	H	$—NO_2$	Cl	–	H	=O
Diazepam (Valium*®)	$—CH_3$	Cl	H	–	H	=O
Flunitrazepam (Rohypnol*®)	$—CH_3$	$—NO_2$	F	–	H	=O
Flurazepam (Dalmane*®)	$—(CH_2)_2—N(C_2H_5)_2$	Cl	F	–	H	=O

TABLE 3.1 (Continued)

Name	R_1	R_2	R_3	R_4	R_5	R_6
Halazepam (Paxipam*®)	$—CH_2CF_3$	Cl	–	–	H	=O
Lorazepam (Ativan*®)	H	Cl	Cl	–	—OH	=O
Medazepam (Nobrium*®)	$—CH_3$	Cl	H	–	H	H
Nitrazepam (Mogadon*®)	H	$—NO_2$	H	–	H	=O
Oxazepam (Serax*®)	▷$—CH_2$	Cl	H	–	—OH	=O
Temazepam (Restoril*®)	$—CH_3$	Cl	H	–	—OH	=O

*® Registered Trademark

new generation of potent compounds which include alprazolam (Xanax*®). This class of compound may possess pharmacologic actions different from the 1,4-benzodiazepines [6]. Alterations in structure that result in changes in potency may be the result of one or more contributing factors. These factors include changes in the pharmacokinetic properties resulting from an alteration in the lipid solubility of the compound or its susceptibility to biotransformation. Structural changes also alter the dynamics of interaction with the site of action.

Among the compounds listed in Table 3.1, the most rapidly absorbed following oral administration are diazepam and clorazepate. The R5 hydroxylated deratives oxazepam, temazepam, and prazepam are absorbed relatively slowly, whereas the remainder of the compounds are intermediate. It must be remembered that absorption depends upon a number of variables, including the physicochemical properties of the drug and its pharmaceutical formulation. Consequently, wide variability among these compounds in the rate of absorption following a single oral dose can be expected. In general, the benzodiazepines are rapidly and completely absorbed. The distribution of the benzodiazepines is in part dependent upon the lipid solubility of the individual compounds.

Diazepam is the most lipophilic among the group (Table 3.1) and has the greatest relative volume of distribution whereas lorazepam and alprazolam have the smallest volume of distribution. These observations are consistent with the rapid onset and short duration of action following an acute dose of diazepam compared with the relatively slower onset and longer duration of action of lorazepam. Thus, redistribution of benzodiazepines to all body tissues (i.e., outside the brain) is an important determinant of the time course of action of these compounds. Plasma binding in excess of 90% of the administered dose of benzodiazepines is observed. A more detailed account of the pharmacokinetics of benzodiazepines and their clinical implications is provided by Greenblatt et. al. [7] and Shader and Greenblatt, [8].

Extensive hepatic biotransformation is a major mechanism involved in the elimination of the benzodiazepines. A number of the benzodiazepines listed in Table 3.1 are metabolized to pharmacologically active compounds. Some of these include chlordiazepoxide, clorazepate, diazepam, halazepam, and prazepam. The presence of active metabolites contributes to the apparent duration of action of these compounds. The three major pathways for biotransformation of benziodiazepines in the liver are oxidation, conjugation, or nitroreduction, depending upon the particular functional groups present on the

---

*® Trademark.

molecule [9]. For example, diazepam is demethylated to nordiazepam followed by hydroxylation at the C-3 position to the active metabolite oxazepam, which is in turn conjugated to glucuronic acid and excreted. Alternatively, diazepam can be hydroxylated at the C-3 position via a minor pathway to yield the active metabolite, temazepam, which is then conjugated and excreted as the glucuronide. Note that some of the active metabolites of diazepam are marketed as well. Thus, it is easy to appreciate the effect of impaired hepatic function upon the clinical efficacy and duration of action of the benzodiazepines when the role of liver metabolism is considered. The benzodiazepines do not appear to induce the hepatic microsomal mixed-function oxidase system. However, a number of drug interactions with benzodiazepines do occur and will either enhance or inhibit the hepatic elimination of these compounds. For example, chronic alcohol, phenobarbital, and antituberculosis drugs will induce hepatic benzodiazepine metabolism. In contrast, acute alcohol, cimetidine, and oral contraceptives will inhibit hepatic elimination. The myriad drug interactions with benzodiazepines have been reviewed recently by Kotz [10]. A summary of the pharmacokinetics and metabolic disposition of some of the commonly prescribed benzodiazepines for the management of anxiety is presented in Table 3.2.

C. Major Applications of the Benzodiazepines in the Treatment of CNS Disorders

The principal indications for the use of benzodiazepines today are in the symptomatic relief of nonpsychotic anxiety, insomnia, and in the treatment of certain types of epilepsy. The use of benzodiazepines in the management of anxiety and insomnia accounts for the majority of the benzodiazepine's clinical applications. Since this discussion is confined to the use of benzodiazepines in the treatment of CNS disorders, the uses of benzodiazepines as muscle relaxants and as anesthetic agents will not be considered. However, reviews of these applications of benzodiazepines can be obtained by referring to the articles by Madorsky and by Dundee and Kawar [11,12].

1. Anxiety

Convincing evidence from numerous well-controlled double-blind experiments indicates that benzodiazepines are significantly more effective than placebo in the symptomatic relief of anxiety of somatic or emotional origins [13,14,15]. On the other hand, benzodiazepines have not been found to be effective in treating anxiety associated with endogenous depressions or with schizophrenia. Thus, for these compounds to produce beneficial effects, a proper diagnosis must be made.

TABLE 3.2 A Summary of the Pharmacokinetics of Selected Benzodiazepines

Drug	Daily dosage range (mg)	Peak plasma concentration time (hr)[a]	$T_{\frac{1}{2}}$ for elimination (hr)	Active metabolites
Chlordiozepoxide	15–100	1.0–2.5	5–30	Yes
Clorazepate	7.5–60	0.5–1.5	30–200	Yes
Diazepam	4–40	0.5–1.5	20–70	Yes
Lorazepam	1–8	1.0–2.5	10–20	No
Oxazepam	30–120	1.5–3.0	5–15	No
Alprazolam	0.5–4	1.0–2.5	8–20	Yes

[a]Values for parent compound following an oral dose in healthy young volunteers. Data from Greenblatt et al. [9].

Based upon the *Diagnostic and Statistical Manual of Mental Disorders* (DSM-III), benzodiazepines are indicated in generalized anxiety disorder, atypical anxiety disorder, anticipatory anxiety, panic disorder, posttraumatic anxiety, adjustment disorder with anxious mood, and somatization disorders [16]. Details of diagnostic methods is beyond the scope of this text and the reader is referred to an excellent monograph edited by Klein and Rabkin [17].

The diagnosis of the disorder and the decision to use benzodiazepine therapy is more difficult than the determination of which benzodiazepine to use. Such a conclusion is based upon the observation that all of the benzodiazepines currently available for the treatment of anxiety have similar pharmacological properties and cannot be differentiated based upon clinical efficacy [13,14,15]. All of these compounds will relieve anxiety, show varying degrees of anticonvulsant and muscle relaxant activity, and produce sedation. Generally, control of anxiety can be accomplished at doses that are nonsedating. The benzodiazepines currently available in the United States for the treatment of anxiety include alprazolam, chlordiazepoxide, clorazepate, diazepam, halazepam, lorazepam, oxazepam, and prazepam. The major considerations in the choice of drug are related to the desired onset and duration of action and propensity toward sedative side effects. Chlordiazepoxide, diazepam, clorazepate, halazepam, and alprazolam have short to intermediate half-lives (Table 3.2). Diazepam has the fastest onset of action following acute oral administration. This property, along with its long half-life with chronic use may in part account for the widespread use of diazepam as an antianxiety agent. In contrast, oxazepam and lorazepam have shorter durations of action and must be taken more frequently. Drugs such as lorazepam and alprazolam are also more potent than diazepam. It is interesting to note that equipotent dosages of alprazolam appear to produce less sedation than the other benzodiazepines [18]. This triazolo-1,4-benzodiazepine also appears to act as an antidepressant [5]. Additional considerations include the presence of active metabolites (Table 3.2), which may be important in situations where impaired hepatic function is present and can be compensated for by using compounds without active metabolites or by reducing the dose or interval between doses of those compounds that can be converted to active metabolites. In summary, the effective management of anxiety can be accomplished by titrating the dose or modifying the regimen of any one of the available benzodiazepines.

It is essential that the efficacy of the therapy with benzodiazepines be assessed early in the treatment program. Some problems associated with lack of response in the first couple of weeks of treatment may include insufficient dose of drug, cross-tolerance, or a misdiagnosis (19). Recently, Rickels and coworkers have described a reliable predictor of patient treatment outcome during a six week treatment program with diazepam [20]. The patient's initial response during the first week of treatment will predict the outcome of the therapy. It was found that 90% of the patients who reported much improvement in the first week of treatment were markedly improved at the end of 6 weeks of treatment. On the other hand, among the patients reporting no improvement or worsening after 1 week of treatment, only 20% were markedly improved after 6 weeks of treatment. Moreover, in the same study it was found that 51% of the patients who showed improvement after 6 weeks of treatment did not show relapse when switched to placebo. This observation suggests that limited-duration benzodiazepine treatment in chronic anxiety is a sound practice that will help reduce the possibility of the development of dependence, often associated with chronic usage of high doses of benzodiazepines. It must be emphasized that benzodiazepines provide only a means to relieve the symptoms of anxiety (not the underlying cause of the anxiety) and should be only one part of the overall therapeutic strategy.

2. Insomnia

As with anxiety, insomnia is a symptom that may have many underlying causes. For example, the complaint of the inability to initiate or maintain sleep may be the result of pain, anxiety, increased sensory stimulation, or the presence of other drugs. Often the pathophysiology of insomnia cannot be traced. Thus, a comprehensive evaluation is necessary before considering the use of hypnotic medication in the treatment of insomnia. Again, the benzodiazepines are only used as adjunctive treatment for symptomatic relief. The diagnosis, classification, and pathophysiology of sleep disorders including insomnia have been reviewed extensively and will not be discussed further [21–24].

Once the decision to use hypnotic medication has been made, the benzodiazepines are preferable to the barbiturates. The primary justifications for this choice are the greater therapeutic index associated with the benzodiazepines and the rapid tolerance that develops to the hypnotic effects of the barbiturates. Currently, there are four benzodiazepines available for use as hypnotics. They are flurazepam, temazepam, nitrazepam (widely used in Europe), and the triazolo-1,4-benzodiazepine, triazolam (Halcion*®). The efficacy of these compounds is well established. All of these drugs except temazepam will facilitate onset of sleep. All of them will prolong sleep time and diminish the number of awakenings. Flurazepam, temazepam, and triazolam will decrease the duration of stages 1, 3, and 4 and increase duration of

---

*®Trademark.

stage-2 sleep. REM sleep is also shortened by these compounds. The net effect is to lengthen total sleep time by increasing the duration of light sleep.

Flurazepam is the most studied and widely prescribed hypnotic. It has been shown to be effective in short-term (1 week), intermediate (2 week) and long-term (4 week) use [25–27]. Abrupt withdrawal of flurazepam following short- or intermediate-term treatment does not appear to result in rebound insomnia [28–30]. Temazepam, because of its slow rate of absorption following oral ingestion, is not very effective in the induction of sleep [31–32]. However, this compound is moderately effective in the maintenance of sleep [31–32]. Some investigators have reported rebound insomnia upon abrupt withdrawal of temazepam. Sleep laboratory studies with triazolam indicate that in short-term use, the efficacy of this compound is comparable to that of flurazepam [33,34]. However, with intermediate-term use, a significant reduction in effectiveness occurs. Rebound insomnia also occurs following withdrawal of triazolam [35]. The phenomenon of rebound insomnia appears to be more intense and prevalent following withdrawal of a benzodiazepine with a short half-life, whereas those with longer half-lives have an infrequent incidence of rebound insomnia that is usually of lesser intensity. To avoid the rebound effect, it is desirable to use benzodiazepines with long half-lives such as flurazepam or gradually withdraw treatment in cases involving benzodiazepines with short half-lives.

3. Seizure Disorders

Currently, two benzodiazepines are available primarily for the therapy of certain seizure disorders. Clonazepam is most effective against absence and myoclonic seizures and is also useful in the treatment of infantile spasms, atypical absence, and atonic seizures [36]. Some evidence also suggests that clonazepam may be effective against simple and complex partial seizures. Clonazepam is indicated in refractory simple and complex absence and atypical absence seizures. Intravenous diazepam is indicated for immediate seizure control in status epilepticus. However, diazepam is not very effective in the long-term control of status epilepticus. As with clonazepam, tolerance develops to the antiepileptic effect. Abrupt withdrawal following chronic treatment with clonazepam will often precipitate tonic-clonic epilepticus. The problem of tolerance limits the usefulness of clonazepam as a drug for long-term treatment of disorders [36]. Approximately 30% of patients who show favorable initial response to clonazepam will develop tolerance. Two-thirds of these patients will respond to higher doses of clonazepam whereas the remainder will not respond to clonazepam at any dose. The tolerance is unrelated to enzyme induction since the elimination half-life of clonazepam during chronic treatment is similar to that observed during initial treatment.

Doses for infants and children are usually 0.01–0.03 mg/kg·day (two to three divided doses) with increments of less than or equal to 0.25–0.5 mg every 3–7 days until a maintenance dose of 0.1–0.2 mg/kg is obtained. Increments are made until seizure control is achieved or until side effects prohibit any further increase. Adult dosages are 1.5 mg/day (three divided doses) initially with increments of 0.5 mg every 3–7 days and a maximum dose of 20 mg. Thus, individual dose regimens can be titrated until effective seizure control is achieved.

D. Mechanism of Action

After the initial observation of the pharmacological effects of the benzodiazepines, the mechanisms of action of these compounds has been extensively studied at the molecular, electrophysiological, and behavioral levels. Early electrophysiological studies in the 1960s identified the limbic system as the primary site of action of the benzodiazepines. The behavioral effects (i.e., antianxiety) were thought to be mediated by the amygdala and hippocampus in particular. Since then evidence has accumulated to suggest that other brain regions are also profoundly affected by the benzodiazepines and that the limbic system appears to be particularly sensitive to these compounds. The next milestone in benzodiazepine research was the discovery that benzodiazepines interacted primarily with a specific neurotransmitter system, the γ-aminobutyric acid (GABA) system [37,38]. The GABAergic synapse is now thought to be the primary and possibly the main site of action of the benzodiazepines in the CNS.

Early behavioral and electrophysiological studies on the structure-activity relationships showed marked differences in pharmacological potencies and profiles of the various benzodiazepine analogs, suggesting that these compounds interacted with a highly specific site on neuronal membranes. In 1977, the discovery of high-affinity, saturable, and specific binding of the radioligand [^{3}H]diazepam to neuronal membranes provided the first evidence for a specific site of action [39–41]. Coupled with the finding that benzodiazepines may produce their effects through the GABA system, research has now focused upon how benzodiazepine modification of GABA function produces the characteristic behavioral effects of these compounds.

It is currently believed that the anxiolytic, anticonvulsant, sedative, and muscle relaxant effects of the benzodiazepines are mediated by the benzodiazepine receptor [42]. This hypothesis is based upon animal studies where the degree of in vivo occupancy of benzodiazepine-binding sites has been correlated with the time course of pharmacological action [43]. Moreover, the binding affinity of individual benzodiazepines is highly correlated with their clinical and pharmacological potencies [44,45].

The benzodiazepine receptor is thought to be part of a supramolecular complex consisting of the GABA receptor and chloride ionophore [45]. The presence of a specific receptor for benzodiazepines suggests the existence of an "endogenous ligand" by analogy to the opiate receptor/endorphin system. However, definitive evidence for such an endogenous compound is not yet available. The exact mechanism by which the occupancy of benzodiazepine receptors will modify GABAergic function is not yet established, but it is believed to involve specific interactions between the benzodiazepine receptor, GABA receptor, and chloride ionophore (Fig. 3.1). The current concepts on the involvement of the benzodiazepine receptor in GABAergic neurotransmission has been recently reviewed [46,47].

The evidence for an essential role of GABA in the antianxiety effects of the benzodiazepines has not been as convincing as for the other pharmacological effects. An additional difficulty in identifying the molecular basis of anxiety is the nature of the relationship between animal models of anxiety such as "approach-avoidance conflict" and human anxiety. Although these models successfully predict antianxiety activity of various drugs in man, the underlying mechanisms may be different despite similar outcomes (i.e., antianxiety). On the other hand, the hypothesis that facilitation of GABA neurotransmission is involved in the anticonvulsant and sedative-hypnotic effects of the benzodiazepines is more compelling. Theoretically, benzodiazepines can act pre- or postsynaptically to enhance the effects of GABA, the primary inhibitory neurotransmitter in the CNS. The bulk of the evidence, both biochemical and electrophysiological, supports a postsynaptic action. Ultimately, facilitation of GABA effects leads to enhanced chloride channel opening and consequent changes in neuronal membrane excitability. The benzodiazepines potentiate the effects of GABA in brain tissue slices and in neuronal cell cultures [48,49]. The effects measured include changes in membrane conductance and the frequency of chloride channel opening. The observation that the benzodiazepines did not increase the

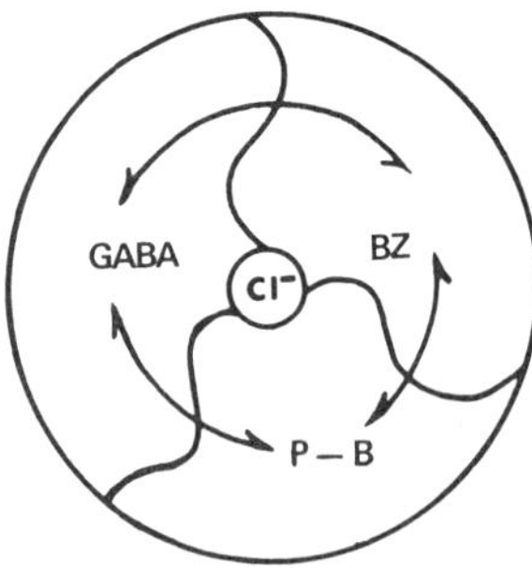

FIG. 3.1 The benzodiazepine (BZ) receptor and its interactions with the picrotoxin/barbiturate (P-B) and GABA sites. Cl^- represents the chloride channel.

maximum increase in membrane conductance produced by GABA supports its neuromodulatory role. At the molecular level, evidence supports an allosteric modulatory role for benzodiazepines in the regulation of the GABA receptor. Benzodiazepines may increase the affinity of the GABA receptor for GABA and thus enhance the coupling between GABA receptor activation and chloride channel opening. These events can then be related to the behavioral effect of the benzodiazepines. For example, in humans, benzodiazepines will suppress most forms of paroxysmal activity and limit the spread of discharge from a focal lesion without suppressing the primary focus. This action may be related to the ability of benzodiazepines to enhance the inhibitory activity of GABA.

There is now evidence from in vitro biochemical studies that more than one subtype of benzodiazepine receptor may exist in the mammalian brain [50]. From these studies, speculation has been raised regarding the possibility that different subtypes of benzodiazepine receptors mediate their pharmacological effects. For example, one subtype may mediate anxiety another sedation. This intriguing possibility has important ramifications in regard to the strategies that can be employed to modify selectively anxiety or sedation. It is therefore, apparent why this area of research is currently receiving a high level of attention.

E. Adverse Effects

In general, the clinically useful benzodiazepines are a safe class of drugs, displaying a high therapeutic index. It is highly improbable that a healthy adult will die as a result of an overdose of a benzodiazepines alone [51]. However, large doses in combination with alcohol, barbiturates, or other depressants can be fatal. Overdoses of benzodiazepines alone result in drowsiness or stupor with only a small decrease in blood pressure and respiration. Most acute reactions to benzodiazepines are dose-related and consist of sedation, lightheadedness, ataxia, and lethargy. These are particular problems for those being treated for anxiety who are expected to perform their normal day-to-day tasks. Upon continued treatment, tolerance will develop to these effects but not to the antianxiety effects. Occasional reactions to hypnotic doses include impaired mental and psychomotor function, dysathria, headache, confusion, euphoria, delayed reaction time, and xerostamia. Responses such as syncope, hypotension, blurred vision, skin rashes, nausea, edema, constipation, agranulocytosis, menstrual irregularities, and lupuslike symptoms have been reported but are rare. The potential teratogenic effects of the benzodiazepines are still under investigation and are controversial.

Chronic use of benzodiazepines presents a special set of problems. After long-term use, tolerance will develop to the sedative-hypnotic and anticonvulsant effects of these compounds. Obviously, this limits their long-term usefulness in many situations. Tolerance to the antianxiety effects of the benzodiazepines following chronic use has not been reported, although the possibility exists [52,53]. The lack of observed tolerance may also be due in part to the episodic nature of anxiety. Both psychological and physical dependence may develop with chronic use of benzodiazepines. Withdrawal responses will occur following abrupt discontinuation of treatment. Serious withdrawal reactions, including convulsions, are observed only following chronic usage at very high doses [54]. Since most patients are maintained at therapeutically relevant doses, the incidence of severe withdrawal responses is low. The length of the treatment regimen is significantly correlated to the occurrence of withdrawal reactions [55]. It was found that 36% of the patients treated for at least a year or more showed definite withdrawal symptoms upon abrupt discontinuation compared with only 6% for those treated for less than a year. To avoid withdrawal reactions, it is recommended that the smallest therapeutic dose be used, that withdrawal of the drug following long-term use be done gradually, and that use in patients with a history of drug abuse be avoided.

III. BARBITURATES

A. Historical Perspective

The first barbiturate synthesized for clinical use was diethylbarbituric acid in 1903. The second barbiturate, phenobarbital, was made available in 1912 and is still important in control of certain convulsive disorders. The use of barbiturates as antianxiety agents and as sedative-hypnotics has largely been supplanted by the benzodiazepines. As indicated earlier, the benzodiazepines are much safer and more effective in such applications, although they are by no means ideal.

B. Chemistry, Biotransformation, and Pharmacokinetics

Barbiturates belong to a class of compounds that are derivatives of barbituric acid. Barbituric acid is formed by the condensation of urea and malonic acid. This compound does not have any observable effect on the CNS. CNS-active barbiturates are those that have alkyl or aryl substituents at position five of the ring (Table 3.3). Structure-activity relationships of the barbiturates have been extensively studied [56]. Polar substituents at C-5 diminish hypnotic activity whereas alkyl side chains of increasing length at C-5 impart convulsant activity. Phenyl groups at the C-5 or N positions will selectively confer anticonvulsant activity. Any modification of structure that alters lipid solubility alters

TABLE 3.3 Names and Structures of Various Barbiturates Commonly Available for Clinical Use

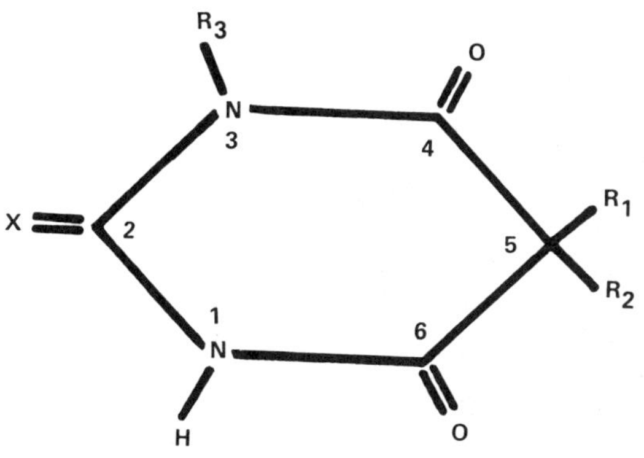

Name	R_1	R_2	R_3	X
Amobarbital	Ethyl	Isopentyl	H	0
Barbital	Ethyl	Ethyl	H	0
Butabarbital	Ethyl	Sec-butyl	H	0
Mephobarbital	Ethyl	Phenyl	CH_3	0
Metharbital	Ethyl	Ethyl	CH_3	0
Pentobarbital	Ethyl	1-Methylbutyl	H	0
Phenobarbital	Ethyl	Phenyl	H	0
Secobarbital	Allyl	1-Methylbutyl	H	0
Thiamylal	Allyl	1-Methylbutyl	H	S
Thiopental	Ethyl	1-Methylbutyl	H	S

the hypnotic potency, onset and duration of action, and the rate of metabolic transformation. For example, thiobarbiturates are more lipid-soluble than oxybarbiturates. The thiobarbiturates are more potent and have faster rates of onset and shorter durations of action than the corresponding oxybarbiturates.

The barbiturates are readily absorbed following oral administration, with the sodium salts being more rapidly absorbed than the free acids. This is the preferred route of administration when these compound are used as anticonvulsants. Intravenous administration is only used in emergencies (e.g., status epilepticus). The major factors affecting the distribution of the barbiturates are protein binding (i.e., plasma protein), lipid solubility, and degree of ionization. For instance, the highly lipid-soluble thiobarbiturates are rapidly distributed and have very short durations of action, with rapid redistribution being the primary mechanism for the termination of the pharmacological effects. The less lipid-soluble oxybarbiturates have slower rates of distribution and metabolism, less protein binding, and longer durations of action. Barbiturates undergo metabolic transformation in the liver by four major routes: (1) oxidation of the larger substituent at C-5; (2) dealkylation when present at position 3; (3) cleavage of the barbiturate ring; and (4) desulfuration in the case of thiobarbiturates. Barbiturates induce hepatic microsomal enzymes and this leads to an increase in the ability of the liver to metabolize barbiturates, thus accounting for part of the tolerance observed with these compounds. Also, most of the drug interactions with the barbiturates are the result of their ability to induce drug-metabolizing enzymes. The pharmacokinetics of the anticonvulsant barbiturate phenobarbital have been reviewed by Wilder and Bruni [57] and they are relevant to the prudent clinical application of this drug.

C. Major Applications of the Barbiturates in the Treatment of CNS Disorders

The marked safety advantage of the benzodiazepines has resulted in a significant reduction in the use of barbiturates as antianxiety and sedative-hypnotic agents. Consequently, application of the barbiturates in the treatment of anxiety and insomnia will not be discussed here. Instead, the discussion will focus upon the use of barbiturates, particularly phenobarbital, in the treatment of specific seizure disorders.

Phenobarbital is one of the most widely prescribed antiepileptic drugs. It is one of four major compounds prescribed in the treatment of generalized tonic-clonic seizures and of simple and complex partial seizures. Phenobarbital is also effective in the treatment and prevention of febrile convulsions, seizures associated with alcohol or drug withdrawal, and in status epilepticus. A detailed classification and description of the seizures susceptible to control with phenobarbital has been provided by Arid and Woodbury [58]. In children, phenobarbital is the drug of choice in the treatment of generalized tonic-clonic seizures and partial seizures. Phenytoin and carbamazepine are preferred in adolescents and adults. The dosage range for the treatment of generalized tonic-clonic seizures and partial seizures (focal) is 1.5–5 mg/kg/day. A therapeutic range of 15–30 μg/ml plasma is considered normal [59]. The exact dosages are adjusted as required for adequate control of seizures and minimal toxicity. Phenobarbital is administered orally when used chronically although it can be given by intramuscular, intravenous, or rectal routes. For oral use, it is normally given as a single daily dose of 2–5 mg/kg. Using this regimen, steady-state plasma levels will be achieved in 20–30 days after initiation. Sedation often occurs in the initial period but tolerance to this effect eventually develops, occurring more readily and to a greater extent than to the anticonvulsant effects. If phenobarbital is discontinued, the withdrawal should be gradual. Otherwise withdrawal seizures may occur.

Phenobarbital is often used in the treatment of alcohol or drug withdrawal seizures. In the case of seizures resulting from withdrawal of short-acting barbiturates, phenobarbital is the drug of choice. This drug is also useful in the treatment of status epilepticus. A dose of 8–15 mg/kg i.v. over a period of 10–15 min is used initially and repeated as necessary to control seizures. It is imperative that vital signs be monitored in these situations.

D. Mechanism of Action

A fundamental property of all barbiturates is their ability to modify the activity of all excitable tissues. In the case of the sedative-hypnotic barbiturates, the activity of neuronal tissue is depressed. Generally, the pharmacological effects of the barbiturates are the result of different degrees of depression of the CNS. However, some selectivity is evident and is reflected by the anticonvulsant effects of phenobarbital occurring at doses that do not produce hypnosis. This discussion will review briefly some of the possible mechanisms underlying the pharmacological effects of the barbiturates. Neurochemical and neurophysiological studies of the possible mechanisms underlying the CNS effects of barbiturates have been reviewed [60–62].

The observations that barbiturates facilitate the fluidization of membrane lipids and block the uptake of calcium in rat brain synaptosomes have formed the basis for the hypothesis that these effects may underly the pharmacological actions of the barbiturates [63,64]. Since the pharmacological specificity of the effects on membrane lipids has not been demonstrated and the calcium uptake effect was only observed at very high concentrations, the pharmacological relevance of these findings has been questioned. Other biochemical and electrophysiological studies regarding the effects of barbiturates on specific neurotransmitter systems have been more promising. Barbiturates appear to inhibit excitatory neurotransmission and facilitate inhibitory transmission [60]. At excitatory synapses, barbiturates appear to decrease the postsynaptic effects of excitatory neurotransmitters and possibly decrease their release [65,66]. Facilitation of inhibitory transmission by barbiturates has been studied primarily at GABAergic synapses. Barbiturates enhance the effects of applied GABA, reverse the effects of GABA antagonists, and mimic the effects of GABA [67—69]. Interestingly, the convulsant barbiturates did not appear to produce these effects and the anticonvulsant barbiturates (i.e., phenobarbital) did not produce GABA mimetic effects at concentrations which produce augmentation of the postsynaptic responses to GABA [70]. These findings suggest that facilitation may be an important mechanism by which barbiturates produce their pharmacological effects and point to the possibility that the anticonvulsant barbiturates such as phenobarbital reduce the spread of paroxysmal activity by the potentiation of inhibitory pathways rather than by a GABA mimetic effect.

The molecular basis of barbiturate modification of GABAergic neurotransmission has been the focus of recent investigations. In vitro studies indicate that the barbiturates do not interact competitively at the postsynaptic GABA receptor [71]. However, the depressant barbiturates allosterically enhance the binding of GABA [72]. Moreover, the interaction is stereospecific and is correlated with the hypnotic and GABA-mediated inhibitory potential of each of the barbiturates studied. Similarly, barbiturates enhance the binding of [^{3}H]diazepam to the benzodiazepine receptor [73]. These observations suggest that the site at which the barbiturates interact is intimately associated with the GABA-benzodiazepine receptor-chloride ionophore complex. Indeed, barbiturates will inhibit the binding of [^{3}H]dihydropicrotoxin to brain membranes; dihydropicrotoxin is a radioligand believed to label the chloride ionophore [74]. Thus, biochemical studies also suggest that the depressant barbiturates modify the binding of GABA at a pharmacologically relevant binding site. Perhaps the enhancement of GABA observed in electrophysiological studies is a result of barbiturate modulation of the GABA receptor. These findings also suggest similarities to the GABA-modifying effects of the benzodiazepines. It is not surprising that both the barbiturates and benzodiazepines share similar therapeutic applications.

E. Adverse Effects

The major side effects of the barbiturates are related to their hypnotic properties. Residual effects (hangover) often occur the day following a hypnotic dose and will have a deleterious effect on intellectual performance and motor skills. Aftereffects can also be manifested as vertigo, nausea, vomiting, diarrhea, and overt excitement. Nightmares may also result and may be related to deprivation of REM and stage-4 sleep.

With chronic use, as may be the case with phenobarbital in treatment of seizure disorders, depression of cognitive function occurs [75]. In children and the elderly, chronic use often results in hyperactivity, irritability, and alterations in sleep patterns. Effects on higher cognitive function in children may have long-term deleterious effects. Animal studies show significant retardation in brain development with chronic phenobarbital treatment [76]. These findings emphasize the importance of using the minimal dose required to achieve therapeutic results. Drug interactions also present problems, these effects are usually related to the ability of barbiturates to induce drug metabolizing enzymes or compete directly with other compounds and thus inhibit their metabolism. Barbiturates have additive effects with other CNS depressants such as alcohol that often result in fatalities.

Tolerance, both pharmacokinetic and pharmacodynamic, develop with chronic use of the barbiturates. Cross-tolerance (pharmacodynamic) do other general CNS depressants such as the benzodiazepines, meprobamate, and the general anesthetics will occur. The symptoms upon withdrawal are amplification of the functions that were originally depressed. Similar to other CNS depressant drugs, the barbiturates can be abused and physical dependence can develop. However, the abuse liability is less that that of the benzodiazepines. The severity of the withdrawal symptoms is dependent upon the degree of tolerance. Barbiturate abuse and dependence has been reviewed in detail by Allgulander [54].

IV. FUTURE DIRECTIONS

The therapeutic importance of the benzodiazepines and the barbiturates can be appreciated when one considers the following statistics: 20% of all medical patients have made the complaint of insomnia, 4% of the population in the United States has seizure disorders, and greater than 10% of the members of a randomly selected group in the United States have taken an antianxiety drug at least once during the year prior to the survey [77–79]. Despite the relative effectiveness of the compounds available today for the treatment of anxiety, insomnia, and seizure disorders, they are far from ideal. The major problems with both the benzodiazepines and the barbiturates are the lack of selectivity (barbiturates more so than benzodiazepines), rapid development of tolerance to some of the therapeutic effects, and the abuse liability.

Common side effects of the benzodiazepines are drowsiness and ataxia. These effects are simply extensions of the pharmacological actions of the benzodiazepines. Often, doses that produce antianxiety effects are not far from those that cause drowsiness. Recently, studies in animal models with a series of novel compounds suggest that antianxiety effects can be achieved without sedation over a broad range of doses [80,81]. Some of these compounds are shown in Fig. 3.2 and are compared with some of the commonly used benzodiazepines. In vitro

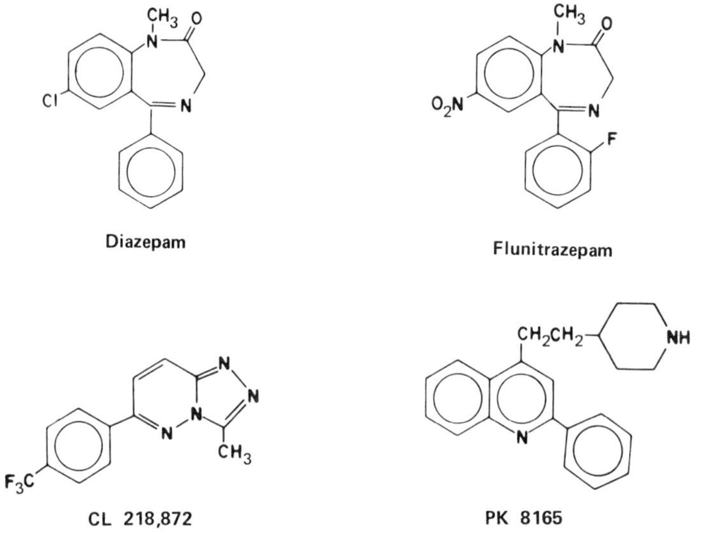

Diazepam

Flunitrazepam

CL 218,872

PK 8165

FIG. 3.2 CL 218,872 and PK 8165 are compounds reported to give antianxiety effects without sedation.

biochemical studies suggest that compounds such as the triazolopyridazine CL 218872 can recognize more than one type of benzodiazepine receptor in the mamalian CNS [82,83]. The ability to discriminate benzodiazepine receptor subtypes and to elicit selective antianxiety effects has led to the hypothesis that the pharmacological effects of the benzodiazepines may be mediated by distinct receptor subtypes [80,84]. If this hypothesis is correct, then it will dramatically alter the therapeutic approach to the problem of selectivity. Drugs can be designed with high selectivity for the benzodiazepine receptor subtype thought to mediate antianxiety effects. Such drugs will be effective against anxiety but will not cause sedation. The ramifications of the concept of multiple benzodiazepine receptor subtypes go beyond drug design since receptor subtypes can be studied in isolation to determine their role in normal and pathophysiological states. These studies may yield insight into various disorders involving anxiety, sleep, and brain excitability.

Some of these novel compounds, including the quinoline derivatives PK 8165 and PK 9084 represent new avenues of approaches to the design of more selective antianxiety agents. Both PK 8165 and PK 9084 produce antianxiety effects in animal models but are neither anticonvulsant nor sedative [81]. The selectivity of these compounds may be related to their partial agonist properties [85]. In other words, these compounds have lower efficacy than the clinically useful benzodiazepines.

Consequently, benzodiazepines that have full efficacy (i.e., full agonists) will produce antianxiety, anticonvulsant, and sedative hypnotic effects whereas compounds that have only partial efficacy only produce a limited spectrum of pharmacological effects. The design of partial agonist compounds may therefore yield a variety of highly selective drugs useful in the treatment of anxiety and related disorders.

REFERENCES

1. L. H. Sternbach, The discovery of CNS active 1,4-benzodiazepines (Chemistry), in *Pharmacology of Benzodiazepines* (E. Usdin, P. Skolnick, J. F. Tallman, D. Greenblatt, and S. M. Paul, Eds.), McMillan Press, London, 1983.
2. L. O. Randall, Discovery of benzodiazepines, in *Pharmacology of Benzodiazepines* (E. Usdin, P. Skolnick, J. F. Tallman, D. Greenblatt, and S. M. Paul, Eds.), MacMillan, London, 1983.
3. J. F. Tallman, S. M. Paul, P. Skolnick, and D. W. Gallagher, *Science*, 207:27 (1980).
4. L. H. Sternbach, Chemistry of 1,4-benzodiazepines and some aspects of the structure activity relationship, in *The Benzodiazepines* (S. Garattini, E. Mussini, and L. O. Randall, Eds.), Raven Press, New York, 1973, pp. 1–26.
5. A. F. Schatzberg, R. I. Altesman, and J. O. Cole, An update of the use of benzodiazepines in depressed patients, in *Pharmacology of Benzodiazepines* (E. Usdin, P. Skolnick, J. F. Tallman, D. Greenblatt, and S. M. Paul, Eds.), MacMillan, London, 1983.
6. J. P. Feighner, Benzodiazepines as antidepressants: a triazolobenzodiazepine used to treat depression, in *Modern Problems in Pharmacopsychiatry*, vol. 18 (H. Lehmann, Ed.), S. Karger, Basel, 1981.
7. D. J. Greenblatt, R. I. Shader, M. Divoll, and J. S. Harmatz, *Br. J. Clin. Pharmacol.*, 11:118 (1981).
8. R. Z. Shader and D. J. Greenblatt, *Am. J. Psychiat.*, 134:652 (1977).
9. D. J. Greenblatt, R. I. Shader, D. R. Abernathy, H. R. Ochs, M. Divoll, and E. M. Sellers, Benzodiazepines and the challenge of pharmacokinetic taxonomy, in *Pharmacology of Benzodiazepines* (E. Usdin, P. Skolnick, V. F. Tallman, D. Greenblatt, and S. M. Paul, Eds.), MacMillian, London, pp. 257–269, 1983.
10. U. Klotz, Drug interactions with benzodiazepines, in *Pharmacology of Benzodiazepines*, (E. Usdin, P. Solnick J. F. Tallman, D. Greenblatt, and S. M. Paul, Eds.), MacMillan, London, pp. 299–311, 1983.
11. J. G. B. Madorsky, *J. Psychoactive Drugs*, 15:45 (1983).

12. J. W. Dundee and P. Kawar, Benzodiazepines in anesthesia, in *Pharmacology of Benzodiazepines* (E. Usdin, P. Skolnick, J. F. Tallman, D. Greenblatt, and S. M. Paul, Eds.), MacMillan, London, 1983 pp. 313–328.
13. D. J. Greenblatt and R. I. Shader, *Benzodiazepines in Clinical Practice*, Raven Press, New York, 1974.
14. K. Rickels, *Psychopharmacology*, 58:1 (1978).
15. M. Lader, *Drug Res.*, 30:910 (1980).
16. American Psychiatric Association, Task Force on Nomenclature and Statistics. Diagnostic and statistical manual of mental disorders (DSM), Amer. Psychiat. Assoc., Washington, D.C., 1980.
17. D. F. Klein and J. G. Rabkin (Eds.), *Anxiety: New Research and Changing Concepts*, Raven, New York, 1981.
18. G. C. Aden and S. G. Thein, *J. Clin. Psychiat.*, 41:245 (1980).
19. L. E. Hollister, *J. Psychoactive Drugs*, 15:41 (1983).
20. R. W. Downing and K. Rickels, *Psychopharm. Bull.*, 18:37 (1982).
21. V. Brezinova, I. Oswald, and J. Loudon, *Br. J. Psychiat.*, 121:439 (1975).
22. R. L. Williams and I. Karacan, (Eds.), *Sleep Disorders: Diagnosis and Treatment*, Wiley, New York, 1978.
23. A. Kales, C. R. Soldatos, and J. D. Kales, *Am. Fam. Physician*, 22:101 (1980).
24. C. R. Soldatos, A. Kales, and J. D. Kales, *Ann. Rev. Med.*, 30:301 (1979).
25. A. Kales, E. O. Bixler, M. B. Scharf, and J. D. Kales, *Clin. Pharmacol. Therap.*, 19:576 (1976).
26. I. Karacan, W. Orr, T. Roth, M. Kramer, J. Thornby, S. Bingham, and D. Kay, *Psychopharmacology*, 73:332 (1981).
27. W. C. Dement, M. A. Carskadon, M. M. Mitler, R. L. Phillip, and V. P. Zarcone, *Behav. Med.*, 5:25 (1978).
28. D. J. Greenblatt, M. Divoll, J. S. Harmatz, D. S. MacLaughlin, and R. I. Shader, *Clin. Pharmacol. Ther.*, 30:475 (1981).
29. M. W. Johns and J. P. Masterson, *Pharmacology*, 11:358 (1974).
30. I. Oswald, K. Adam, S. Borrow, and C. Idzikowski, The effects of two hypnotics on sleep, subjective feelings and skilled performance, in *Pharmacology of the States of Alertness* (P. Passouant and I. Oswald, Eds.), Pergammon, New York, 1979, pp. 51–63.
31. E. O. Bixler, A. Kales, C. R. Soldatos, M. B. Scharf, and J. P. Kales, *J. Clin. Pharmacol.*, 18:110 (1970).
32. M. M. Mitler, M. A. Carskadon, R. C. Phillips, W. R. Sterling, V. P. Zarcone, R. Speigel, C. Gulleminault, and W. C. Dement, *Br. J. Clin. Pharmacol.*, 8:635 (1979).
33. T. Roth, M. Kramer, and T. Lutz, *J. Int. Med. Res.*, 4:59 (1976).
34. V. Pegram, P. Hyde, and P. Linton, *J. Int. Med. Res.*, 8:224 (1980).

35. A. Kales, M. B. Scharf, J. D. Kales, and C. R. Soldatos, *J. Am. Med. Assoc.*, 241:1692 (1979).
36. T. R. Browne, *N. Engl. J. Med.*, 299:812 (1978).
37. W. Haefely, A. Kulcsar, H. Mohler, L. Pieri, P. Polc, and R. Schaffner, *Adv. Biochem. Psychopharmacol.*, 14:131 (1975).
38. E. Costa, A. Guidotti, and C. C. Mao, *Adv. Biochem. Psychopharmacol.*, 14:113 (1975).
39. H. B. Bosmann, R. Case, and P. Disterfano, *FEBS Lett.*, 82: 368 (1977).
40. H. Mohler and T. Okada, *Life Sci.*, 20:2101 (1977).
41. R. F. Squires and C. Braestrup, *Nature*, 266:734 (1977).
42. S. M. Paul, P. J. Syapin, M. Paugh, V. Monacada, and P. Skolnick, *Nature*, 281:688 (1979).
43. L. Pieri, R. Schaffner, R. Scherschlicht, P. Polc, J. Sepinwall, A. Davidson, H. Mohler, R. Cumin, M. DaPrada, W. P. Burkard, H. H. Keller, R. K. M. Muller, M. Gerold, M. Pieri, L. Cook, and W. Haefely, *Drug Res.*, 31:2180 (1981).
44. H. Mohler and T. Okada, *Science*, 198:849 (1977).
45. R. W. Olsen, *Ann. Rev. Pharmacol. Toxicol.*, 22:245 (1982).
46. G. Biggio and E. Costa (Eds.), Benzodiazepine recognition ligands: Biochemistry and pharmacology, in *Adv. Biochem. Psychopharmacol*, vol. 38, Raven, New York, 1938.
47. F. J. Ehlert, W. R. Roeske, K. W. Gee, and H. I. Yamamura, *Biochem. Pharmacol.*, 32:2375 (1983).
48. D. W. Choi, D. H. Farb, and G. D. Fishbach, *Neurophysiology*, 45:621 (1981).
49. R. L. MacDonald and J. L. Barker, *Brain Res.*, 167:323 (1979).
50. R. F. Squires, *Neuropharmacology*, 22:1443 (1983).
51. L. E. Hollister, Psychiatric disorders, in *Drug Treatment*, 2nd ed., ADIS Press and Churchill Livingston, Edinburgh, 1980, pp. 1057–1121.
52. D. J. Greenblatt, T. P. Laughren, M. D. Allen, J. S. Harmatz, and R. I. Shader, *Br. J. Clin. Pharmacol.*, 11:35 (1981).
53. L. E. Hollister, F. K. Conley, R. H. Britt, and L. Suer, *J. Am. Med. Assoc.*, 246:1568 (1981).
54. C. Allgulander, *Suppl. Acta. Psychiatr. Scand.*, 270:1 (1978).
55. K. Rickels, W. G. Case, and R. W. Downing, *Psychopharm. Bull.*, 18:38 (1982).
56. A. Vida and E. H. Gerry, Cyclic ureides, in *Anticonvulsants*, (J. A. Vida, Ed.), Academic Press, New York, 1977, pp. 152–284.
57. B. J. Widler, and J. Bruni, *Seizure Disorders: A Pharmacological Approach to Treatment*, Raven, New York, 1981.
58. R. B. Arid, and D. M. Woodbury, *Management of Epilepsy*, Charles C. Thomas, Illinois, 1974.

59. F. Buchthal and M. A. Lennox-Buchthal, Phenobarbital: relation of serum concentration to control of seizures, in *Antiepileptic Drugs* (D. M. Woodbury, J. K. Penry, and R. P. Schmidt, Eds.), Raven, New York, 1972, pp. 335–343.
60. R. A. Nicoll, Differentiated post-synaptic effects of barbiturates on chemical transmission, in *Neurobiology of Chemical Transmission* (M. Otsuka and Z. Hall, Eds.), Wiley, New York, 1979, pp. 267–278.
61. S. H. Roth, *Ann. Rev. Pharmacol. Toxicol.*, 19:159 (1979).
62. I. K. Ho and R. A. Harris, *Ann. Rev. Pharmacol. Toxicol.*, 21:83 (1981).
63. A. G. Lee, *Biochim. Biophys. Acta*, 455:102 (1976).
64. W. F. Hood and R. A. Harris, *Biochem. Pharmacol.*, 28:3075 (1979).
65. R. A. Nicoll, *Science*, 199:451 (1978).
66. J. A. Richter, and M. B. Waller, *Biochem. Pharmacol.*, 26:609 (1977).
67. J. L. Barker and H. Gainer, *Science*, 182:720 (1973).
68. W. Schlosser and S. Franco, *Neuropharmacology*, 18:377,381 (1979).
69. N. G. Bowery, and A. Dray, *Br. J. Pharmacol.*, 63:197 (1978).
70. R. L. MacDonald and J. L. Barker, *Science*, 200:775 (1978).
71. R. W. P. Cutler, D. Markowitz, and D. S. Dudzinski, *Brain Res.*, 81:189 (1974).
72. T. Asano and N. Ogasawara, *Brain Res.*, 225:212 (1981).
73. F. Leeb-Lundberg, A. Snowman, and R. W. Olsen, *Proc. Natl. Acad. Sci. USA.*, 77:7468 (1980).
74. M. K. Ticku, and R. W. Olsen, *Life Sci.*, 22:1643 (1978).
75. S. J. Hutt, P. M. Jackson, A. Belsham, and G. Higgins, *Dev. Med. Child. Neurol.*, 10:626 (1968).
76. R. J. Schain and K. Watanabe, *Exp. Neurol.*, 50:806 (1976).
77. E. O. Bixler, A. Kales, and C. R. Soldatos, *Behav. Med.*, 6:1 (1979).
78. Epilepsy Foundation of America: Basic statistics on the epilepsies. F. A. Davis, Philadelphia, 1975.
79. H. J. Parry, M. B. Palter, and G. D. Mellinger, *Arch. Gen. Psychiatry.*, 28:769 (1973).
80. A. S. Lippa, J. Coupet, E. N. Greenblatt, C. A. Klepner, and B. Beer, *Pharmacol. Biochem. Behav.*, 11:99 (1979).
81. G. LeFur, J. Mizoule, M. C. Burgenin, O. Ferris, A. Heauline, A. Gaultier, C. Gueremy, and A. Uzan, *Life Sci.*, 28:1439 (1981).
82. R. F. Squires, D. I. Benson, C. Braestrup, J. Coupet, C. A. Klepner, V. Myers, and B. Beer, *Pharmacol. Biochem. Behav.*, 10:825 (1979).
83. H. I. Yamamura, T. Mimaki, S. H. Yamamura, W. D. Horst, M. Morelli, G. Bautz, and R. A. O'Brien, *Eur. J. Pharmacol.*, 77:351 (1982).

84. C. A. Klepner, A. S. Lippa, D. I. Benson, M. C. Sano, and B. Beer, *Pharmacol. Biochem. Behav.*, 11:457 (1979).
85. K. W. Gee, R. E. Brinton, and H. I. Yamamura, *Brain Res.*, 264:168 (1983).

4
Neuroleptic Agents: Acute and Chronic Receptor Actions

PETER JENNER and C. DAVID MARSDEN *University Department of Neurology, Institute of Psychiatry, King's College Hospital Medical School, London, England*

I. INTRODUCTION

The introduction of chlorpromazine into clinical practice provided the first effective drug management of schizophrenia and marked the start of the neuroleptic era [1]. The drug controlled psychiatric hallucinations and thought disorders without producing sedation, a combination of properties that warranted the introduction of a new term to describe this class of drugs, namely "neuroleptics" ("that which grips the nerve"). Since that time the use of neuroleptic drugs has formed the mainstay of the treatment of schizophrenia, replacing all previous treatments.

In the short term, neuroleptics act to control acute schizophrenic episodes and toxic confusional states and, as maintenance therapy, reduce the rate of relapse and the need for rehospitalization [2–7]. Initially, benefit was thought to occur in all measures of psychopathology, but it is now accepted that neuroleptics are more effective in the abolition of the positive symptoms of the disease, as opposed to the treatment of negative symptoms [8].

As with all major advances in the drug treatment of disease, the discovery of chlorpromazine led to the introduction of many other groups of neuroleptic agents that also possessed antipsychotic activity. However, it was soon discovered that virtually all such drugs also caused a number of unwanted motor side effects [9,10]. These included akathisia, acute dystonia, Parkinsonism, and, eventually, tardive dyskinesia [11–14]. Of these, tardive dyskinesia has given rise to most concern for it only appears after prolonged periods of treatment and may persist following drug withdrawal. At first it was thought that antipsychotic activity was inevitably linked to the ability to produce motor disturbances but, subsequently, this has been shown to be untrue [15]. Much research has gone into discovering how neuroleptic drugs produce antipsychotic activity, and how they induce extrapyramidal motor disturbances, particularly tardive dyskinesia.

It is commonly accepted that while neuroleptic drugs exert actions on a number of neuronal systems, their critical action is to cause blockade of cerebral dopamine receptors. However, dopamine systems in some brain areas rapidly adapt to the actions of neuroleptic drugs, such that tolerance occurs to the acute dopamine receptor blockade, and dopamine receptor supersensitivity may even supervene. So neuroleptic action in brain must be considered in relation to both the acute and chronic actions of this class of psychotropic drugs.

Before proceeding to discuss acute and chronic pharmacological actions of neuroleptic drug on dopamine systems, we will summarize briefly the evidence that suggests involvement of dopamine in schizophrenia and in tardive dyskinesias.

A. The Dopamine Hypothesis of Schizophrenia

At the present time, there is no established morphological or biochemical cause for schizophrenia. However, one of the major theories advanced in recent times to explain the disease, the dopamine hypothesis of schizophrenia, has received most attention. The idea that brain dopamine systems may be involved is based on three major pieces of evidence:

1. Amphetamine, which acts by releasing dopamine (and noradrenaline), induces a psychosis that may resemble acute paranoid schizophrenia in susceptible subjects [16].
2. The symptoms of schizophrenia and amphetamine-induced psychosis can be reversed by the administration of neuroleptic drugs, all of which have in common the property of antagonizing cerebral dopamine function [17,19].
3. Postmortem examination of dopamine-containing areas of brain from schizophrenics has shown increased numbers of dopamine receptors in drug-treated and apparently drug-free patients [20–23].

From these observations it was suggested that schizophrenia might be due to overactivity of cerebral dopamine mechanisms, and that the benefical effects of neuroleptic drugs are due to blockade of cerebral dopamine receptors. The hypothesis subsequently was refined to suggest that schizophrenia results from overactivity of cerebral dopamine mechanisms in specific regions of the brain, perhaps the mesolimbic and/or the mesocortical dopamine systems [24]. This suggestion was based on the following evidence:

1. All effective antipsychotic drugs can produce a range of extrapyramidal side effects that are attributed to blockade of dopamine receptors in the corpus striatum.
2. But effective antipsychotic action can be obtained in schizophrenia with doses of drugs not necessarily causing extrapyramidal disturbances.

Accordingly, it was deduced that striatal dopamine receptor blockade was not necessary for antipsychotic action which then was attributed to blockade of dopamine receptors in the other known dopamine containing brain regions, in particular the mesolimbic and mesocortical regions.

B. Tardive Dyskinesia

Chronic tardive dyskinesias become apparent after months or years of neuroleptic treatment and may persist even though the offending drug may be withdrawn [25–27]. The incidence of tardive dyskinesias in those on chronic neuroleptic therapy is believed to be greatly in excess of that of similar spontaneous oro-facial dyskinesias. Chronic tardive dyskinesias occur in between 5–40% of those on long-term neuroleptic drugs. A recent survey suggested an overall incidence of approximately 20% [27]. The risk of permanent tardive dyskinesias has been estimated to be somewhere around 30% of those who develop the problem.

The evidence suggesting that tardive dyskinesias involve dopamine mechanisms in the brain [28] is as follows:

1. Tardive dyskinesias are induced by all classes of neuroleptic drugs whose common action is believed to be blockade of dopamine receptors.
2. The cessation of neuroleptic drug therapy may result in the appearance of tardive dyskinesia or the exacerbation of existing movements.
3. The movements characterizing tardive dyskinesia closely resemble movements sometimes induced by L-dopa in patients with Parkinson's disease.
4. Tardive dyskinesia can be suppressed, at least partially and temporarily, by increasing the dose of the offending drug or by the introduction of another neuroleptic.
5. Drugs which cause a depletion of brain dopamine, for example oxypertine or tetrabenazine, can decrease the severity of tardive dyskinesia.
6. The movements of tardive dyskinesias are enhanced by administration of high doses of dopamine agonists.

From this evidence a paradox is immediately apparent. Tardive dyskinesias appear to exhibit the pharmacological sensitivity characteristic of dopaminergic overactivity, yet they are produced by drugs whose prime mode of action is to antagonize dopamine receptors. For this reason, the hypothesis has been put forward that striatal dopamine receptor supersensitivity may develop during continued neuroleptic administration, and that this may be the pathophysiological mechanism responsible for tardive dyskinesias [9,29]. However, at the present time there is no direct evidence to support this hypothesis. No post-mortem studies have been carried out.

It is obvious from this description of dopamine involvement in schizophrenia, and in extrapyramidal movement disorders, why much of the research effort applied to the understanding of neuroleptic drug action has dealt with their ability to interact and alter brain dopamine function. It is for this reason that this chapter will concentrate on the ability of neuroleptic drugs to interact with dopamine receptors. It is proposed to compare and contrast the ability of neuroleptic drugs to alter dopamine receptor function on acute and chronic administration. It is also our purpose to then look again at mechanisms by which neuroleptic drugs might exert their antipsychotic action and produce extrapyramidal movement disorders.

II. CLASSES OF NEUROLEPTIC AGENTS

As with all therapeutic innovations, the production of the first neuroleptic drug molecule led to the synthesis of novel structures on a massive scale with the introduction of a number of new classes of antipsychotic agents. In this section we will briefly review the compounds available and summarize their development and clinical uses. All the drug groups described have been shown to possess antipsychotic activity, and the use of most, if not all, such compounds is associated with the production of extrapyramidal motor disorders.

A. Phenothiazine Derivatives (Fig. 4.1)

The original phenothiazine compounds were developed almost a 100 years ago in connection with the advent of aniline dyestuffs such as methylene blue [see Ref. 30]. Their modern history starts with the synthesis in the 1930s of promethazine which was found to exert antihistaminic activity and to be a potent sedative compound [31]. The synthesis and introduction of chlorpromazine for the treatment of schizophrenic illness in the 1950s was the most critical innovation in the modern treatment of this disorder [32]. Subsequent synthesis of related compounds has led to the introduction of a wide range of effective antipsychotic neuroleptic phenothiazines which can be divided into distinct subclasses:

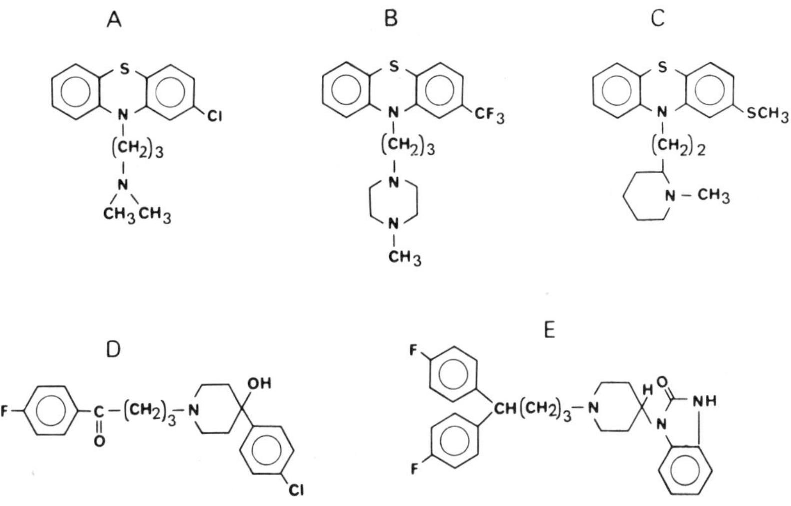

FIG. 4.1 Structural formulae of some phenothiazine, butyrophenone, and diphenylbutylpiperidine neuroleptic drugs. A. Chlorpromazine. B. Trifluoperazine. C. Thioridazine. D. Haloperidol. E. Pimozide.

1. Phenothiazines with an aliphatic side-chain, e.g., chlorpromazine, trifluopromazine, and promazine.
2. Phenothiazines containing a piperidine moiety in the side chain, e.g., thioridazine, mesoridazine, and piperacetazine.
3. Phenothiazines with a piperazine moiety in the side-chain, e.g., fluphenazine, trifluoperazine, perphenazine, and butaperazine.

Phenothiazine drugs have undergone extensive evaluation in the treatment of schizophrenia, and there is overwhelming evidence to support the therapeutic benefit that can be derived from these compounds. Despite the introduction of a wide range of derivatives, there appears to be little difference between subclasses of phenothiazines and their efficacy or therapeutic profile in the treatment of schizophrenia. Drugs of the aliphatic and piperidine subclasses possess marked sedative properties which make them particularly useful in the treatment of patients with psychotic illness in which anxiety and excitation are prominent.

All phenothiazine neuroleptics induce extrapyramidal disturbances. Those phenothiazine derivatives with high inherent anticholinergic activity, for example thioridazine, may produce a lower incidence of movement disorders, although much of the evidence appears anecdotal. Phenothiazine drugs also differ in the extent to which they produce autonomic side effects and this has recently been reviewed by McKay [33].

Phenothiazines also have been introduced as depot neuroleptic therapy. Fluphenazine decanoate and fluphenazine enanthate administered by intramuscular injection provided a relatively simple means of providing maintenance therapy that avoided the risk of noncompliance. Even so, approximately 20% of patients receiving such depot medication default due to an awareness of the occurrence of acute extrapyramidal symptoms, akathisia, Parkinsonism, and acute dystonia, concurrent with each depot administration [34].

B. Butyrophenone Compounds (Fig. 4.1)

Butyrophenone derivatives were not discovered through research designed to produce novel neuroleptic compounds. They emerged from a systematic search for 4-phenylpiperidine compounds related to pethidine [35]. However, some compounds produced were devoid of morphinomimetic properties but were almost indistinguishable from chlorpromazine in pharmacological tests. The largest group of butyrophenones includes substituted piperidine compounds that are analogs of the most successful compound, haloperidol. Among those in present usage are benperidol, bromperidol, oxiperomide, and trifluperidol.

Haloperidol is as effective as chlorpromazine in the management of schizophrenia [36]. Another major therapeutic application is in the management of manic illness, since motor hyperactivity appears particularly susceptible to this drug. Recently, haloperidol decanoate has been introduced as depot maintenance therapy for chronic psychosis. Haloperidol decanoate injected every 4 weeks appears to be as effective as orally administered haloperidol [37].

C. Diphenylbutylpiperidine Derivatives (Fig. 4.1)

Modification of the butyrophenone side-chain by replacement of the keto function with a 4-flurophenylmethene moiety resulted in the production of diphenylbutylpiperidine derivatives such as pimozide, penfluridol, fluspirilene, and chlopimozide. The diphenylbutylpiperidines differ from butyrophenone drugs in ther long duration of action. All are effective in the control of schizophrenia and in particular, pimozide has been shown to be useful in treating acute schizophrenia and in reducing the rate of relapse in chronic schizophrenic patients [38]. The long duration of action of penfluridol and fluspirilene allows their use as once weekly maintenance drug treatment.

D. Thioxanthene Derivatives (Fig. 4.2)

Thioxanthene derivatives were derived by the simple replacement of the phenothiazine nucleus with a thioxanthene nucleus. This led to

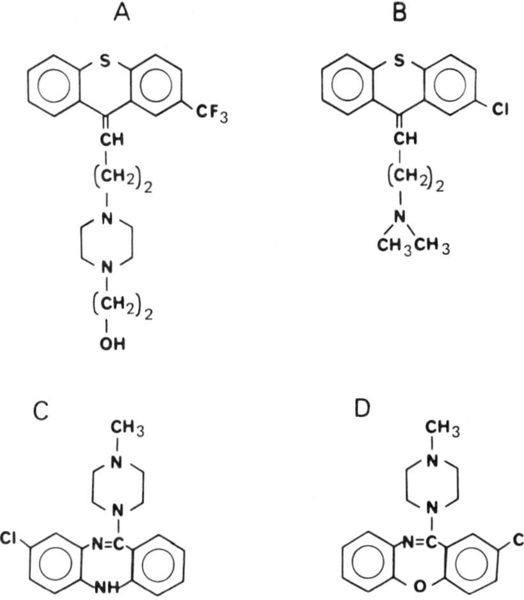

FIG. 4.2 Structural formulae of some thioxanthene and piperazinyldibenzoxazepine and neuroleptic drugs. A. Flupenthixol. B. Chlorprothixene. C. Clozapine. D. Loxapine.

the introduction of the early thioxanthene derivatives, chlorprothixene, chlopenthixol, and thioxene, all of which were effective antipsychotic agents [39]. More recently, the widely used thioxanthene derivative, flupenthixol, has been introduced. Chlorprothixene, thioxene, and flupenthixol are effective antischizophrenic drugs which to a large extent appear to resemble phenothiazine derivatives.

Flupenthixol decanoate is an effective depot maintenance therapy for schizophrenia [40]. The clinical efficacy and prevalence of side effects are essentially equivalent to those produced by fluphenazine decanoate.

E. Piperazinyldibenzoxazepine Derivatives (Fig. 4.2)

The dibenzoazepines are tricyclic structures that differ from the phenothiazenes and thioxanthene neuroleptics in having a central seven-membered ring. Variation of the structure has led to the introduction of perlapine, loxapine, chlothiapine, and clozapine [41]. Loxapine and chlothiapine possess the pharmacological profile of classical neuroleptic compounds, but perlapine is only partially effective in such tests. Clozapine, while exhibiting sedative properties, is not active in classical tests for neuroleptic activity. However, all such compounds have been shown to be antipsychotic in man, and the atypical profile clozapine will be highlighted in later sections. Clozapine is of particular interest because its use does not appear to be associated with the production of extrapyramidal disturbances [42]. Unfortunately, clozapine caused agranulocytosis in some initial clinical trials, which limited its use. However, new nontoxic derivatives are under development. The major problem with clozapine like compounds is their powerful sedative properties and anticholinergic activity.

F. Substituted Benzamide Drugs (Fig. 4.3)

Substituted benzamide drugs were first derived by the synthesis of derivatives of *para*-aminobenzoic acid and the analogous derivative, *para*-aminosalicylic acid [see Ref. 43]. This produced *ortho*-methoxyprocainamide, a compound with local anaesthetic properties and potent antiemetic action. Further structural alteration produced metoclopramide which possesses antiemetic activity but limited local anaesthetic properties. Metoclopramide was found to possess central dopamine antagonist properties and subsequently has been shown to be antipsychotic [44,45]. Further derivatives of these original molecules have given rise to the pyrrolidinyl-containing benzamides sulpiride and sultopride, which also are antipsychotic agents [45–47]. Sultopride more closely resembles phenothiazine-type neuroleptics in that it has pronounced sedative properties and produces an appreciable incidence of extrapyramidal disturbances. In contrast, sulpiride has no marked sedative properties in man and may produce disinhibitory effects in low doses [48]. Its use has been associated with production of acute

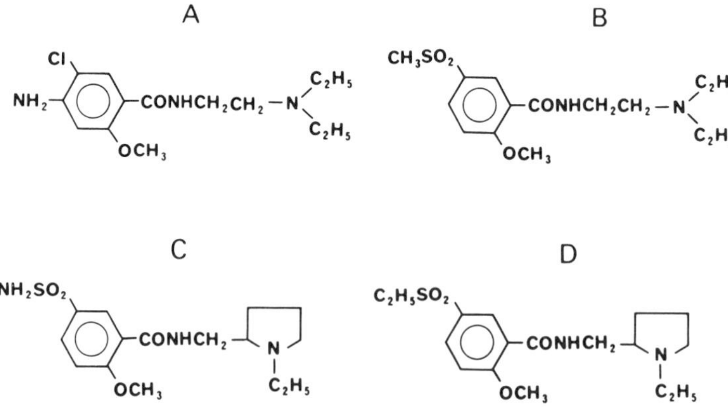

FIG. 4.3 Structural formulae of some substituted benzamide neuroleptic drugs. A. Metoclopramide. B. Tiapride. C. Sulpiride. D. Sultopride.

extrapyramidal disturbances, Parkinsonism, acute dystonia, and akathisia, but its propensity to induce tardive dyskinesia remains unclear. More recently, a further derivative of the series, tiapride, which is a weak dopamine antagonist, has been found useful in the treatment of dyskinesias [49].

III. ACUTE PHARMACOLOGICAL ACTIONS OF NEUROLEPTICS ON BRAIN DOPAMINE FUNCTION

Dopamine-containing neuronal cell bodies give rise to fibers ascending to innervate many different areas of the forebrain (Table 4.1). The data to be discussed in this chapter will be concerned with those dopamine tracts that innervate the neostriatum, the mesolimbic area, and the mesocortical region. The cell bodies, presynaptic terminals, and postsynaptically located receptors each provide a potential target for neuroleptic drug action.

Neuroleptic drugs exert a single common property on acute administration to animals or man, namely the blockade of dopamine receptors. This action occurs at all levels of dopamine neuronal organization within the brain and peripheral nervous system and it can be detected using electrophysiological, biochemical, and behavioral tests. Many of these actions are not of direct relevance to the main theme of this volume, namely the psychotropic effects of drugs, so we have summarized the acute pharmacological actions of typical neuroleptic compounds in Table 4.2 We will only deal in detail with the ability of neuroleptics to alter motor behavior and to interact with brain dopamine receptors, since this would seem to be of most relevance to the actions of these agents in causing movement disorders and in controlling schizophrenia.

A. Motor Inhibitory Properties

Neuroleptic drugs inhibit motor phenomena associated with cerebral dopamine function and those induced by the administration of known dopamine agonists, such as apomorphine or amphetamine.

The administration of neuroleptics alone to rodents depresses spontaneous locomotion and exploration and causes a general cataleptic immobility such that the animals will maintain an abnormal posture, for example holding on to a raised bar. Catalepsy and the decrease in locomotion, however, are not specific examples of the interaction of neuroleptics with dopamine receptors, for other classes of centrally active compounds, for example opiates, antihistaminics and anticholinergics, may induce similar behavioral changes.

The administration of dopamine agonists to rodents induces characteristic behavioral changes. Low doses of apomorphine or *N*,*n*-propylnorapomorphine produce inhibition of locomotion [66]. This is believed

TABLE 4.1 Dopamine Pathways that Innervate Rat Forebrain

System	Cells of origin	Projections
Mesostriatal system	Substantia nigra	Striatum
Mesocortical system	Ventral tegmental area	Prefrontal and cingulate cortex
Mesolimbic system	Substantia nigra and ventral tegmental area	Nucleus accumbens, tuberculum olfactorium, and amygdala
Tubero-infundibular system	Arcuate and periventricular hypothalamic nuclei	Median eminence

Source: Refs. 51, 52 and 53.

TABLE 4.2 Neuroleptic Drugs Block Cerebral Dopamine Receptors on Acute Administration

---

Behavior

Produce catalepsy [53]

Inhibit spontaneous locomotion [54]

Inhibit apomorphine-induced locomotor activity [55]

Inhibit apomorphine-induced stereotyped behavior [56]

Inhibit apomorphine-induced climbing behavior [57]

Inhibit apomorphine-induced rotation in rodents with unilateral nigro-striatal lesions [58]

Inhibit locomotor activity induced by bilateral injection into nucleus accumbens [59]

Inhibit apomorphine-induced vomiting in dogs [60]

Biochemistry

Increase dopamine turnover [27]

Inhibit dopamine-induced stimulation of adenylate cyclase formation [61]

Displace [^{3}H]-labeled neuroleptic and [^{3}H]dopamine agonist ligands from specific binding sites [29,62]

Increase circulating prolactin levels [63]

Electrophysiology

Increase nigral cell firing [64]

Inhibit dopamine-induced inhibition of nigral cell firing [65]

---

to be due to a preferential interaction of these agonists with presynaptic dopamine receptors, such as to decrease cerebral dopamine function. Higher doses of the same agonists produce an increase in locomotion. Still higher doses produce characteristic stereotyped responses composed of sniffing, licking, and biting. These latter effects are more prevalent in rats than in mice, in which locomotion appears to predominate. Apomorphine and other dopamine agonists also may induce climbing behavior in both rats and mice when these animals are presented with a vertical grid.

All of these motor phenomena induced by dopamine agonists can be inhibited by the administration of neuroleptic compounds. Some neuroleptics may have a preferential ability to inhibit one rather than another of these behaviors. For example, thioridazine is more potent in inhibiting apomorphine-induced motor events than in inducing catalepsy. In this case, the difference may reflect the high inherent anticholinergic activity of this molecule (see later).

The behavioral changes described so far occur after peripheral administration of both dopamine agonists and neuroleptic compounds. The question arises as to where in the brain such drugs act to alter motor behavior and in particular which dopamine-containing brain areas are involved. Bilateral injection of dopamine into the nucleus accumbens produces locomotor hyperactivity which can be prevented by either the peripheral or focal injection of neuroleptic agents [67]. Bilateral injection of dopamine into the prefrontal cortex produced locomotor hyperactivity, which also can be reversed by the administration of neuroleptic drugs either peripherally or focally [68]. Bilateral administration of dopamine agonists into the striatum results in a combination of locomotor hyperactivity and perioral biting movements [69]. The intensity of the two behaviors depends on the topographical location of the injection site within the striatum, and the two behaviors are differentially inhibited by neuroleptic compounds [70]. Locomotor hyperactivity is potently inhibited by the peripheral administration of a range of typical neuroleptic agents, but these compounds have little effect on the perioral biting movements. In contrast, some atypical compounds, such as tiapride and oxiperomide, are only moderately affective in inhibiting locomotor hyperactivity, but can suppress the chewing movements produced by the intrastriatal administration of dopamine agonists. The action of dopamine agonists within the various dopamine-containing areas of the brain and the reversal of their action by the administration of neuroleptic drugs reflects the function of dopamine systems attributed to the individual areas.

The circling rodent model also provides a potent test for detection of neuroleptic acitivity [71,72]. Such animals with unilateral 6-hydroxydopamine lesions of one nigrostriatal pathway show contraversive rotation to directly acting dopamine agonists, such as apomorphine, and ipsiversive rotation to the administration of indirectly acting compounds, such as amphetamine. The postural component of circling is generated from the striatum whereas locomotor drive originates from the nucleus accumbens [73,74]. Administration of neuroleptic drugs inhibits both drug-induced ipsiversive and contraversive rotation.

The general conclusion is that neuroleptic drugs are potent inhibitors of spontaneous and dopamine agonist-induced motor phenomena. Such actions provide a proven test bed for the development of new neuroleptic drugs, but selection of molecules with motor inhibitory properties may only provide a further generation of antipsychotic compounds that induce extrapyramidal disturbances.

B. Actions on Adenylate Cyclase Systems

The finding that dopamine-containing areas of the brain contained a dopamine-specific adenylate cyclase provided one of the first opportunities to study the interaction of drugs with dopamine receptors directly [61,75]. It was rapidly established that many neuroleptic drugs potently inhibited dopamine stimulation of adenylate cyclase in striatal preparations in vitro. Compounds belonging to the phenothiazine and thioxanthene classes of neuroleptics were particularly potent in this respect (Fig. 4.4). However, other neuroleptics, in particular the butyrophenones, were much less potent than was expected from their ability to inhibit dopamine function in animals [76]. Furthermore, members of the substituted benzamide class of neuroleptics turned out to be almost inactive [77,78]. Accordingly, the receptor through which dopamine stimulates production of cyclic AMP could not be the only receptor involved in cerebral dopamine function. The ability of neuroleptic drugs to alter adenylate cyclase activity is thought to be due to their interaction with the recognition site for the enzyme system. However, the adenylate cyclase system consists of a number of components (GTP-sensitive protein, calmodulin, phosphodiesterase) which potentially could be altered by the action of neuroleptic drugs. Particular attention has been paid to the interaction of neuroleptics, such as

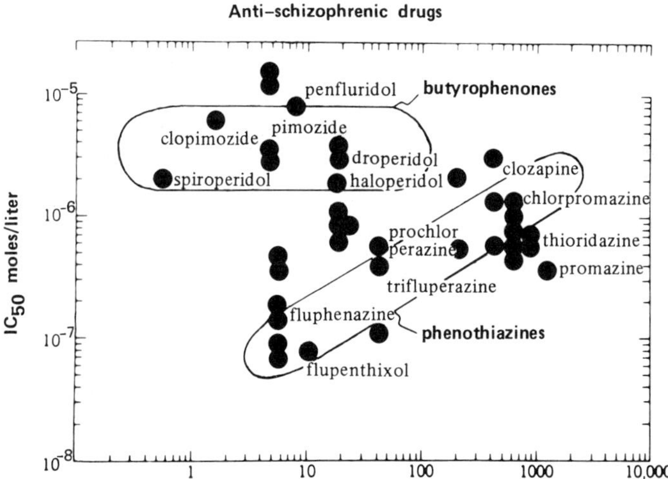

FIG. 4.4 Correlation between clinical potency of neuroleptics and their ability to inhibit dopamine-stimulated adenylate cyclase activity in striatal or caudate homogenates. (From Ref. 76.)

trifluoperazine, with calmodulin but the relevance of this to drug action is not clear [79,80].

Calmodulin activates several calcium-dependent enzymes, in particular phosphodiesterase and adenylate cyclase. In the synaptic membrane, calmodulin in believed to catalyze calcium-dependent activation of adenylate cyclase to cause an increase in cyclic AMP formation. In cytosol, however, calmodulin catalyzes calcium-dependent activation of phosphodiesterase to its high-affinity form, thereby reducing the availability of cyclic AMP. The acute administration of neuroleptic drugs causes a decrease in the spontaneous release of calmodulin from striatal membranes, although there is no change in total calmodulin content [81]. Neuroleptics may interact directly with calmodulin. Thus, trifluoperazine has been reported to show saturable, reversible and calcium-dependent binding to calmodulin preparations [82]. This effect occurs with a range of neuroleptic drugs. However, it occurs only in micromolar concentrations and not in the nanomolar concentrations commonly associated with synaptic transmission. In addition, the rank order of potency in binding of neuroleptics to calmodulin does not parallel their known potency as dopamine antagonists. Butyrophenones usually are weak in displacing [^{3}H]trifluoperazine from calmodulin. In addition, there is little difference between the ability of *cis*- and *trans*-flupenthixol to displace [^{3}H]trifluoperazine and there is only a four- to 5-fold difference between the isomers of butaclamol [83]. An examination of the phenothiazine antagonism of calmodulin-stimulated magnesium-calcium ATPase activity in erythrocyte ghosts showed four analogs of chlorpromazine to be equally potent inhibitors, but only one of these compounds, namely chlorpromazine, possessed neuroleptic activity or antagonized dopamine-sensitive adenylate cyclase activity [84]. Recently, phenothiazines were shown to be inhibitors of calmodulin sensitive calcium phosphokinase system that phosphorylates several proteins in cerebral cortex [85]. Phenothiazines also similarly affect a phospholipid-sensitive, calcium-dependent phosphokinase system. All these findings imply that the interaction of neuroleptics with such calcium-dependent systems is not a specific phenomenon related only to their ability to interact with dopamine-sensitive adenylate cyclase.

C. Displacement of Dopamine Receptor Ligands

A most important advance made in the study of neuroleptics was the introduction of ligand binding assays [29,86]. By using highly labeled tritiated derivatives of dopamine, dopamine agonists, or neuroleptic agents, it has been possible to examine specific interactions with populations of dopamine receptors and the alterations that occur in the nature of these dopamine receptors in response to pharmacological or other manipulation (Table 4.3).

TABLE 4.3 Ligands Currently Available for Labeling Brain Dopamine Receptors

Agonist ligands	Antagonist ligands
[^{3}H]Dopamine	[^{3}H]Piflutixol
[^{3}H]ADTN	[^{3}H]*cis*-flupenthixol
[^{3}H]Apomorphine	[^{3}H]Haloperidol
[^{3}H]*N*,*n*-propylnorapomorphine	[^{3}H]Spiperone
[^{3}H]Bromocriptine	[^{3}H]Domperidone
[^{3}H]Lisuride	[^{3}H]Pimozide
[^{3}H]Pergolide	[^{3}H]Sulpride
[^{3}H]ET 495	[^{3}H]Sultopride
[3H]S 3608	[^{3}H]Tiapride
	[^{3}H]Trifluoperazine

The sites labeled by tritiated neuroleptic ligands, such as [^{3}H]spiperone, in in vitro preparations of rat brain have the characteristics of dopamine receptors. The number of sites to which [^{3}H]spiperone, for example is specifically bound are limited and saturable by nanomolar concentrations of ligand. Suitable ligands exhibit a high affinity for such saturable binding sites. The ligand can be displaced from its specific binding site in a stereospecific manner by the isomers of compounds such as (+)- and (–)-butaclamol, or *cis*- and *trans*-flupenthixol (Table 4.4). The pharmacologically active isomer of each of these drugs causes the greatest displacement. Specific saturable binding of a neuroleptic ligand is displaced by dopamine in concentrations at which other neurotransmitters are ineffective. Such binding sites are in the subcellular fraction containing synaptic vesicles. The regional distribution of such specific binding throughout the brain correlates with the known terminal projection areas of dopamine fibres.

The ability of a wide range of neuroleptic drugs to displace tritiated neuroleptic ligands from their specific binding sites correlates with their known pharmacological potency in behavioral and clinical models (see below).

The interpretation of receptor binding data, however, has pitfalls (Fig. 4.5). Nonspecific, but saturable, binding sites exist, for example of spirodecanone sites which are labeled by close structural analogs of [^{3}H]spiperone [87]. Most neuroleptic drugs are not specific for dopamine receptors (see later). [^{3}H]Spiperone, for example, labels 5-hydroxytryptamine (5HT) receptors in frontal cortex preparations

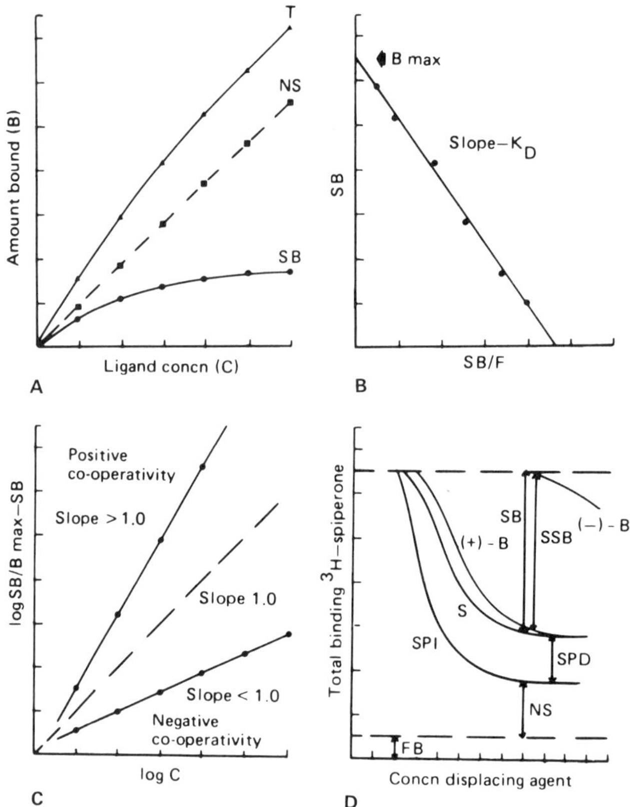

FIG. 4.5 Schematic diagrams to illustrate: A. saturation of specific binding; B. Scatchard analysis of specific binding data; C. Hill plot analysis; and D. the definition of specific binding to show spirodecanone sites. T, total binding; NS, nonspecific binding; SB, specific binding; F, free ligand concentration; FB, filter binding; SPD, spirodecanone site; SSB, stereoselective binding; SPI, spiperone, S, sulpiride; (+)-B, (+)-butaclamol (active); and (−)-B, butaclamol (inactive). A. The linear increase in total and nonspecific binding of ligand to tissue compared with the saturable specific component defined using an appropriate displacing agent. In B the saturable component has undergone linear transformation by Scatchard analysis to give the kinetic constants B_{max} and K_D. C. Further analysis of specific binding data using Hill plot to detect multiplicity of binding sites or cooperativity, D shows the difficulties inherent in the definition of specific binding using [^{3}H] spiperone as an example. Total binding consists of a number of components. Binding to filters is relatively

TABLE 4.4 The Displacement of Specific [^{3}H]Spiperone Binding to Striatal Membranes by Drugs and Transmitter Substance

Displacing Agent	IC_{50}	Displacing Agent	IC_{50}
(+)-Butaclamol	22	Spiperone	2
(−)-Butaclamol	9,000	Haloperidol	6
		Domperidone	29
cis-flupenthixol	23	Pimozide	25
trans-flupenthixol	298		
(−)-Sulpiride	360	Apomorphine	1,200
(+)-Sulpiride	2,000	ADTN	1,300
Trifluoperazine	22	Dopamine	3,000
Thioridazine	120	Noradrenaline	44,000
Chlorpromazine	110	5-HT	>100,000
		Acetylcholine	>100,000
		GABA	>100,000

[88]. Much evidence now exists to suggest that more than one type of dopamine receptors exists within the brain, and different neuroleptics show different propensities to interact with the various receptor populations (see later).

Radioactively labeled neuroleptic drugs also may be used to identify dopamine receipts in vivo. Thus, the in vivo administration of ligand such as [^{3}H]haloperidol or [^{3}H]spiperone leads to an accumulation of

---

small, but note that spiperone itself cannot displace [^{3}H]-spiperone from the nonspecific sites. In addition, note that the component defined as specific binding using sulpiride is smaller than that obtained using spiperone. The difference represents the binding of [^{3}H]-spiperone to a saturable nonphysiological spirodecanone site, from which it can only be displaced by close structural analogs. Last, not also, the definition of stereoselective binding by the isomers of butaclamol as the difference between the displacement caused by the active and inactive enantiomers at a minimally effective concentration of the inactive isomer.

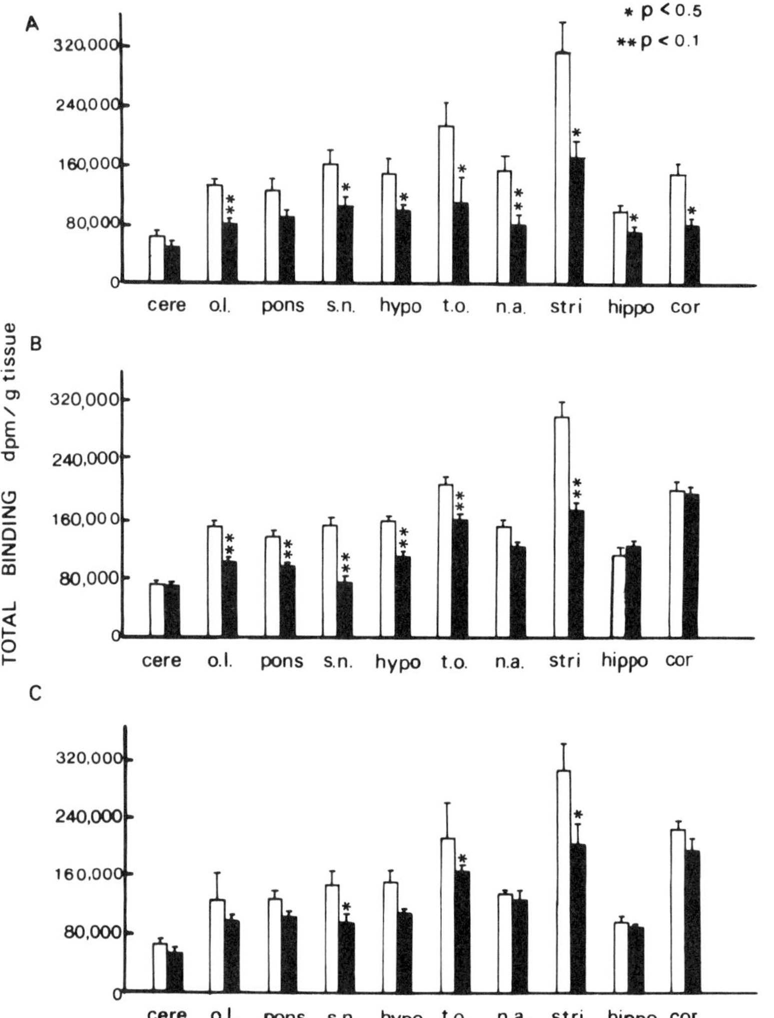

FIG. 4.6 In vivo binding of [^{3}H]spiperone (25 μCi) to various areas of rat brain as defined using 5 mg/kg (+)-butaclamol (A), 0.5 mg/kg haloperidol (B), and 40 mg/kg sulpiride (C). (□) Radioactivity following [^{3}H]spiperone alone; (■) radioactivity in the presence of displacing drug. cere, Cerebellum; o.l., olfactory lobes; pons, pons-medulla; s.n., substantia nigra; hypo, hypothalamus; t.o., tubercullum olfactorium; n.a., nucleus accumbens; str, striatum; hipps, hippocampus; cor, frontal cortex.

radioactivity in brain dopamine-containing areas that can be displaced selectively by dopamine-active drugs (Fig. 4.6) [89,90]. Such in vivo studies also can be combined with autoradiographic techniques to provide detailed localization of neuroleptic binding sites within a given brain area [91,92]. In vivo binding assays also can be employed to give some index of receptor occupancy by an unlabeled neuroleptic drug administered in doses producing behavioral changes.

D. Actions of Atypical Neuroleptic Drugs

Since neuroleptic drugs were introduced in the 1950s, the drugs produced have, to a large extent, closely resembled each other, particularly in their actions of brain dopamine function. In recent times, interest has centered on the production of a neuroleptic compound that possesses antipsychotic actions but does not induce extrapyramidal motor disturbances. Only two compounds have been introduced that are thought to induce a lesser incidence of extrapyramidal disturbances. These are clozapine and sulpiride. We will now briefly compare the acute pharmacological properties of these neuroleptic drugs with those of more typical neuroleptic compounds.

1. Sulpiride

Sulpiride is a proven antipsychotic agent [48,93], and its action in man may be associated with a lower incidence of extrapyramidal disturbances than that seen with classical neuroleptic compounds. In man, sulpiride acts as a typical dopamine receptor antagonist as shown by antiemetic activity, antipsychotic activity, and the elevation of circulating prolactin levels (Table 4.5). In animal models of cerebral dopamine function, however, sulpiride appears to exert only a part of the spectrum of activity of classical neuroleptic compounds. In behavioral experiments, sulpiride inhibits climbing behavior in mice but does not produce pronounced catalepsy. Sulpiride is ineffective against apomorphine- or amphetamine-induced stereotyped behavior in rats, particularly the higher-grade components. Sulpiride does not antagonize apomorphine-induced circling in rats with a unilateral 6-hydroxydopamine lesion of the nigro-striatal pathway, although it does appear able to inhibit the same behavior in mice. Sulpiride poorly inhibits the apomorphine-induced reversal of reserpine induced akinesia in mice, and does not antagonize apomorphine-induced behavioral changes such as checking, locomotion, and inactivity in marmosets.

The direct dopamine antagonist properties of sulpiride are apparent in electrophysiological experiments where it prevents dopamine-mediated inhibition of nigral cell firing. In biochemical experiments,

Table 4.5 Typical and Atypical Neuroleptic Properties of Sulpiride in Animals and Man

Typical dopamine receptor antagonist actions	Atypical actions
Animals	
Antiemetic [46]	Induces weak catalepsy [77,96, 102]
Inhibits climbing behavior in rats and mice [57,94,95]	Weak antagonism of stereotypy [95,96,102–104]
Inhibits rotational behavior in mice [197]	Weak antagonism of apomorphine-induced locomotion in mice [105]
Increases brain dopamine turnover [96–100]	No inhibition of rotational behavior in rats [103]
Inhibits dopamine-induced depression of nigral cell firing [101]	No inhibition of apomorphine-induced checking and locomotion in marmosets [106]
Displaces radioactive ligands from dopamine receptors [77]	No inhibition of dopamine-stimulation of adenylate cyclase [78,96,99]
Man	
Antiemetic [107]	"Disinhibitory" [112]
Antipsychotic [93]	No sedation [112]
Extrapyramidal side effects [108]	
Elevated plasma prolactin levels [109,110]	
Increased homovanillic acid levels in cerebrospinal fluid [111]	

sulpiride increases dopamine turnover in all dopamine-containing areas of the rodent brain. Sulpiride also displaces tritiated dopamine ligands from their specific binding sites. However, sulpiride does not inhibit dopamine stimulation of adenylate cyclase activity in brain homogenates. The actions of sulpiride on cerebral dopamine function are stereoselective. The (−)-isomer possesses far greater pharmacological activity than (+)-sulpiride [105].

Atypical actions of sulpiride may be at least partially due to the selectivity of its interaction with brain dopamine receptors. Thus, sulpiride does not inhibit dopamine stimulation of adenylate cyclase activity in vitro using slice or homogenate preparations from various dopamine-containing areas of the brain including striatum, nucleus accumbens, and tuberculum olfactorium. The failure of sulpiride in vitro to inhibit dopamine-stimulated adenylate cyclase systems might suggest involvement of active metabolites in vivo. However, no increase in basal striatal cyclic AMP concentration can be detected after peripheral sulpiride administration [113]. These findings suggest that sulpiride does not act on that dopamine receptor responsible for the stimulation of the adenylate cyclase enzyme. This distinguishes sulpiride from the phenothiazine and thioxanthene classes of neuroleptics which are potent inhibitors of dopamine-stimulated adenylate cyclase, and also from the butyrophenone class of neuroleptics which, although weakly active on the adenylate cyclase system, can cause maximal inhibition. The interaction of sulpiride directly with dopamine receptors can, however, be shown by its ability to displace ligands such as [^{3}H]spiperone and [^{3}H]haloperidol from their specific binding sites on rat striatal preparations. In contrast, sulpiride shows little or no ability to displace a ligand such as [^{3}H]piflutixol which also binds to the recognition site for adenylate cyclase [114].

The availability of [^{3}H]sulpiride as a ligand has allowed examination of the nature of the dopamine receptor population with which this compound interacts [115-117]. Scatchard analysis of specific saturable [^{3}H]sulpiride binding in rat striatal preparations has revealed the existence of two binding sites, a high-affinity site and a low affinity site. Examination of the ability of a range of compounds to displace [^{3}H]sulpiride from its high affinity site showed that of all the transmitter substances examined only dopamine was effective in causing displacement (Table 4.6). This suggests that sulpiride binds to dopamine receptors, a conclusion verified by the ability of a range of enantiomeric pairs of dopamine active drugs to stereoselectively displace [^{3}H]sulpiride from striatal preparations. At first sight, the binding of the [^{3}H]sulpiride to rat striatal preparations is almost identical to that of [^{3}H]spiperone or [^{3}H]haloperidol. However, the interaction of [^{3}H]sulpiride with brain dopamine receptors differs in one critically important manner from that of other neuroleptic ligands. Thus, the interaction of [^{3}H]sulpiride with its binding site is critically dependent on the presence of sodium ions within the incubation media [118,119]. In a similar manner, the ability of sulpiride to

TABLE 4.6 Displacement of the Specific Binding of [^{3}H]Sulpiride (10 nM) from Rat Striatal Preparations by a Range of Transmitter Substances and Neuroleptic Drugs

Drug	IC_{50}
(−)-Sulpiride	9
(+)-Sulpiride	355
(−)-Sultopride	3
(+)-Sultopride	370
Metoclopramide	57
Tiapride	135
(+)-Butaclamol	2
(−)-Butaclamol	3,800
cis-flupenthixol	5
trans-flupehthixol	21
Haloperidol	250
Thioridazine	48
Clozapine	750
Dopamine	6,700
Noradrenaline	70,000
5-Hydroxytryptamine	19,000
Acetylcholine	>100,000
GABA	>100,000

Source: Ref. 117.

displace ligand such as [^{3}H]spiperone or [^{3}H]haloperidol also depends on the presence of physiological concentrations of sodium ions [120]. The effect of sodium is a specific action since it cannot be replaced by other monovalent or divalent cations. The reason for the sodium dependency of [^{3}H]sulpiride binding is not understood, but it may provide further evidence for the existence of multiple dopamine receptors within the brain (see later).

Another reason for the atypical actions of sulpiride may be due to its ability to exert a differential action on dopamine receptors in different areas of the brain, studies carried out by ourselves and by Kohler and colleagues [89], have shown that sulpiride may preferentially show an action on dopamine receptors in substantia nigra and that that much higher doses are required for it to interact with striatal dopamine receptors. Only when toxic levels are approached was there any evidence for an interaction with dopamine receptors in the nucleus accumbens. This latter fact, in particular, clearly differentiates sulpiride from (+)-butaclamol which strongly displaces [^{3}H]spiperone from nucleus accumbens, and also from haloperidol which causes a small but significant displacement in this region. The conclusion must be that sulpiride administered systemically does not have a major action on dopamine receptors located in the nucleus accumbens. The direct injection of sulpiride into this region, however, causes potent inhibition of locomotor hyperactivity induced by the focal injection of dopamine [121]. Sulpiride in vivo either does not penetrate into the region of the nucleus accumbens or the dopamine receptors on which it acts in this region are not labeled to any significant extent by [^{3}H]spiperone in vivo.

2. Clozapine

Clozapine is an effective antipsychotic but, unfortunately, it also occasionally produces a bone marrow toxicity which has prevented its widespread use. New derivatives for clozapine possess the same clinical actions but not the toxicity, so that the profile of clozapine in acute pharmacological experiments has gained importance. Clozapine is the only neuroleptic compound for which there is good evidence that it does not induce extrapyramidal side effects.

Examination of clozapine in a range of tests associated with alterations of cerebral dopamine function reveals that this compound, like sulpiride, only exerts part of the spectrum of activity of a typical neuroleptic drug (Table 4.7).

Clozapine decreases spontaneous locomotor activity and inhibits apomorphine-induced locomotion, climbing behavior, and circling behavior. It does not however, produce catalepsy and has little or no ability to inhibit apomorphine- or amphetamine-induced stereotyped behavior. Clozapine, does decrease hyperactivity induced by the bilateral injection of dopamine into striatum, nucleus accumbens, or tuberculum olfactorium of the rat, albeit weakly.

In contrast to other neuroleptic drugs, clozapine only increases dopamine turnover in relatively high dosage as judged by metabolite levels or by turnover studies. This occurs in all dopamine-containing areas of the brain. In contrast to other neuroleptic compounds, there is evidence that clozapine in low doses decreases dopamine turnover; the reasons for this are not known. In high doses, clozapine also induces an increase in the dopamine content of forebrain; this is

TABLE 4.7 Typical and Atypical Neuroleptic Properties of Clozapine in Animals and Man

Typical dopamine receptor antagonist actions	Atypical actions
Animals	
Inhibits spontaneous locomotor activity [122]	Does not induce catalepsy [128]
Inhibits apomorphine-induced locomotion [123]	Little or no inhibition of apomorphine-induced stereotypy [129]
Inhibits apomorphine-induced climbing [124]	No inhibition of nigral cell firing [130]
Inhibits rotational behavior in mice [125]	No inhibition of dopamine or apomorphine-induced depression nigral cell firing [130]
Increases brain dopamine turnover [126]	Reverses haloperidol-induced increases in nigral cell firing [130]
Inhibits dopamine-stimulated adenylate cyclase [75]	Potent anticholinergic activity [131]
Displaces radioactive ligands from dopamine receptors [127]	
Man	
Antipsychotic	No extrapyramidal side effects [133]
	Weak elevation of prolactin levels [134]

thought to occur because of relatively greater ability to increase dopamine synthesis conpared with transmitter utilization. Again, in contrast to other neuroleptics, clozapine only elevates circulating prolactin levels when administered in very high doses.

These biochemical and behavioral data suggest a relatively weak and somewhat selective action of clozapine on brain dopamine function. There are obvious differences between the spectrum of effects initiated by clozapine and those of typical neuroleptic drugs.

Clozapine does interact with adenylate cyclase-linked dopamine receptors, and in high concentrations, it inhibits dopamine stimulation of adenylate cyclase. Clozapine also weakly interacts with nonadenylate cyclase-linked receptors, for in high concentrations it can displace [^{3}H]haloperidol or [^{3}H]spiperone from their specific binding sites in rat striatal preparations. However, in all these in vitro assay systems, clozapine only exhibits weak dopamine-active properties.

Electrophysiological experiments also suggest differences between clozapine and other typical neuroleptic agents. Peripheral administration of clozapine does not inhibit decreased nigral cell firing induced by iontophoretic application of dopamine. Clozapine only weakly prevents the inhibition of nigral cell firing caused by apomorphine, but it does reverse the inhibitory actions of amphetamine. This contrasts with the action of typical neuroleptics and, indeed, of sulpiride which reverses the inhibitory actions of dopamine and dopamine agonists. Unexpectedly, clozapine reverses the haloperidol-induced increase in nigral cell firing. The mechanism underlying these changes is not understood. In contrast to its atypical actions in substantia nigra, clozapine, like haloperidol, increases firing of both striatal and mesolimbic neurones [130].

So, in these respects the actions of clozapine not only differ from typical neuroleptics such as haloperidol, but also distinguish the drug from sulpiride. Clozapine does not appear to affect dopamine function in a classical manner, and does not appear to be selective for one dopamine receptor population.

IV. ACUTE PHARMACOLOGICAL ACTIONS OF NEUROLEPTIC DRUGS ON NONDOPAMINE SYSTEMS

Most neuroleptic drugs do not act only on cerebral dopamine receptors, but also exert a range of effects on other neurotransmitter systems. This is either the result of their actions on dopamine systems causing secondary effects on other neurotransmitter pathways or because the neuroleptics also act directly on other neurotransmitters' receptors.

We will now briefly consider the actions of neuroleptics on a range of neurotransmitter systems other than dopamine.

A. Noradrenaline

Some neuroleptic drugs (e.g., thioridazine, haloperidol) interact directly with brain noradrenaline receptors. This is shown by their ability to displace ligands such as [^{3}H]WB 4101 from their specific binding sites to α-1 receptors (Table 4.8). Similarly, some neuroleptic drugs cause displacement of [^{3}H]clonidine from its specific binding site to α-2 receptors; the affinity for this site appears to be

TABLE 4.8 Drug Displacement of Ligand Binding to Brain Adrenergic Receptors

	K_i (nM)		
Displacing agent	[^{3}H]WB 4101 (α-1)	[^{3}H]Clonidine (α-2)	Ratio-activity
Oxymetazoline	24	1.9	13
Clonidine	430	5.7	75
Phentolamine	3.6	22	0.16
WB 4101	0.6	200	0.003
Thioridazine	5.1	520	0.010
Chlorpromazine	6.2	590	0.011
Haloperidol	11	1200	0.009
Trifluoperazine	44	4400	0.010

Source: Ref. 135.

approximately 100-fold less than for the α-1 site [135]. In contrast to the actions of neuroleptic drugs on α-adrenoreceptors, their ability to displace ligands such as [^{3}H]dihydroalprenolol from β-adrenergic sites is weak or nonexistent [136].

Some neuroleptic compounds (e.g., chlorpromazine, thiethylperazine) also inhibit noradrenaline-sensitive cyclic AMP generating systems in homogenates of limbic forebrain [137–138]. However, the correlation between activity in this model and neuroleptic effects is poor. Indeed, some neuroleptic molecules (e.g., metoclopramide, sulpiride) do not block the action of noradrenaline in stimulating cyclic AMP formation.

Administration of neuroleptic drugs to rodents enhances noradrenaline synthesis and turnover, presumably by a receptor-mediated feedback mechanism [18]. The ability of phenothiazine and thioxanthene neuroleptics to increase noradrenaline turnover correlates with their ability to antagonize the inhibitory effects of noradrenaline on cerebellar Purkinje cells [139]. Neuroleptics also may enhance potassium-evoked noradrenaline release from cortical slices by an action on presynaptic adrenoreceptors. However, they have little effect on noradrenaline reuptake mechanisms.

In general, neuroleptic drugs may be seen as acting on postsynaptically located α-1 receptor sites, but as having a lesser effect on the α-2 receptor population, which is thought to be located predominantly presynaptically. Sulpiride may be an exception to this rule since it appears to exert only weak andrenoreceptor antagonist actions at the postsynaptic site, but in some models it is able to antagonize the presynaptic actions of clonidine. Indeed, binding studies have shown sulpiride to exert a higher affinity for [^{3}H]clonidine binding sites than for [^{3}H]WB 4101 sites.

B. 5-Hydroxytryptamine

There is surprisingly little evidence to suggest a major action of neuroleptic drugs on 5-HT function.

Ligand-binding assays show that neuroleptic drugs interact directly with 5-HT receptors. Receptor binding assays using [^{3}H]5-HT or [^{3}H]LSD have shown neuroleptic drugs to possess some ability to displace these ligands from their specific binding sites to 5-HT receptors, particularly in cerebral cortex [88]. A 5-HT-sensitive adenylate cyclase system exists in rat synaptic membranes. There has been no comprehensive study of the actions of neuroleptics on this system. However, there is evidence to suggest that chlorpromazine, fluphenazine, and *cis*-flupenthixol can inhibit AMP formation in concentrations that are not different from those of 5-HT antagonists [140,141]. There may be no correlation between the ability of neuroleptics to act at 5-HT receptors, as demonstrated by ligand-binding assays and their in vivo actions. Thus, in vitro haloperidol and (+)-butaclamol displace [^{3}H]spiperone from both 5-HT and dopamine receptors, but in vivo they accelerate forebrain dopamine turnover but not 5-HT turnover [142].

Neuroleptic drugs can alter 5-HT turnover. Butyrophenone compounds, such as spiperone, haloperidol, and pimozide, decrease 5-HT utilization in the rat brain stem but cause only minor changes in 5-HT concentrations in other areas of rat brain [143]. These changes are likely to be secondary to the interaction of neuroleptic drugs with dopamine receptors, since apomorphine increased 5-HT turnover. More recently, Rastogi and colleagues [144] have shown that haloperidol and chlorpromazine increase 5-HT and 5-hydroxyindoleacetic acid (5-HIAA) concentrations in the mid-brain, and chlorpromazine has a similar effect in the striatum. These changes are accompanied by an increase in midbrain tryptophan hydroxylase activity suggesting a discrete enhancement of 5-HT synthesis and utilization. It has also been demonstrated that a range of phenothiazine drugs (with the exception of chlorpromazine), increase brain tryptophan content, and increase brain 5-HT levels [145]. The increase in 5-HT has been interpreted as being due to increased 5-HT synthesis rather than to decreased utilization. Interestingly, both antipsychotic phenothiazines and nonantipsychotic drugs (promethiazine, trimeprazine) produce the same effects, suggesting no relationship of neuroleptic activity to change in 5-HT function.

However, all the above studies contrast with the findings of Carlsson [146] who was unable to show any consistent effect of neuroleptic drugs, with the exception of chlorprothixene, on the accumulation of 5-hydroxytryptophan following decarboxylase inhibition. It is evident that the effect of neuroleptic drugs on 5-HT function is not simple. The actions produced by neuroleptic drugs on this system may not be necessary for antipsychotic action. Neuroleptics such as haloperidol have little effect on behaviors induced by the administration of *L*-5-hydroxytryptophan, for example hyperextension and athetoid movements of the hindlegs in the acute spinal rat or myoclonus evoked in guinea pigs [147].

C. Histamine

Many neuroleptic drugs, for example phenothiazines, possess marked antihistaminic activity, and such drugs may interact directly with histamine receptors.

Receptor binding studies have shown phenothiazines to be potent H-1 antagonists, displacing [^{3}H]mepyramine from its specific binding site. *cis*- and *trans*-Flupenthixol also were potent in displacing this ligand, but (+)-butaclamol and the butyrophenones, haloperidol and spiperone, were markedly weaker than other neuroleptic agents [148]. A range of neuroleptic drugs also inhibit histamine-sensitive adenylate cyclase in guinea pig hippocampus and rabbit cerebral cortex [149,150]. Thioridazine was extremely potent in this respect, but other phenothiazines, thioxanthenes, dibenzodiazepines, and butyrophenones also were effective.

There appears to be little relation between antipsychotic activity and antihistamine action. Nonantipsychotic phenothiazines, such as promazine, also are potent antihistamines.

Chlorpromazine inhibits the activity of *N*-methyltransferase in vitro and in vivo so reducing methylation of histamine in the cat and mouse [151]. The results of this inhibition is an increase in the levels of histamine observed in the cat hypothalamus and in the rat brain following chlorpromazine administration. However, the doses of chlorpromazine required to produce such changes are far higher than those necessary to alter dopamine function.

D. Acetylcholine

In striatum, at least, many dopamine receptors are thought to lie on the cell bodies of cholinergic interneurons. Therefore, neuroleptic drugs can exert an indirect influence on cholinergic function through their dopamine antagonist properties. However, some neuroleptic drugs also possess direct actions on cholinergic receptors.

TABLE 4.9 Anticholinergic Activity of Neuroleptic Drugs as Measured using Displacement of [^{3}H]PrBCM Binding and Antagonism of Acetylcholine-Induced Contraction of Guinea Pig Ileum

Drug	[^{3}H]PrBCM	Guinea pig Ileum
Phenothiazine		
acepromazine	350	840
chlorpromazine	1,010	490
fluphenazine	8,000	1,900
thioridazine	84	620
Thioxanthenes		
cis(Z)-chlorprothixene	110	160
trans(E)-chlorprothixene	56	220
cis(Z)-clopenthixol	6,000	5,400
cis(Z)-flupenthixol	3,900	4,500
methixene	49	42
piflutixol	2,050	5,800
Butyrophenones and related drugs		
haloperidol	8,600	8,100
piroside	2,550	550
spiperone	17,000	10,000
Dibenzodiazepines		
clozapine	49	610
loxapine	450	10,000
Substituted benzamides		
sulpiride	160,000	>23,500
Anticholinergics		
benztropine	2.3	4.7
atropine	4.7	8.4
trihexyphenidyl	18	22

Source: Ref. 131.

TABLE 4.10 Receptor Binding Profiles of Sulpiride and Clozapine Compared

Receptor	Ligand	Brain area	Sulpiride	Clozapine
Dopamine	[^{3}H]Spiperone	Striatum	51	73
5-HT	[^{3}H]Spiperone	Frontal cortex	>10,000	16
H_1-histamine	[^{3}H]Mepyramine	Cerebellum	>10,000	4.3
α_1-Adrenergic	[^{3}H]WP 4101	Forebrain	>1,000	7.3
α_2-Adrenergic	[^{3}H]Clonidine	Cortex	>10,000	120
Acetylcholine	[^{3}H]Dexetemide	Striatum	>10,000	31

Source: Ref. 164.

Receptor binding assays using 3-propylbenzylcholine mustard, [^{3}H]-3-quinuclidinyl benzylate or [^{3}H]dexetemide have shown neuroleptic drugs to vary considerably in their inherent anticholinergic activity (Table 4.9). Compounds such as thioridazine and clozapine exhibit marked anticholinergic activity but in general, butyrophenones are weak in this respect [131].

Dopaminergic action in the striatum is inhibitory on cholinergic function. Administration of dopamine agonists such as apomorphine causes a decrease in acetylcholine neuronal firing and a corresponding decrease in acetylcholine turnover, with subsequent accumulation of acetylcholine in this area [152,153]. In contrast, the administration of neuroleptic compounds decreases striatal acetylcholine content, due to increased utilization and turnover of the transmitter [154,155]. They do not change choline accumulation in striatal tissue preparations. The increased turnover of acetylcholine is reflected by a corresponding increase in the potassium-evoked release of acetylcholine from striatal slices [156]. Such effects are produced by a wide range of neuroleptics including haloperidol, spiperone, fluphenazine, pimozide, and chloromazine. In contrast to the effects in the striatum, no similar changes in acetylcholine have been elicited by neuroleptic drugs in the nucleus accumbens or cortical dopamine-containing areas.

E. γ-Aminobutyric Acid

There is no direct evidence of an interaction of neuroleptic drugs with γ-aminobutyric acid (GABA) or benzodiazepine receptor binding sites.

with Typical Neuroleptic Drugs

K_i (nM) values for drug displacement			
Haloperidol	Trifluoperazine	Pimozide	Thioridazine
1.2	3.9	0.9	13
48	41	211	36
4390	51	>10,000	41
8.1	20	41	3.2
>10,000	>10,000	>10,000	1385
4370	>10,000	1022	78

However, because of the intimate connections between dopamine and GABA systems within basal ganglia, it is not surprising that such drugs elicit alterations in GABA function.

Administration of neuroleptic drugs, including haloperidol, pimozide, chlorpromazine, clozapine, and thioridazine, increases GABA turnover in both the nucleus accumbens and globus pallidus [157,158]. Clozapine and thioridazine also increase GABA turnover in the substantia nigra and striatum, but this is not observed with the other neuroleptic compounds. Increased GABA turnover is thought to be secondary to dopamine receptor blockade since it is observed following the administration of (+)-butaclamol but not the inactive (−)-isomer [157].

F. Peptides

The effects of neuroleptics on brain peptide function are uncertain. Single doses of neuroleptics, for example, do not alter substance P levels in substantia nigra [159], but Pettibone and Wurtman [160] observed that a single dose of amphetamine caused a dose-dependent reduction in substance P in rat striatum, an action that was prevented by haloperidol administration. Hansen and colleagues [161] recently have confirmed this finding; acute apomorphine treatment lowered nigral substance P, an effect that could be blocked by acute pretreatment with haloperidol. Subacute administration of haloperidol does reduce nigral substance P immunoreactivity [161]. Substance P levels in other brain regions examined were unchanged following drug administration. A single dose of haloperidol has been reported not to change striatal met-enkephalin content [162,163] and we recently have found that the acute administration of *cis*-flupenthixol also is ineffective.

Perhaps the failure of neuroleptic drugs to alter peptide concentrations lies in the relatively slow rate of turnover of these substances. In any case, only absolute levels of peptide neurotransmitters have been studied, and these may give no indication of turnover or utilization. Even where changes are observed, it is not known whether they reflect increases or decreases in peptide turnover. The close anatomical relationship that appears to exist between dopamine innervation of striatum and cholecystokinin and neurotensin suggests that further reports of interactions between neuroleptic drugs and peptide substances will soon appear.

G. Receptor Profiles of Neuroleptics

From the previous discussion, it is apparent that neuroleptic drugs may exert many actions on cerebral neurotransmitter systems. It is also apparent that the ability of neuroleptics to act at different receptor sites varies enormously. Leysen and colleagues [164] recently have carried out a substantial study on the effects of many neuroleptics in ligand-binding assays for dopamine, noradrenaline, 5-HT, histamine, and acetylcholine receptors (Table 4.10). There are very wide variations in the range of neuronal activity shown by various neuroleptic drugs using these ligand-binding techniques. Compounds from different neuroleptic classes do not exhibit any general pattern. For example, although haloperidol is a potent dopamine receptor antagonist, it also interacts potently with α-adrenergic receptors and with 5-HT receptors. Similarly, pimozide also potently antagonizes dopamine receptor function and is active at α-1 adrenergic and 5-HT receptors but, in addition it has actions at acetylcholine receptors. The phenothiazine derivative, trifluoperazine, shows interaction with dopamine receptors, but also possesses activity at 5-HT and α-1 adrenergic receptors, and interacts with histamine receptors. Even more complex is the receptor profile of thioridazine which, while showing moderate action at dopamine receptors, interacts also with 5-HT, histamine, α-1 adrenergic, and acetylcholine receptors.

In contrast to these typical neuroleptic drugs, the receptor profile of sulpiride shows a weak ability to interact with dopamine receptors, which is a selective effect, for the drug has little or no ability to interact with radioactive ligands labeling other neurotransmitter receptor sites. The other atypical neuroleptic of interest, clozapine, also shows a weak interaction with dopamine receptors, but has potent interactions with 5-HT, histamine, α-adrenergic, and acetylcholine receptors. This is reflected by the binding of [^{3}H]clozapine to rat brain membranes which show a large muscarinic component and a smaller component comprising an interaction with dopamine, 5-HT, and noradrenaline receptors [165].

The pharmacological action of neuroleptic drugs not only reflects the receptor profile of the parent drug but that of metabolites formed in vivo. Two recent studies have explained the importance of differences in the receptor profile of neuroleptic drug metabolites compared with that of the parent drug [166,167] (Table 4.11).

For example, thioridazine-5-sulfoxide (mesoridazine) and the sulfone (sulforidazine) are more potent at dopamine and α-1 adrenergic receptors than thioridazine itself but less active at cholinergic sites. On the other hand, northioridazine and northioridazine-5-sulphoxide are 10 times less active on dopamine receptors but have the same or greater activity on α-1 and cholinergic receptors. A similar pattern of changes is found for chlorpromazine metabolites. Clearly, changes in the levels of metabolites in brain during the use of chronic neuroleptic therapy might be of considerable pharmacological consequence.

V. MULTIPLE SITES OF ACTION WITHIN THE STRIATAL COMPLEX

Neuroleptic drugs may act at dopamine receptors in different brain regions. Within each of these dopamine-containing systems, dopamine receptors may be located presynaptically either on dopamine neuronal cell bodies and dendrites or on dopamine nerve terminals, or postsynaptically either on the cell bodies of other neurons or on the terminals of afferent fiber projections. In the striatal complex, at least five different locations for dopamine receptors have been proposed. Each of these might provide a target for neuroleptic drug action. The major evidence supporting the existence of these various dopamine receptor populations is shown in Table 4.12. In addition to the post-synaptic dopamine receptor thought to lie on cell bodies of cholinergic and probably GABA interneurons, there is evidence for the existence of dopamine receptors on presynaptic dopamine terminals within striatum which regulate dopamine synthesis and release. It is currently believed that low concentrations of dopamine agonists preferentially interact with this presynaptic receptor population so as to decrease dopaminergic action [76]. There is also some evidence to suggest that low concentrations of certain neuroleptics such as sulpiride act preferentially on these sites to cause dopamine release [185,186]. However, there is considerable controversy over any such preferential neuroleptic action. Indeed, it is not clear whether such autoreceptors represent surface receptors or whether they are within nerve terminals associated with tyrosine hydroxylase. Raiteri and his colleagues [187] demonstrated in superfused synaptosomal preparations that the ability of dopamine to interact with autoreceptors is prevented by blockade of reuptake mechanisms, suggesting that they lie within nerve terminals.

TABLE 4.11 Comparison of the Receptor Profiles of Thioridazine and Chlorpromazine with That of Their Metabolites

Compound	[^{3}H]Spiperone (dopamine)	[^{3}H]WB 4101 (α-2)	[^{3}H]QNB (acetylcholine)
		K_i (nM)	
Thioridazine	9.8	74	6.1
Thioridazine-S-sulfoxide	4.2	21	26
Thioridazine-S-sulfone	4.2	2.7	21
Northioridazine	110	54	11
Northioridazine-S-sulfoxide	150	4.7	3.4
Thioridazine-R-sulfoxide	2700	160	50
Thioridazine disulfone	5000	3200	580
Thioridazine disulfoxide	21000	900	580

		IC_{50}	
Chlorpromazine	18	10	170
Nor_1chlorpromazine	40	23	450
7-Hydroxychlorpromazine	56	120	700
7-Hydroxynor_1chlorpromazine	80	50	1800
Nor_2chlorpromazine	200	180	2000
7-Hydroxynor_2chlorpromazine	320	130	9000
8-Hydroxychlorpromazine	620	40	400
7-Hydroxychlorpromazine sulfoxide	3500	5000	3000
7-Hydroxynor_1chlorpromazine sulfoxide	5600	>10000	>10000
Chlorpromazine sulfoxide	>10000	950	5500
Nor_2chlorpromazine sulfoxide	>10000	1100	>10000
7-Hydroxynor_2chlorpromazine sulfoxide	>10000	>10000	>10000
Nor_1chlorpromazine sulfoxide	>10000	600	>10000

Source: Ref. 166 and 167.

TABLE 4.12 Evidence for Different Locations of Dopamine Receptors within the Striatal Complex

---

(a) *Dopamine receptors located on the striatal cells*

Neuroleptics enhance and dopamine depresses striatal cell firing [168].

Destruction of nigro-striatal fibers increases dopamine receptor numbers in striatum [169].

Kainic acid lesions of striatum decrease both dopamine-stimulated adenylate cyclase activity and adenylate-independent receptor numbers [170].

(b) *Dopamine receptors located on presynaptic dopamine terminals in striatum*

Neuroleptic-induced increase in dopamine turnover persists following destruction of strio-nigral pathway [171].

Neuroleptic-induced increase in dopamine turnover persists following kainic acid lesions of striatum [172].

Neuroleptic-induced increase in dopamine turnover persists following hemisection of cessation of impulse flow using γ-butyrolactone [173,174].

Neuroleptic-induced increase in dopamine turnover occurs in striatal slices and synaptosomes [175–177].

(c) *Dopamine receptors located on terminals of cortico-striate fibers*

Decortication to remove cortico-striate glutamate fibers decreases the number of adenylate cyclase-independent receptors in striatum [170].

Neuroleptics alter glutamate release in synaptosomal preparations [178].

(d) *Dopamine receptors located on dopamine cell bodies in substantia nigra*

Neuroleptics cause dendritic release of dopamine [179].

Neuroleptics inhibit nigral cell firing [64,65].

Local application of dopamine inhibits cell firing, an effect reversed by systemic neuroleptic administration [180].

Intranigral amphetamine (presumably releasing dopamine) causes a marked inhibition of neuronal activity in pars compacta of substantia nigra [181].

TABLE 4.12 (Continued)

Destruction of nigro-striatal pathway reduced neuroleptic binding sites in nigra [182].

(e) *Dopamine receptors located on the terminals of strio-nigral feedback pathway*

Dopamine dendrites do not possess dopamine receptors linked to adenylate cyclase [183], but lesions of the strio-nigral dopamine-stimulated adenylate cyclase [184].

Most of the evidence for the existence of autoreceptors comes from indirect behavioral or biochemical studies. Attempts to label presynaptic dopamine receptors using ligand binding assays have been only partially successful. Such receptors apparently can be labeled by dopamine agonist ligands, but neuroleptic ligands have not been demonstrated to identify this site. How neuroleptic drugs might act preferentially at such sites if they are not labeled by neuroleptic compounds is unclear. The striatum also receives an extensive glutamate pathway from areas of motor cortex; other dopamine receptors may be located on the terminals of these cortico-fugal fibers. Dopamine acts to inhibit glutamate release from striatal slices, an action that can be reversed by neuroleptic drugs [50]. Neuroleptic drugs alone appear to have no effect on glutamate release, suggesting normally low inhibitory tone.

Other dopamine receptors are found within the substantia nigra. There is considerable evidence to support the release of dopamine from dendrites. This release may act on dopamine receptors located on dopamine cell bodies in substantia nigra, so as to regulate nigral cell firing, or on dopamine receptors on the terminals of the strio-nigral feedback pathway, which may be concerned with the regulation of GABA release. There also is some electrophysiological evidence to support the existence of dopamine receptors on cell bodies of the nigro-thalamic GABA pathway [188]. The role dopamine may play at this site is unknown.

This brief description of the distribution and function of dopamine receptors in the strio-nigral complex illustrates the number of potential sites at which neuroleptic drugs might act to produce their varying behavioral and biochemical effects. It should not be considered that neuroleptics have a single action at a single postsynaptic dopamine receptor.

A. Classification of Sites of Action

Neuroleptic drug action is further complicated by the abundant evidence for more than one type of brain dopamine receptor at each

TABLE 4.13 Current Classification of Brain Dopamine Receptors Based on Ligand Binding Experiments

Classification		Definition
D-1		Adenylate cyclase-linked dopamine receptors
D-2		Adenylate cyclase independent dopamine receptors
Agonist sites		High affinity for dopamine agonist but low affinity for antagonists
Antagonist sites:		Low affinity for dopamine agonists but high affinity for dopamine antagonists
	D-1	Adenylate cyclase-linked dopamine receptors
	D-2	Adenylate cyclase-independent dopamine receptors
	α	-guanine nucleotide regulated
	β	-guanine nucleotide independent
	D-3	Adenylate cyclase-independent dopamine receptors with high affinity for dopamine agonists but low affinity for antagonists
	D-1	Adenylate cyclase-linked dopamine receptors
	D-2	Adenylate cyclase-independent dopamine receptors with high affinity for both agonists and antagonists
	D-3	Adenylate cyclase-independent dopamine receptors with high affinity for agonists but low affinity for antagonists
	D-4	Adenylate cyclase-independent dopamine receptors with low affinity for agonists but high affinity for antagonists
Sodium-dependent sites		Adenylate cyclase-independent dopamine receptors where neuroleptic interaction is critically dependent on presence of sodium ions

TABLE 4.13 (Continued)

Classification	Definition
Sodium-independent sites	Adenylate cyclase-independent dopamine receptors where neuroleptic interaction is independent of sodium ions.

Source: Refs. 118, 120 and 189–195.

particular neuronal site. The evidence is based on a compilation of histochemical, electrophysiological, biochemical, and behavioral experiments. Most of the classifications of dopamine receptors are based on biochemical evidence and, in particular, on ligand binding studies. A number of different classifications of dopamine receptors have appeared in recent years (Table 4.13).

1. Division of Dopamine Receptors Based on Linkage to Adenylate Cyclase

One hypothesis of multiple dopamine receptors has had a considerable effect on the concepts of neuroleptic drug action. This was that advanced by Kebabian and Calne [189], and it proposed that dopamine receptors may be divided into those linked to the enzyme adenylate cyclase (D-1) and those acting independent of this enzyme (D-2).

The differentiation of dopamine receptors on the basis of their linkage to a dopamine-sensitive adenylate cyclase stems from the discovery that not all dopamine agonists stimulate cyclic AMP formation, and not all dopamine antagonists inhibit dopamine's capacity to stimulate adenylate cyclase activity (see Table 4.14).

Some dopamine agonists, particularly ergot derivatives such as bromocriptine, not only do not stimulate basal adenylate cyclase activity in tissue preparations from dopamine containing brain regions but also inhibit enhancement of cyclic AMP formation induced by dopamine [197].

Neuroleptic drugs of the thioxanthene and phenothiazine classes inhibit dopamine-induced stimulation of adenylate cyclase with a potency consistent with their known antidopamine activity and clinical actions. In contrast, members of the butyrophenone series, such as haloperidol or spiperone, are much weaker antagonists of dopamine-stimulated adenylate cyclase preparations that would be expected from their behavioral or clinical potency [76]. Substituted benzamide drugs, such as sulpiride and metoclopramide, are inactive in blocking adenylate cyclase activity, suggesting that these compounds are selective D-2 antagonists [77,78].

TABLE 4.14 Criteria for D-1 and D-2 Division of Dopamine Receptors

Criteria	D-1	D-2
Cyclase linkage	Yes	No
Occupancy by agonist	Enhances cyclic AMP formation	No enhancement of cyclic AMP formation
Occupancy by antagonist	Inhibits cyclic AMP formation	Enhances cyclic AMP formation
Dopamine	Agonist (uM potency)	Agonist (nM potency)
Apomorphine	Partial agonist (uM potency)	Agonist (nM potency)
Dopaminergic ergots	Antagonist (uM potency)	Agonist (nM potency)
Selective antagonists	None	Substituted benzamides
Radiolabeled ligand	[^{3}H]-cis-flupenthixol or [^{3}H]piflutixol (in presence high concentration sulpiride or domperidone)	[^{3}H]spiperone [^{3}H]sulpiride [^{3}H]domperidone

Source: Modified from Refs. 189 and 196.

The existence of adenylate cyclase-linked and adenylate cyclase-independent receptors is supported by differential labeling by different dopamine ligands. [^{3}H]Haloperidol and [^{3}H]spiperone can be used to label D-2 receptors in concentrations that are 1000 times lower than those required to inhibit adenylate cyclase activity [98]. Newer ligands such as [^{3}H]sulpiride and [^{3}H]domperidone can be used to label D-2 receptors even more selectively, for they do not inhibit adenylate cyclase. No selective ligands are available to identify D-1 receptors specifically but [^{3}H]*cis*-flupenthioxol and [^{3}H]piflutixol label both D-1 and D-2 receptors with more or less equal affinity [199, 200]. Using a selective D-2 antagonist, such as domperidone or sulpiride, in high concentrations to mask D-2 receptors, it is possible to examine selectively D-1 receptors with [^{3}H]*cis*-flupenthixol or [^{3}H]-piflutixol. The ability of neuroleptic drugs to inhibit adenylate cyclase activity correlates with their ability to displace [^{3}H]*cis*-flupenthixol or [^{3}H]pifluxtiol from their specific binding sites in rat striatal preparations [98].

The division of dopamine receptors into those linked to adenylate cyclase and those acting independently of this enzyme allows the opportunity for selective drug action. Recently, a selective D-1 agonist (SKF 38393) and a selective D-2 agonist (LY 141685) have been introduced [201,202]. A number of selective D-2 receptor antagonists are available (see above). However, at the present time there is no selective D-1 receptor antagonist. Why it should be possible to produce drugs selective at one site and not the other is not clear, but some indications of the parameters necessary for selective drug action have been evolved recently. This evidence is based mainly on the use of sulpiride and other substituted benzamide drugs which, in general, appear to be selective antagonists of those receptors not linked to adenylate cyclase.

The inability of sulpiride to inhibit adenylate cyclase may be related to its difficulty in transversing a lipid barrier beyond which adenylate cyclase lies [203]. This would be consistent with current concepts of the adenylate cyclase enzyme being at least partially embedded into the lipid membrane [204]. This idea is based on the poor penetration of the blood-brain barrier by sulpiride and its relatively low lipid solubility. On this basis, larger, more lipophilic substituted benzamide drugs would be expected to inhibit cyclic AMP formation. However, increasing the lipid solubility of substituted benzamide to an extent that is equivalent to that of classical neuroleptic compounds does not necessarily confer action at D-1 receptors. When the neuroleptic drugs are ranked in order of lipid solubility and compared for their actions at D-1 and D-2 receptors, it is clear a log P value of greater than 2 is required for actions at D-1 receptors; therefore, lipid solubility is important to some extent [205]. However, beyond this critical point, there is no absolute correlation between lipid solubility and the ability to interact with D-1 receptors. This suggests that other structural features of the molecules are critical for action at D-1 sites. Using such characteristics, it may become feasible to produce a drug acting selectively at adenylate cyclase-linked receptors.

Recent evidence also suggests that D-1 and D-2 receptors may not be completely independent entities. In some circumstances, activation of D-2 receptors is inhibitory on D-1 receptor function. Stimulation of cyclic AMP formation in striatal prisms by apomorphine or by a selective D-1 agonist SKF 38393 is potentiated by the selective blockade of D-2 receptors using sulpiride [206]. This suggests that an intimate relationship exists between the function of D-1 and D-2 receptors such that they serve to regulate each other's functions. This idea is consistent with evidence from the pituitary where a D-2 receptor is able to decrease the activity of isoprenaline-sensitive adenylate cyclase systems [207].

2. Division of Adenylate Cyclase-Independent Receptors Based on Agonist-Antagonist Sensitivity

Various other concepts of the division of brain dopamine receptors have been proposed. All recognize the existence of the dopamine receptor linked to adenylate cyclase. These schemes differ from each other in the manner in which they further divide adenylate cyclase-independent receptors. In general terms, there are three types of adenylate cyclase independent dopamine receptors:

1. A population of receptors with high affinity for dopamine antagonists and low affinity for dopamine agonists
2. A population of receptors with high affinity for dopamine agonists but low affinity for dopamine antagonists
3. A population of receptors with high affinity for both dopamine agonists and antagonists

All classifications recognize a class of receptor site with high affinity for dopamine agonists but low affinity for antagonist compounds (class 2). These sites are, in general, termed D-3 receptors and are thought to lie selectively on presynaptic dopamine terminals in the striatum.

The other sites recognized differ in their affinity for agonists but show high affinity for antagonists. These sites have received varying terminology, as shown in Table 4.14. The main differences of opinion lie in whether such receptors are affected by guanine nucleotides or whether they might exist in interconvertible high- and low-affinity forms [208,209].

At the present time, there is no clear consensus of opinion as to whether these different binding sites represent dopamine receptors or not (see below).

One of the major difficulties in differentiating between the various adenylate cyclase-independent sites is the lack of selective drugs for such receptors. In general, it does not appear that compounds are available that show sufficient selectivity to allow differentiation of binding sites. However, Sokoloff and colleagues [194] have claimed that sulpiride may show up to five times greater affinity for the D-4 site compared with their D-2 site, whereas classical neuroleptics such as haloperidol show equal affinity for both binding sites. These data, however, remain to be replicated.

A major argument has ensued from the subdivision of brain dopamine receptors as to whether agonist and antagonist ligands label different sites. Comparison of the specific binding of antagonist ligands such as [^{3}H]spiperone with that of agonist ligands such as [^{3}H]*N*,*n*-propylnorapomorphine, have yielded variable results [210,211]. Unfortunately, the technique of agonist binding requires precise methodology, and the variations in techniques utilized have led to a state of confusion. Our own studies would suggest that agonist and antagonist binding sites may be distinct if not independent entities. However, whether the antagonist and agonist forms are functionally distinct dopamine receptors or whether they represent different subunits of a single dopamine receptor, as suggested by Leysen [212], remains to be resolved.

3. Division of Dopamine Receptors Based on the Role of Sodium Ions

One further subclassification of dopamine receptors in striatum is worthy of mention, namely, that based on the sodium dependency of the interaction of neuroleptic ligands with striatal preparations. This division is based on two fundamental observations. First the interaction of [^{3}H]sulpiride with its specific binding site shows an absolute requirement for the presence of sodium ions in the incubation buffer [118,119]. This effect is specific for sodium ions; it cannot be replaced by other ions in equimolar concentrations. Second, the ability to displace specific binding of [^{3}H]spiperone by sulpiride (and substituted benzamide drugs in general) is decreased by the omission of sodium ions from the incubation buffer [120] (Table 4.15). The ability of other classes of neuroleptic drugs to displace the specific binding of [^{3}H]spiperone is unaffected by sodium. The effect of sodium is to cause an alteration in the number of available [^{3}H]sulpiride-binding sites rather than a change in receptor affinity [119]. Why this is so

TABLE 4.15 The Ability of Drugs to Displace [^{3}H]Spiperone (0.5 nM) Striatal Membranes in the Presence and Absence of 120 nM Sodium Chloride

	K_1 (nM)	
Drug	120 mM Sodium chloride	No sodium chloride
Fluphenazine	5.4 ± 1.4	7.9 ± 1.7
(+)-Butaclamol	2.8 ± 0.9	4.0 ± 0.8
Haloperidol	13.1 ± 3.0	15.7 ± 2.6
Clebopride	36 ± 11	6400 ± 1100
Sultopride	116 ± 42	21,900 ± 4600
(−)-Sulpiride	203 ± 21	>40,000
Tiapride	249 ± 72	>40,000
(−)-Butaclamol	16,900 ± 4300	29,000 ± 5000
(+)-Sulpiride	18,700 ± 4900	>40,000

Source: Ref. 120.

is not understood. It is possible that [^{3}H]sulpiride labels a different portion of the dopamine receptor complex from that identified by [^{3}H]-spiperone. The existence of different sites is suggested also by the differing ontogeny of [^{3}H]spiperone-binding sites in rat striatum and the sodium dependency of sulpiride displacement of this ligand [213]. In addition, although a progressive loss of striatal [^{3}H]spiperone-binding sites occurs with age in the rat, no such decrease is apparent in [^{3}H]sulpiride binding [214]. Whatever the mechanism underlying sodium effects, they may be of critical importance in understanding how substituted benzamide drugs such as sulpiride interact with their receptor sites in vivo.

These data at least might suggest that one class of neuroleptic drugs can exert a selective action on one population of the adenylate cyclase-independent dopamine receptors. There is at least some evidence to suggest that the sodium-dependent binding sites may be related to those of D-2 receptor population that are inhibitory on adenylate cyclase activity, even though they do not act directly through this enzyme system. Thus, guanine nucleotides that are involved in the coupling of D-1 receptors to adenylate cyclase also act in vitro to reduce the affinity of dopamine agonists for D-2 sites in a sodium-dependent manner [215]. It is possible that there is a distinct sodium-dependent population of D-2 receptors present in brain that exerts inhibitory control on adenylate cyclase activity. At the present time, this is a hypothesis that remains to be tested.

B. Location of Dopamine Receptors within the Nigrostriatal Complex

The division of dopamine receptors into distinct classes may be of importance to neuroleptic drug action if such receptors can be shown to be located at different anatomical sites within the dopamine-containing areas of the brain. So far, only the striatum and substantia nigra have been investigated to any extent so we will confine ourselves to what is known of this area of the brain. It is perhaps surprising that the type of study to be described has not been applied to either the mesolimbic or mesocortical dopamine containing regions.

Schwarcz and his colleagues [170] first demonstrated a differential localization of dopamine receptors within the striatum. They found that kainic acid lesions of the striatum to destroy dopamine receptors lying on striatal cell bodies caused a loss of both [^{3}H]haloperidol binding and of dopamine-sensitive adenylate cyclase activity (Table 4.16). In contrast, they found that removal of parietal and frontal areas of the cerebral cortex to destroy cortico-striate glutamate fibers led to a loss of [^{3}H]haloperidol binding in striatum but no change in adenylate cyclase activity. These results were interpreted as showing the existence of dopamine receptors linked to adenylate cyclase on striatal cell bodies, and dopamine receptors acting independently of adenylate cyclase located on the terminals of cortico-striate fibers. However, the concentrations of [^{3}H]haloperidol that were employed would preferentially have labeled D-2 receptors. So a reappraisal of their data suggests that both D-1 and D-2 receptors are located on striatal cell bodies. Subsequently, Creese and colleagues [169] showed that 6-hydroxydopamine lesions of the medial forebrain bundle to remove presynaptic dopamine terminals led to an increase in binding of [^{3}H]-haloperidol, from which they surmised that D-2 receptors were located postsynaptically and increased in number as a result of development of denervation supersensitivity. The results of other investigations have, in general, confirmed this distribution of neuroleptic ligand binding sites, as portrayed in Fig. 4.7.

More recent evidence has been produced to support the idea that D-1 and D-2 receptors are located on striatal cell bodies. Comparison was made of the effects of kainic acid lesions of striatum on the specific binding of [^{3}H]*cis*-flupenthixol to D-1 and D-2 receptors compared with the specific binding of [^{3}H]spiperone to D-2 receptors only [216]. Lesions resulted in the greater loss of [^{3}H]*cis*-flupenthixol

TABLE 4.16 The Effect of Kainic Acid Lesions of Striatum and Cortical Ablation on Dopamine Receptors in Rat Striatum

Lesion (time after lesion)	$[^3H]$haloperidol binding	% Control values			
		Adenylate cyclase	Tyrosine hydroxylase	Choline acetyl transferase	Glutamic acid decarboxylase
Kainic acid (22 days)	64 ± 3[a]	13 ± 8[a]	97 ± 4[a]	49 ± 4[a]	42 ± 7[a]
Cortical ablation (5 days)	68 ± 5[a]	84 ± 12	101 ± 3	73 ± 4[a]	99 ± 7
Kainic acid and cortical ablation	30 ± 5[a]	–	120 ± 9	39 ± 6[a]	41 ± 6[a]

[a] $p < 0.05$ compared with control animals.
Source: Ref. 170.

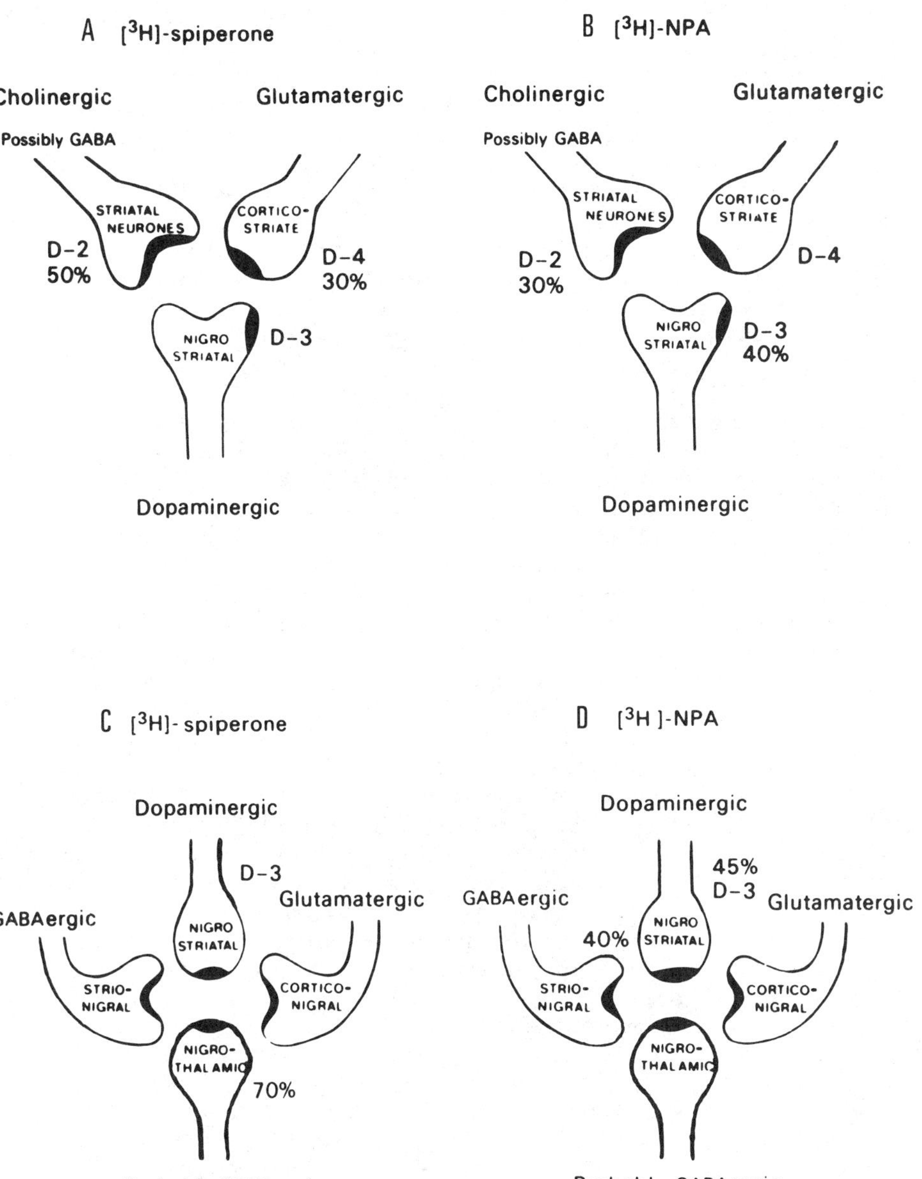

FIG. 4.7 Summary diagram of the possible anatomical location of [^{3}H]spiperone and [^{3}H]NPA binding sites in rat striatum (A and B) and in rat substantia nigra (C and D) as determined from the binding data. (From Ref. 222.)

binding sites than [^{3}H]spiperone-binding sites. The greater loss of [^{3}H]*cis*-flupenthixol-binding sites suggests this ligand to identify sites other than those labeled by D-2-selective ligands such as [^{3}H]-spiperone. The 73% fall in [^{3}H]*cis*-flupenthixol binding corresponds closely to the percentage loss of adenylate cyclase activity reported by Schwarcz and colleagues [170]. The conclusion from these experiments must be that both D-1 and D-2 receptors are located on striatal cell bodies.

In contrast to neuroleptic binding sites, there is considerable debate as to the exact location of dopamine agonist binding sites within the striatal complex. Destruction of striatal cells with kainic acid is reported to cause a loss of [^{3}H]apomorphine or [^{3}H]*N,n*-propylnorapomorphine (NPA) binding sites, suggesting that these lie partially at this location[217,218]. However, the effect of removal of the nigrostriatal dopamine fibers using the neurotoxin 6-hydroxydopamine has been controversial. Some studies have suggested that the removal of the presynaptic dopamine terminal leads to a marked reduction of the number of agonist-binding sites [219]. Others claim that such lesions have no effect on agonist binding [220]. Many of these differences appear to be related to the in vitro binding technique employed. Our own use of [^{3}H]*N,n*-propylnorapomorphine showed labeling of at least two different sites of striatal dopamine receptors in the experimental conditions we employ [221]. When we carried out lesions of the medial forebrain bundle using 6-hydroxydopamine or kainic acid or of the striatum using kainic acid, we obtained a loss of [^{3}H]NPA binding sites [222], suggesting that at least part of the population labeled by [^{3}H]NPA is located presynaptically (Table 4.17).

More recently, interest has centered on the location of D-2, D-3, and D-4 populations of adenylate cyclase-independent receptors. A comprehensive study of the effects of lesions on these sites has been carried out by Sokoloff and his colleagues [194] (Table 4.18). They found that D-2 receptors were localized on striatal cells since their numbers were decreased following kainic acid lesions of the striatum and increased after 6-hydroxydopamine-induced degeneration of nigrostriatal fibers. In contrast, D-4 receptors were only slightly reduced after kainic acid lesions in the striatum, and a small increase was observed following 6-hydroxydopamine lesions. This suggests that a significant fraction of D-4 receptors are localized on terminals of extrinsic neurons such as the cortico-striate fibers. In contrast, D-3 receptors appear to be, at least in part, autoreceptors. Their numbers were decreased in striatum after 6-hydroxydopamine lesions and were not modified following kainic acid lesions. Where the remaining populations lie is not clear. Sokoloff and colleagues [194] suggested the remaining D-3 receptors are located on the terminals of extrinsic neurons or on intrastriatal cells resistant to kainic acid, but there is no evidence to support either suggestion. Of the adenylate cyclase-

TABLE 4.17 The Effect of Lesions on the Number of Binding Sites (B_{max}) and Equilibrium Dissociation Constants (K_D) for Specific Striatal [^{3}H]N,n-Propylnorapomorphine (0.05–2.0 nM) Binding

Lesion	B_{max} (pmoles/g wet weight tissue)		K_D (nM)	
	Intact	Lesioned	Intact	Lesioned
Unlesioned	17.4 ± 2.0	–	1.10 ± 0.10	–
6-OHDA lesion of MFB	18.9 ± 2.6	11.4 ± 1.3[a] (68%)	1.08 ± 0.11	0.74 ± 0.07[a] (69%)
KA lesion of SN	17.3 ± 1.9	10.4 ± 2.4[a] (59%)	0.88 ± 0.10	0.58 ± 0.13[a] (66%)
KA lesion of striatum	16.3 ± 1.7	11.6 ± 1.4[a] (71%)	0.94 ± 0.10	0.90 ± 0.07 (96%)

Results are expressed as the mean (±1 SEM) of the estimates of B_{max} and K_D from tissue pools of 10 animals performed at least three independent experiments. The values in parentheses represent the data for lesioned hemisphere expressed as a percent of values obtained from intact forebrain. Tissue from lesioned and intact forebrains from the same animals was always compared on the same occasion and in strict parallel.

[a] $p < 0.01$ compared with striatal preparations from the intact forebrain using a two-tailed Student's t-test.

Source: Ref. 222.

TABLE 4.18 The Effect of Kainic Acid and Lesions of Striatum and 6-Hydroxydopamine (6-OHDA) Lesion of the Medial Forebrain Bundle on Specific Binding of [^{3}H]Apomorphine or [^{3}H]Domperidone to D-2, D-3, and D-4 Receptors in Striatal Preparations

	% Control values			
	[^{3}H]Apomorphine		[^{3}H]Domperidone	
Lesion (time after lesion)	D-2	D-3	D-2	D-4
Kainic acid (10–15 days)	43 ± 9[a]	97 ± 13	45 ± 12[a]	83 ± 3[a]
6-OHDA	139 ± 10[a]	71 ± 4[a]	100 ± 6	117 ± 5[a]

[a] $p < 0.05$ compared with control animals.
Source: Ref. 194.

independent receptor sites, only D-2 and D-4 receptors show high affinity for neuroleptic drugs, suggesting that these are the major sites of action of neuroleptic agents.

The localization of dopamine receptors within the substantia nigra is less clear. A major difficulty is the small amount of tissue that can be utilized for ligand-binding experiments, so that, in general, only a single ligand concentration can be employed rather than a range of concentrations so as to obtain an accurate estimation of the number of binding sites present. Early studies suggested that 6-hydroxydopamine lesions of the medial forebrain bundle or substantia nigra decreased [^{3}H]spiperone binding, suggesting an association between D-2 sites and dopamine-containing cell bodies [223,224]. However, our own findings [222] on the effects of lesions on [^{3}H]spiperone binding in nigral tissue are not in agreement with these previous reports (Table 4.19). Thus, after destruction of dopamine cell bodies using 6-hydroxydopamine, we obtained a 75% increase in specific [^{3}H]spiperone binding. There are differences, however, between the earlier studies and our own work that might explain this discrepancy. We used a saturating concentration of [^{3}H]spiperone to detect changes in B_{max}, whereas other studies used subsaturation ligand concentrations that would more readily detect alterations in the dissociation constant, K_D, than changes in receptor numbers. Whether such changes occur is unknown. Differences in the time allowed following the lesion for neuronal adaptation also might be of importance. The study showing decreased binding was performed at 7 or 14 days following surgery, whereas we allowed 21 days which had previously been shown effective in striatum. It is conceivable that 6-hydroxydopamine lesions did cause a loss of [^{3}H]spiperone binding sites on nigral cell bodies but that this was compensated for by proliferation of dopamine receptors at other sites within nigra due to loss of nigral dopamine release. An alternative explanation is that a change in dopamine receptor numbers and dissociation constant occurs within nigra with time after lesioning, as has been demonstrated in striatum following 6-hydroxydopamine lesions.

Whatever the explanation, the present results suggest that considerable numbers of dopamine receptors in substantia nigra are to be found at locations other than on dopamine cell bodies. Following kainic acid lesions in the striatum, we observed an increase in nigral [^{3}H]spiperone binding. This suggests that few dopamine receptors labeled by [^{3}H]spiperone are found on the terminals of the strio-nigral fibers and that a considerable number have another anatomical location within substantia nigra. This is supported by the dramatic decrease in specific [^{3}H]spiperone binding caused by kainic acid lesions of substantia nigra. Such lesions destroy the dopamine-containing cell bodies of zona compacta as well as nondopamine cell bodies in both zona compacta and reticulata. We observed no loss of [^{3}H]-spiperone binding after 6-hydroxydopamine lesions, so the conclusion must be that the majority of these binding sites are located on non-dopamine-containing cell bodies. These might either be the cell bodies of GABA-containing outflow pathways to the thalamus and reticular formation, or GABA interneurons within substantia nigra.

Cortical ablation did not decrease [^{3}H]spiperone binding in nigral tissue, but did cause an increase. This result suggests that the majority of nigral dopamine receptors do not lie on such terminals, in contrast to significant proportion found on the terminals of corticofugal fibers in striatum. Why dopamine receptors should increase in number in response to the apparent loss of cortical efferents is not clear.

Specific [^{3}H]NPA binding in nigra showed a different pattern of change following the various lesions. Destruction of the medial forebrain bundle using 6-hydroxydopamine caused a loss of specific [^{3}H]-NPA binding, which would be consistent with location of agonist-labeled dopamine receptors on dopamine neurons. Kainic acid lesions of substantia nigra caused a similar loss of specific [^{3}H]NPA binding. This also may represent loss of agonist sites on dopamine cell bodies, but the possibility that some sites may lie on nondopamine cell bodies in nigra cannot be excluded. Some [^{3}H]NPA-binding sites appear to lie on the terminals of strio-nigral fibers for kainic acid lesions of striatum caused a loss of specific [^{3}H]NPA binding. In contrast, decortication failed to alter [^{3}H]NPA binding in nigra, again suggesting

TABLE 4.19 The Effects of Lesions on Specific [^{3}H]Spiperone (4.0 nM) or [^{3}H]NPA (2.0 nM) Binding to Tissue Preparations of Substantia Nigra from Lesioned and Intact Forebrain

	[^{3}H]Spiperone specific binding (pmoles/g wet weight tissue)			[^{3}H]NPA specific binding (pmoles/g wet weight tissue)		
	Intact	Lesioned		Intact	Lesioned	
6-OHDA lesion of MFB	2.11	3.77	(179%)	5.78	2.56	(44%)
	2.32	4.05	(175%)	4.87	2.77	(57%)
	2.76	4.90	(177%)	5.45	3.64	(67%)
	2.40 ± 0.19	4.25 ± 34[a]	(177%)	6.37 ± 0.27	2.99 ± 0.33[a]	(56%)
Kanic acid lesion of SN	1.89	0.59	(31%)	4.72	2.74	(58%)
	2.70	1.06	(39%)	4.71	3.37	(72%)
	3.68	1.12	(30%)	5.74	3.72	(65%)
	2.76 ± 0.52	0.92 ± 0.17[a]	(33%)	5.06 ± 0.34	3.28 ± 0.29[a]	(65%)

Kanic acid lesion of striatum	2.69	4.54	(169%)	5.16	3.06	(59%)
	2.60	3.79	(146%)	5.04	2.99	(59%)
	2.42	3.74	(155%)	6.05	3.65	(60%)
	2.57 ± 0.08	4.02 ± 0.26[a]	(156%)	5.42 ± 0.32	3.23 ± 0.21[a]	(60%)
Decortication	3.09	4.23	(137%)	5.97	5.87	(90%)
	2.62	3.45	(132%)	5.00	4.68	(94%)
	2.86	3.84	(134%)	5.49	5.28	(96%)

Results given are from three individual experiments; also shown are the mean (±1 SEM) for binding to substantia nigra from lesioned and intact forebrain. Each determination was the mean of triplicate estimates on pooled substantia nigra tissue from 10 animals per experiment. For decortication, only two experiments were performed. The values in parentheses represent the data from lesioned hemispheres expressed in percent of values obtained for the intact forebrain.

[a] $p < 0.05$ compared with substantia nigra preparations from intact forebrain using a two-tailed Student's *t*-test.

Source: Ref. 222.

that dopamine agonist receptors do not lie on the terminals of cortico-nigral fibers. The conclusion from the studies of the anatomical location of dopamine receptors within the striatum and substantia nigra, based on lesioning techniques, must be that agonist and antagonist binding sites do not lie at identical sites. Dopamine receptors exist at a number of different sites within each of these two brain regions, but the distribution of agonist and antagonist binding sites is not identical within these two areas. The function of the various binding sites remains uncertain and further study is required to determine whether the binding technique identified physiological receptors. Lastly, the effects of lesions on the number of binding sites may not necessarily reflect only the removal of the particular element for, as pointed out by Hattori and Fibiger [225], adaptive changes may occur so as to mask the true effect on receptor population.

C. Relative Involvement of Different Neuroleptic Receptor Populations in Behavioral Change Induced by Neuroleptic Drugs

As pointed out previously, different dopamine-mediated behaviors may originate from different dopamine-containing regions of the brain. However, only within the striatum has any attempt been made to correlate the action of neuroleptics on subclasses of specific dopamine receptors with their behavioral effects. There is no correlation between the ability of neuroleptic drugs to inhibit dopamine-mediated behaviors and their actions on D-1 adenylate cyclase-linked receptors [195]. An obvious correlation exists between the acute motor inhibitory properties of neuroleptics, both in animals and in man, and activity at D-2 receptors as measured by [^{3}H]spiperone or [^{3}H]haloperidol binding (Fig. 4.8) [164,226].

Attempts have been made to relate neuroleptic actions to the different adenylate cyclase-independent receptor populations within the striatal complex. Neuroleptic-induced catalepsy is thought to originate from striatum, and lesions of this area have been carried out to localize the neuronal elements involved (Table 4.20). However, no agreement has been reached as to whether it is dopamine receptors located on the striatal cells or those on the terminals of cortico-striate glutamate fibers that are responsible for catalepsy. Sanberg [229,230] showed gross kainic acid lesions of the striatum to virtually abolish haloperidol-induced catalepsy whereas the more discrete lesions of Zarkovsky and colleagues [232] did not prevent haloperidol-induced catalepsy.

Sokoloff and colleagues [194,233] have employed a different approach to dissect out the receptor populations involved in various dopamine-mediated behaviors. They compared the ability of a range of neuroleptic drugs to inhibit binding of radioactive ligands to D-2 and D-4 receptors,

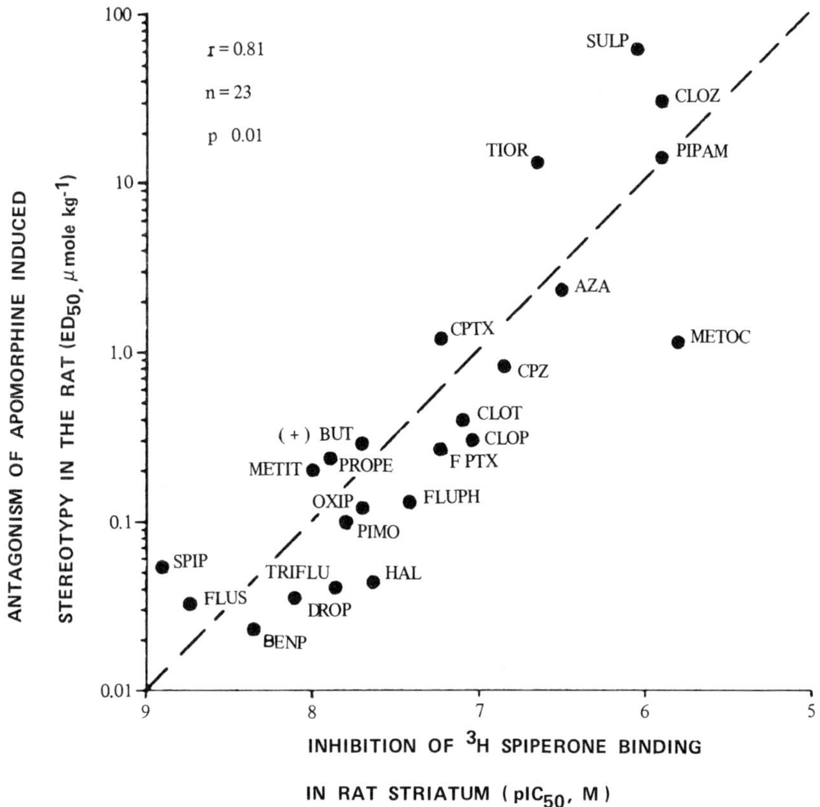

FIG. 4.8 Comparison of the ability of a range of neuroleptic drugs to inhibit apomorphine-induced sterotyped behavior and to displace [^{3}H]spiperone from specific binding sites in rat striatal preparations. (From Ref. 164.)

which are those with a high affinity for neuroleptics (Table 4.21). Although the neuroleptics such as haloperidol have equivalent activity in displacing ligands from both D-2 and D-4 sites, sulpiride exhibited a five times greater ability to interact with D-4 than with D-2 receptors. They then compare the ability of sulpiride and haloperidol to inhibit two dopamine-mediated behaviors, namely apomorphine-induced stereotypy and apomorphine-induced climbing in rats. Haloperidol was equally active in inhibiting both behaviors, but sulpiride was five times more effective in inhibiting climbing behavior. The correlation between sulpiride's action on D-4 receptors and its ability to inhibit climbing behavior suggests that the latter

TABLE 4.20 Effect of Lesions of Striatal Components on the Production of Catalepsy by Neuroleptic Drugs

Author	Lesion	Effect on neuroleptic-induced catalepsy
Costall and Naylor [227]	Electrolytic lesion striatum	Reduced
Carter and Pycock [228]	Electrolytic cortical lesion	Reduced
Sandberg et al. [229,230]	Kainic acid lesion of striatum	Reduced
	Decortication	Enhanced
Bartholini et al. [231]	Decortication	Reduced
Zarkovsky et al. [232]	Kainic acid lesion of striatum	No effect

is mediated by D-4 dopamine receptors lying on the terminals of the cortico-striate glutamate fibers. Stereotyped behavior, on the other hand, may be due to stimulation of postsynaptic D-2 dopamine receptors on the striatal cells. Our own studies have shown that following kainic acid lesions of the striatum, to leave cortico-glutamate

TABLE 4.21 Comparison of the Ability of Haloperidol and Sulpiride to Interact with D-2 and D-4 Receptors with Inhibition of Dopamine-Mediated Behavior

	K_i (nM)			ID_{50} (mg/kg)		
Drug	D-2	D-4	Ratio/ D-2 D-4	Stereotypy	Climbing behavior	Ratio
Haloperidol	6	4	1.5	0.10	0.07	1.4
Sulpiride	94	17	5.5	90	19	4.7

Source: Refs. 194 and 233.

fibers intact, the remaining dopamine receptor populations have an unchanged affinity for haloperidol but a greater affinity for [^{3}H]-sulpiride.

Sokoloff and colleagues [234] recently have extended these findings by comparing other properties of sulpiride as a dopamine antagonist to those of typical neuroleptic compounds. Sulpiride is relatively weak in inhibiting gnawing, licking, and sniffing and in inducing catalepsy so these behaviors are classified as D-2 receptor responses. In contrast, sulpiride inhibits locomotor activity and climbing behavior, so these are classified as D-4 receptor responses.

VI. ADAPTATIONS OF DOPAMINE RECEPTOR FUNCTION TO NEUROLEPTIC DRUG ADMINISTRATION

The acute administration of neuroleptic drugs causes blockade of cerebral dopamine receptors. Repeated administration of neuroleptic drugs to rodents for several weeks continues to antagonize many effects of dopamine agonists, although some tolerance to both the acute behavioral and biochemical actions of such compounds occurs (Table 4.22). Studies in the striatal, mesolimbic, and mesocortical dopamine-containing areas suggests tolerance, at least to the compensatory increase in dopamine turnover, occurs in all regions [240,244].

Interest in the adaptation of dopamine neuronal function to the presence of neuroleptic drugs has centered on the development of dopamine receptor supersensitivity. Studies with rodents have shown that supersensitivity can occur after:

1. A single dose of neuroleptic drug
2. After brief periods of repeated neuroleptic administration and subsequent drug withdrawal
3. During chronic continuous neuroleptic treatment

This response to neuroleptic treatment may be looked upon as compensation for receptor blockade. Ultimately, it is a result of change in the nature of the dopamine receptor population so as to produce an exaggeration of the responses elicited by the application of agonist compounds. Such changes may be of importance not only to the antipsychotic action of neuroleptic drugs but also to the subsequent appearance of extrapyramidal disturbances.

A. Acute Neuroleptic Administration

The development of acute adaptive changes to neuroleptic drugs has been demonstrated behaviorally both in rats and mice. Normal mice

TABLE 4.22 Tolerance to the Acute Dopamine Receptor Blocking Properties of Neuroleptic Drugs on Repeated Neuroleptic Administration

Behavior

Inhibition of catalepsy reversed [235]

Inhibition of apomorphine-induced stereotypy decreased [236]

Inhibition of apomorphine-induced locomotion reversed [237]

Inhibition of apomorphine-induced climbing reversed [238]

Inhibition of apomorphine-induced circling reversed [239]

Biochemistry

Tolerance to increased dopamine turnover [240,241]

Tolerance to initial inhibition of dopamine-stimulated adenylate cyclase [242]

Electrophysiology

Tolerance to increased spontaneous firing of dopamine neurons [245]

given methylphenidate show a stereotyped gnawing response, but normal mice given apomorphine show no gnawing response. In animals treated with a single dose of a variety of neuroleptic drugs, there is initial inhibition of methylphenidate-induced gnawing while apomorphine remains ineffective. After some 2 days, at a time when inhibition of methylphenidate-induced gnawing disappears, apomorphine then induces a gnawing response in these animals [245]. Similarly, following the administration of a single dose of haloperidol to mice, the initial inhibition of apomorphine-induced climbing behavior is followed some 3 days later by an exaggerated response to the administration of apomorphine [246] (Fig. 4.9). In rats, the development of single dose supersensitivity is less marked. However, we and others [247,248] have demonstrated that the administration of a single dose of neuroleptic drugs, such as haloperidol or butaperazine, to rats results in initial inhibition of apomorphine-induced stereotyped behavior which is followed, 2 days later, by a transient increase in the behavioral response of these animals to apomorphine.

The supersensitivity appearing after a single dose of neuroleptic drug is associated with a reduction in the ability of neuroleptic agents to antagonize postsynaptic dopamine receptors. In mice treated 4 days previously with a single dose of teflutixol [249], the doses of a range

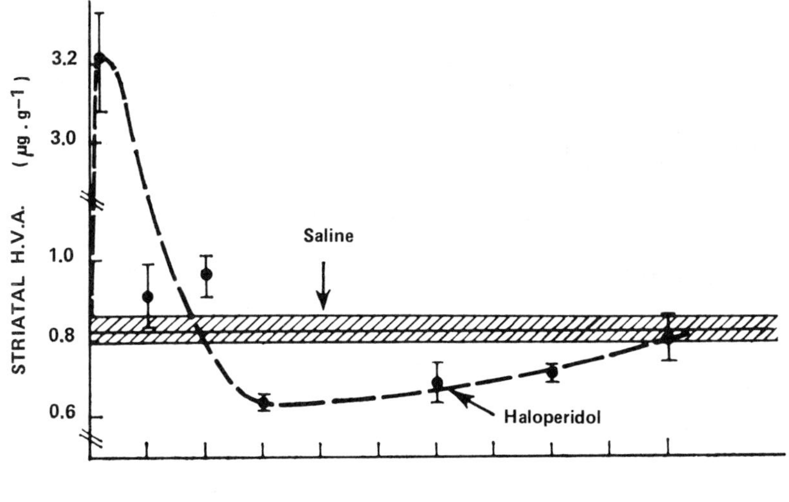

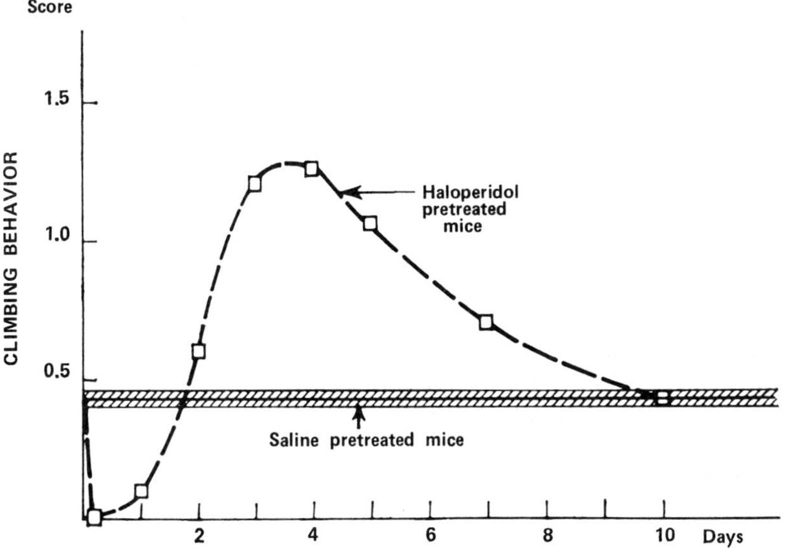

FIG. 4.9 Time course of behavioral and biochemical changes after a single administration of haloperidol [246]. (*Upper curve*) Striatal HVA level measured at different time intervals after a single i.p. injection of 4 mg/kg haloperidol. Means ± SEM of 6–12 determinations. The shaded area represents the mean ± SEM of HVA levels in 20–30 control mice. (*Lower curve*) The climbing behavior scored (quantal mode) after the S.C. injection of a test dose of 0.45 mg/kg apomorphine at various time intervals after the treatment by 4 mg/kg haloperidol. Means of 15–30 experiments. The shaded area represents the mean ± SEM of responses in 20–30 controls.

of neuroleptic drugs that were required to antagonize methylphenidate-induced gnawing were approximately 10-fold greater than required in saline-treated animals. There is some evidence to suggest that a change in the postsynaptic dopamine receptor population occurs under such conditions. Thus, following the administration of α-methyl-*p*-tyrosine 16 hr previously (so producing dopamine depletion), mice exhibited an enhanced climbing response following administration of apomorphine. This enhanced response decayed progressively over the following 3 days. Administration of either cycloheximide or anisomycin, both of which are protein synthesis inhibitors, prevented this α-methyl-*p*-tyrosine-induced increase in behavioral responsiveness to apomorphine [246]. Although these data are open to criticism on the grounds that the protein synthesis inhibitors employed have a wide spectrum of activity, they suggest that the synthesis of a new receptor protein is necessary for the expression of enhanced behavioral response to apomorphine.

There have been various attempts made to detect the biochemical correlate of the increased behavioral response occurring following acute neuroleptic administration (Table 4.23). During the period of acute receptor blockade, increased dopamine turnover occurs, but at the time when supersensitivity to apomorphine is apparent

TABLE 4.23 Striatal Biochemical Parameters Unchanged following Administration of a Single Dose of Haloperidol, Butaperazine, or Teflutixol to Rats or Mice (24–96 hr after drug treatment) and at a Time When Animals Exhibit Behavioral Supersensitivity

[^{3}H]Haloperidol binding [250]
[^{3}H]Spiperone binding [251]
[^{3}H]Domperidone binding [252]
[^{3}H]Piflutixol binding [251]
Dopamine-stimulated adenylate cyclase activity [250,251]
[^{3}H]Acetylcholine release [251]
[^{3}H]Dopamine release [251]
[^{3}H]Glutamate release [251]
[^{3}H]QNB binding [250]
[^{3}H]GABA binding [250]

there is decreased dopamine synthesis and release [252]. This rebound decrease in dopamine synthesis may be due to the development of postsynaptic dopamine receptor supersensitivity. Attempts to demonstrate change in the number and sensitivity of post-synaptic dopamine recetpors have been singularly unsuccessful. No change occurs in the specific binding of [^{3}H]haloperidol or [^{3}H]spiperone to D-2 receptors or of [^{3}H]piflutixol to D-1 receptors, at the time of behavioral supersensitivity. Similarly, there is no evidence of change in either basal or dopamine-stimulated adenylate cyclase activity. It could be that changes in the influence of other neurotransmitter systems upon dopamine function are altered by single-dose neuroleptic treatment. However, no changes in muscarinic or GABA receptor binding have been found, and we have recently demonstrated that striatal [^{3}H]dopamine, [^{3}H]acetylcholine, and [^{3}H]-glutamate release from striatal preparations was unaltered in animals treated acutely with haloperidol. If changes in receptor numbers cannot be demonstrated then some subtle change in receptor affinity must occur (although this is yet to be detected), or there might be changes in the degree of receptor occupancy that have yet to be measured.

Lastly, one must consider the possibility that the enhanced behavioral response to apomorphine seen in rats and mice has nothing to do with a change in neuronal function. It is feasible that the administration of a single dose of a neuroleptic might enhance the cerebral penetration of dopamine agonists such as apomorphine so as to produce apparently an enhanced behavioral response. Nobody appears to have measured apomorphine levels in the brains of rodents treated using the protocols described in the above experiments. The only evidence available, however, suggests that neuroleptics might prevent the entry of apomorphine into brain [253].

B. Brief Periods of Repeated Neuroleptic Administration (with or without Subsequent Drug Withdrawal)

The development of dopamine receptor supersensitivity following administration of neuroleptic drugs in most rodent species is seen after repeated administration of neuroleptic agents for a period of some weeks followed by a few days drug withdrawal. Under these conditions, there is much evidence to suggest proliferation of dopamine receptors at the time when the animals show exaggerated behavioral responses to dopamine agonists [see Ref. 254]. There is also some evidence to suggest that some of these adaptive changes can occur while neuroleptic administration continues over a period of a few weeks. In this section, we will review the evidence supporting the ability of brief periods of repeated neuroleptic administration to alter dopamine receptor function.

In the rat, following brief repeated neuroleptic treatment and subsequent drug withdrawal, a pattern of enhancement of spontaneous and apomorphine-induced motor behaviors is observed (Table 4.24). Rats treated in this manner show enhanced spontaneous and apomorphine-induced locomotion, enhanced apomorphine-induced stereotyped behavior (in particular licking, gnawing, and biting), and enhancement of apomorphine-induced rotation in animals with a prior 6-hydroxydopamine lesion of the nigro-striatal pathway.

The increase in the higher-grade components of stereotyped behavior is taken as an index of increased dopamine receptor sensitivity within the striatal complex. This is verified by the fact that kainic acid lesions of the striatum prevent the increase in apomorphine-induced stereotypy [264], whereas direct bilateral injection of dopamine into striatum induced a stereotyped gnawing behavior that is not seen in naive animals [265]. Supersensitivity also appears to occur in mesolimbic areas, particularly the nucleus accumbens. Bilateral injection of dopamine into the nucleus accumbens produced a greater locomotor response in animals pretreated with neuroleptic

TABLE 4.24 Evidence for the Development of Dopamine Receptor Supersensitivity following Repeated Neuroleptic Administration and Subsequent Drug Withdrawal

Behavior
Enhanced apomorphine-induced stereotypy [255]
Enhanced apomorphine-induced locomotion [256]
Enhanced apomorphine-induced climbing behavior [257]
Enhanced apomorphine-induced circling in rats with unilateral 6-OHDA lesions of the nigro-striatal pathway [258]
Biochemistry
Decreased dopamine turnover [259]
Increased numbers of dopamine receptors [260]
Increased dopamine stimulation of adenylate cyclase activity [257][a]
Electrophysiology
Increased inhibition of striatal cells by iontophoretic application of dopamine or apomorphine [263]

[a]Not found in all studies [261,262].

drugs than it does in control animals [266]. At the present time, there would appear to be no information on the effect of repeated neuroleptic administration on the sensitivity of cortical dopamine receptors.

Behavioral supersensitivity in mice is apparent without withdrawal of neuroleptic treatment. Thus, administration of apomorphine to animals undergoing daily teflutixol administration resulted in compulsive gnawing [267]. This effect was even more marked in animals examined 24 hr after the last dosage of teflutixol. When considering the implications of these experiments, it must be remembered that apomorphine in normal circumstances will not induce stereotyped gnawing in the mouse, unlike the rat. The implication of this is that the change represents the induction of a new behavior rather than the exaggeration of an existing behavior.

The apparent behavioral supersensitivity to dopamine receptor agonists is accompanied by changes in either the number or affinity or the dopamine receptors present in the brain. There have been numerous reports that the brief repeated administration of neuroleptic drugs, in particular haloperidol, for some weeks and subsequent drug withdrawal for a few days results in increased specific binding of tritiated neuroleptic ligands to dopamine receptors in rat striatal preparations (Table 4.25).

There is general agreement that brief repeated neuroleptic administration and subsequent drug withdrawal causes an increase in D-2 receptor populations. Receptor affinity appears unaltered provided drug removal is complete. Such changes have been reported in the striatal and mesolimbic area but a recent report suggests that cortical dopamine receptors may not increase in number in response to such pharmacological manipulation [274].

The ability of neuroleptics to elevate striatal dopamine receptor numbers is a function of the dose administered. However, the increase in the number of receptors is only approximately twofold over a 100-fold dose range [275]. The duration of neuroleptic administration is also important, since continuing increases in binding occur with increasing duration of treatment. The extent to which the increase in receptor numbers persists following drug withdrawal is a function of the duration of treatment. Calculation has been made from two separate studies that supersensitivity will persist for 0.6 days/day of drug treatment [254,275].

In contrast to the increase in D-2 receptor numbers, there is no clear-cut evidence for change in D-1 adenylate cyclase-dependent receptors in response to brief repeated neuroleptic administration and subsequent drug withdrawal. Claims of both an increase and no change in adenylate cyclase activity in response to similar treatment have appeared (Table 4.23). In our studies, we have been unable to find any consistent change in the ability of dopamine to stimulate

TABLE 4.25 Alterations in the Specific Binding of Tritiated Neuroleptic Ligands to Striatal Dopamine Receptors following Repeated Haloperidol Administration

Drug	Dose (mg/kg)	Duration of treatment (days)	^3H-labeled ligand	Conditions	% Change	Reference
Haloperidol	1.0	70	[^3H]Spiperone	β_{max}	+128%	[268]
Haloperidol	10.0	21	[^3H]Spiperone	1.0 nM	+ 45%	[269]
Haloperidol	4.0	7	[^3H]Domperidone	β_{max}	+ 38%	[270]
Haloperidol	1.5	21	[^3H]Spiperone	β_{max}	+ 37%	[271]
Haloperidol	5.0	21	[^3H]Spiperone	0.8 nM	+ 36%	[272]
Haloperidol	5.0	7	[^3H]Haloperidol	0.8 nM	+ 36%	[260]
Haloperidol	10.0	21	[^3H]Haloperidol	2.0 nM	+ 34%	[273]
Haloperidol	4.0	7	[^3H]Pimozide	β_{max}	+ 30%	[270]
Haloperidol	0.2	21	[^3H]Spiperone	2.0 nM	+ 19%	[211]

adenylate cyclase in animals pretreated with neuroleptics for a few weeks and subsequently withdrawn. However, the neuroleptic most commonly administered has been haloperidol, which is selective for D-2 receptors. Alterations of adenylate cyclase may depend on the relative D-1/D-2 actions of the drug administered. In a recent study [276], we have shown that *cis*-flupenthixol, which acts equally on D-1 and D-2 receptors, only produces a small increase in the number of binding sites for [^{3}H]piflutixol and enhancement of cyclic AMP formation in response to dopamine (Table 4.26). Comparison of the abilities of sulpiride (D-2), haloperidol (D-2 > D-1), and *cis*-flupenthixol (D-2 ≡ D-1) to alter dopamine receptor function on repeated administration showed that all three drugs increased D-2 receptor numbers whereas only *cis*-flupenthixol increased D-1 receptor numbers, despite the fact that all three drugs caused behavioral supersensitivity. The implication is that this behavioral change is a D-2 receptor response.

For changes in adenylate cyclase activity to occur, there need not ben an alteration in the number or affinity of the D-1 recognition site. Changes would occur in a component of the adenylate cyclase system lying beyond the dopamine receptor. Gnegy and colleagues [277] have looked for changes in the calmodulin content of striatal membranes and in protein phosphorylation in rodents pretreated with haloperidol and subsequently withdrawn. These animals exhibited enhanced apomorphine-induced stereotypy and a decrease in the K_a for dopamine stimulation of adenylate cyclase activity, indicating the development of receptor supersensitivity. This effect, like acute neuroleptic treatment, was accompanied by a decrease in the spontaneous release of calmodulin from striatal membranes. However, in contrast to acute neuroleptic treatment, there was an increase in the total calmodulin content of the particulate fraction of the striatum. This effect became evident between 2 and 9 days following the cessation of haloperidol intake. In the same tissue there was a marked increase in calcium-dependent protein phosphorylation; protein kinase activity was 3.5 times greater in haloperidol-treated animals than in saline-treated controls. These changes may either be relevant to the development of dopamine receptor supersensitivity or may indeed be a consequence of enhanced receptor activation.

The repeated administration of neuroleptic drugs to rodents and their subsequent withdrawal causes not only an increase in the number of D-2 receptors labeled by antagonist ligands such as [^{3}H]spiperone, but also causes an increase in the number of sites labeled by tritiated agonist ligands such as [^{3}H]apomorphine or 2-amino-6,7-dihydroxy-1,2,3,4-tetrahydro-naphthalene. There is, however, some controversy on this matter. Goldstein and his colleagues [278] found that brief repeated administration of haloperidol caused an increase in the number of binding sites for [^{3}H]spiperone but not for [^{3}H]-*N*,*n*-propylnorapomorphine (NPA). There is no apparent reason for this discrepancy, but it should be remembered that the binding of agonist ligands appears extremely susceptible to the experimental conditions employed, and it has yet to be resolved whether such agonist

TABLE 4.26 Alteration in Apomorphine-Induced Stereotypy, Specific Striatal [^{3}H]Piflutixol Binding and Dopamine (50 μM)-Stimulated Striatal Adenylate Cyclase Activity following Repeated Administration of Haloperidol, Sulpiride, or *cis*-Flupenthixol for 21 Days following 3 Days Withdrawal

Drug Treatment	Stereotypy score	B_{max} (pmoles/g tissue)		Adenylate cyclase (pmoles cyclic AMP formed 2.5 min · 2 mg tissue)
		[^{3}H]Spiperone	[^{3}H]Piflutixol	
Saline	1.4 ± 0.2	17.8 ± 0.2	70 ± 5	32.4 ± 5.3
Haloperidol	3.0 ± 0.2[a]	29.0 ± 2.3[a]	83 ± 4	36.4 ± 5.3
cis-Flupenthixol	3.1 ± 0.2[a]	27.8 ± 1.2[a]	86 ± 5[a]	52.7 ± 7.5[a]
Sulpiride	3.1 ± 0.2[a]	25.5 ± 1.5[a]	77 ± 5	36.8 ± 8.3

Source: Ref. 246.

ligands label a single site or a number of sites with different anatomical locations within the striatal complex. In our own studies [279] using [^{3}H]NPA under controlled conditions, we have found that the administration of a range of neuroleptic drugs to animals for a few weeks plus drug withdrawal leads to an increase in [^{3}H]NPA- and [^{3}H]spiperone-binding sites in striatal prepations. However, this does not mean that the sites labeled by [^{3}H]spiperone and [^{3}H]NPA are identical. Measurement of binding sites for these ligands after 1, 2, or 4 weeks continuous haloperidol administration (and without subsequent drug withdrawal) showed a reciprocal relationship to exist between changes in [^{3}H]spiperone and [^{3}H]NPA binding sites (Table 4.27). The results suggested that agonist and antagonist binding sites might be distinct but not independent entities.

The site(s) at which dopamine receptors become supersensitive within the striatal complex is unclear. Limited lesion studies suggest involvement of those receptors lying on striatal cell bodies since kainic acid lesions of striatum reduced the increase in receptor numbers observed using [^{3}H]spiperone [280]. In contrast, cortical ablation enhances [^{3}H]spiperone binding in haloperidol-treated rats.

The overall conclusion from these studies is that brief periods of repeated administration of neuroleptic drugs (and subsequent withdrawal) results in the development of behavioral supersensitivity to the administration of dopamine agonists such as apomorphine with tolerance to the effects of neuroleptic drugs themselves. Such animals develop agonist supersensitivity, and antagonist subsensitivity, despite an increase in the number of dopamine receptors labeled by neuroleptic ligands such as [^{3}H]spiperone or [^{3}H]haloperidol. One interpretation of these results would be that the nature of the dopamine receptor has undergone a fundamental change that accounts for these characteristics.

We have so far concerned ourselves with talking mainly about forebrain dopamine systems. This does not, however, mean that all dopamine systems respond to brief repeated neuroleptic treatment in an identical manner. Thus, there is no evidence to suggest that dopamine receptors in the pituitary and/or hypothalamus show tolerance to the effects of neuroleptic drugs on repeated administration since serum prolactin levels are unchanged following the brief repeated administration of neuroleptic drugs. Receptor binding studies carried out in rats pretreated with haloperidol and then withdrawn showed an increase in both [^{3}H]haloperidol and [^{3}H]apomorphine binding in the striatum but a decrease in the binding of these ligands in the pituitary [281]. Although this study was carried out using a single ligand concentration, it might appear that the regulation of pituitary and striatal dopamine receptors differs.

Those dopamine receptors located in the area postrema also may be different. Following brief repeated administration of penfluridol to dogs for 12 days, apomorphine-induced stereotyped running was enhanced but the ED_{50} values of apomorphine-induced vomiting were not different

TABLE 4.27 The Effect of Continuous Administration of Haloperidol for up to 4 Weeks on the B_{max} (pmoles/g tissue) And K_D (nM) for Specific Binding of [^{3}H]Spiperone and [^{3}H]NPA to Striatal Membranes

	[^{3}H]Spiperone				[^{3}H]NPA			
	Control		Haloperidol		Control		Haloperidol	
Week	B_{max}	K_D	B_{max}	K_D	B_{max}	K_D	B_{max}	K_D
1	25 ± 2	0.26 ± 0.03	38 ± 5[a]	0.73 ± 0.10[a]	12 ± 1	0.53 ± 0.01	8 ± 1[a]	0.40 ± 0.01[a]
2	27 ± 3	0.30 ± 0.04	33 ± 4	0.38 ± 0.07	12 ± 2	0.55 ± 0.11	12 ± 2	0.62 ± 0.11
4	21 ± 2	0.20 ± 0.02	33 ± 2[a]	0.41 ± 0.03[a]	12 ± 2	0.43 ± 0.06	6 ± 1[a]	0.56 ± 0.12

[a] $p < 0.05$ compared with control animals.
Source: Ref. 279.

from those obtained in these animals prior to drug treatment [282]. This would suggest that the nigro-striatal dopamine system in the dog exhibits supersensitive receptors after repeated penfluridol administration but that the dopamine receptors of the emetic chemoreceptor trigger zone do not.

C. Supersensitivity Following the Repeated Administration of Sulpiride or Clozapine

The ability of atypical neuroleptics, such as sulpiride and clozapine, to produce dopamine receptor supersensitivity following brief periods of repeated administration and subsequent withdrawal may be of use in assessing the propensity of a compound to induce extrapyramidal disturbances in man. Alternatively, if antispychotic compounds such as clozapine and sulpiride produce dopamine receptor supersensitivity, then this phenomenon may be related to more antipsychotic efficacy rather than to the production of neurological side effects.

There is controversy over the effects of brief repeated administration of sulpiride. In our own study [283], the repeated administration of sulpiride for 21 days followed by a 3-4 day withdrawal period caused an increase in apomorphine-induced stereotyped behavior and an increase in striatal dopamine receptors as measured by increases in the specific binding of [^{3}H]spiperone, [^{3}H]sulpiride, and [^{3}H]NPA (Table 4.28). These effects of sulpiride were similar to those produced by haloperidol given for the same period of time. This suggests that sulpiride, at least on repeated administration, acts in a manner typical of neuroleptic compounds. It was of interest that while the acute administration of sulpiride did not antagonize apomorphine-induced stereotypy, in a repeated dosage experiment apomorphine-induced stereotypy was enhanced in agreement with previous findings by Fuxe and his colleagues [284]. This suggests that the acute pharmacological profile of sulpiride is not a true reflection of its in vivo activity on brief repeated administration. The study we have presented, however, is in contrast to findings of others (Table 4.28). Trabucchi and colleagues [285] showed sulpiride did not enhance [^{3}H]spiperone binding and that haloperidol did not increase the high-affinity binding of [^{3}H]sulpiride. There is no apparent reason for these discrepancies between the various studies, but differences in dosage might be one explanation.

Sulpiride, however, may produce selective changes in dopamine-mediated behavior on brief repeated administration. Seven days following administration of (−)-sulpiride (50 mg/kg i.p.) for 21 days, apomorphine-induced hypermotility was enhanced but apomorphine-induced stereotypy was unchanged [287]. In the same experiments, repeated haloperidol (1 mg/kg i.p.) administration enhanced both behaviors. This might suggest differential effects of sulpiride on dopamine receptors compared with haloperidol. Alternatively, it may reflect a greater

TABLE 4.28 Comparison of Studies Carried Out to Investigate the Effect of Repeated Sulpiride Administration, and Subsequent Withdrawal on Striatal Dopamine Function in the Rat

Authors	Dose	Treatment period	Behavior
Jenner et al. [283]	2 × 100 mg/kg i.p.	21 days 3-4 days withdrawal	Enhanced apomorphine-induced stereotyped behavior
Trabucchi et al. [284]	20 mg/kg i.p.	16 days 4 days withdrawal	—
Fuxe et al. [285]	2 × 20 mg/kg i.p.	14 days 2 days withdrawal	Enhanced apomorphine-induced stereotyped behavior and hyperactivity
Banet et al. [286]	50 or 70 mg/kg p.o.	21 days 4 days withdrawal	—

[a]*Note*: No change found either after administration of haloperidol 0.2 mg/kg for 14 days.

ability of sulpiride to alter mesolimbic dopamine receptors controlling locomotion compared with striatal receptors initiating stereotyped behavior.

The low dopamine antagonist activity and high inherent anticholinergic activity of clozapine might be expected to prevent the onset of striatal dopamine receptor supersensitivity on brief repeated drug administration and subsequent drug withdrawal. The evidence to date is mixed. There are reports of both no effects and clear striatal dopamine receptor supersensitivity (Table 4.29).

There is no apparent reason for the differences between these studies. Those studies finding no behavioral change perhaps overall used lower dosage regimes. Also the time of observation after drug withdrawal might appear crucial. Perhaps the most pertinent point is the

Ligand	Concentration	Definition	Result
[^{3}H]Spiperone	0.125-4.0 nM	5 × 10^{-6} M (+)-Butaclamol	23% increase
[^{3}H]-(±)-sulpiride	5-40 nM	5 × 10^{-6} M (−)-Sulpiride	40% increase
[^{3}H]*N*,*n*-propyl-norapomorphine	0.0625-2.0 nM	10^{-6} M (+)-Butaclamol	43% increase
[^{3}H]Spiperone	?	10^{-7} M (+)-Butaclamol	No change
[^{3}H]-(−)-sulpiride	?	10^{-6} M (−)-Sulpiride	Increased
[^{3}H]Spiperone	0.05-2 nM	10^{-6}M (+)-Butaclamol	No change[a]
[^{3}H]ADTN	2-24 nM	10^{-6} (+)-Butaclamol	No change
[^{3}H]Spiperone	?	?	No change

failure of all studies to date to demonstrate any change in dopamine receptor numbers as judged by ligand binding assays. This in itself may be the crucial parameter deciding whether extrapyramidal disturbances will occur or not.

In a recent study [293] where animals were treated with clozapine or haloperidol for 3 weeks and then remained drug free for a further 5 days, haloperidol enhanced apomorphine-induced stereotyped behavior but clozapine selectively enhanced apomorphine-induced locomotor activity and cage floor crossing. This suggests that clozapine acts selectively on those dopamine receptors located in the mesolimbic area rather than on those located within the striatum. Indeed, haloperidol enhanced [^{3}H]spiperone binding in the striatum and in the mesolimbic area, but clozapine did not. It seems that the enhanced behavioral

TABLE 4.29 Summary of Studies Investigating the Effect of Repeated Clozapine Administration and Subsequent Withdrawal on Striatal Dopamine Function in Rat

Author	Dose	Treatment period	Behavioral change	Receptor change
Sayers et al [239]	20 or 80 mg/kg p.o.	6 days 3 days withdrawal	No change in apomorphine-induced stereotyped behavior	—
			No effect on apomorphine-induced rotation in rats with unilateral electrolytic striatal lesions	
Gnegy et al. [288]	5 mg/kg s.c.	20 days 14-17 days withdrawal	No change in apomorphine induced stereotyped behavior	No increase in dopamine-stimulated adenylate cyclase

Kobayashi et al. [289]	30 mg/kg i.p.	21 days 7 days withdrawal	—	No change [^{3}H]-spiperone binding to striatal preparations
Racagni et al. [290]	10 mg/kg i.p.	21 days 2 days withdrawal	No change in apomorphine-induced stereotyped behavior	—
Creese and Snyder [291]	30 mg/kg s.c.	21 days 3 days withdrawal	—	No change [^{3}H]-spiperone binding
Smith and Davis [292]	25 mg/kg i.p.	6-7 weeks 6 or 8 days withdrawal	Increase in apomorphine-induced stereotypy and locomotor activity	—
Gianutsos and Moore [256]	0.075% diet	8-10 days 2 days withdrawal	Increase in apomorphine-induced locomotor activity	—

actions in clozapine-treated animals can occur independently of altered postsynaptic dopamine receptor function.

A recent study of our own has shown another facet of the actions of clozapine which may help explain its atypical neuroleptic profile [294]. Animals received continuous intake of haloperidol, sulpiride, or clozapine. Both haloperidol and sulpiride caused increases in [^{3}H]-spiperone binding and reciprocal decreases in [^{3}H]NPA binding (Table 4.30). In contrast, clozapine had no effect on [^{3}H]spiperone binding but caused a fall in [^{3}H]NPA-binding sites. This suggests that clozapine exerts a differential action on agonist and antagonist binding sites within the striatum.

D. Pituitary Involvement in the Development of Dopamine Receptor Supersensitivity

The supersensitivity that results from brief periods of repeated neuroleptic administration is presumed to be due to the persistent blockade of the postsynaptic dopamine receptor leading to adaptive changes. However, there has been debate recently as to the role pituitary factors might play in this phenomenon.

Hruska and his colleagues [295] found that hypophysectomy prevented the ability of brief repeated administration of haloperidol to induce striatal dopamine receptor supersensitivity. Since the administration of prolactin itself could also induce an increase in striatal [^{3}H]spiperone binding sites, this was taken as evidence to support the role of prolactin in the induction of striatal dopamine receptor supersensitivity [296]. However, in our own study [297], using higher doses of haloperidol and using sulpiride, we were unable to show any effect of hypophysectomy on the development of striatal dopamine receptor supersensitivity (Table 4.31). Subsequently Hruska and colleagues [298], using a range of doses of haloperidol, suggested that the pituitary may not prevent the development of supersensitivity but may alter the level of drug dosage required to induce this effect. One important question that has not been answered is whether hypophysectomy causes any changes in the pharmacokinetic handling of the neuroleptic so as to alter the brain levels achieved.

An increase in the level of circulating prolactin alone is not sufficient to induce dopamine receptor supersensitivity following neuroleptic administration. Thus, in a recent study [299], we have compared the effects of repeated administration of haloperidol with those of a low dose of sulpiride and of domperidone. The latter doses were shown to have peripheral effects but not central actions (Table 4.32). After 3 weeks administration, each drug treatment had caused a marked elevation in circulating prolactin levels. However, only

TABLE 4.30 The Effect of Continuous Administration of Haloperidol or Clozapine for up to 4 Weeks on Apomorphine-Induced Stereotypy and the B_{max} (pmoles/g tissue) and K_D (nM) for Striatal [^{3}H]Spiperone and [^{3}H]NPA Binding

Drug treatment (dose mg/kg·day)	Duration of treatment (weeks)	Apomorphine-induced stereotypy score	[^{3}H]Spiperone		[^{3}H]NPA	
			B_{max}	K_D	B_{max}	K_D
Controls	1	3.0 ± 0.4	24.8 ± 3.9	0.22 ± 0.04	11.0 ± 1.5	0.50 ± 0.11
	2	2.5 ± 0.3	29.8 ± 2.8	0.26 ± 0.03	10.7 ± 2.3	0.54 ± 0.07
	4	3.0 ± 0.3	24.1 ± 0.8	0.12 ± 0.01	11.7 ± 0.9	0.46 ± 0.04
Haloperidol (0.8-1.0)	1	0.8 ± 0.3[a]	42.7 ± 2.4[a]	0.77 ± 0.03[a]	7.7 ± 1.1[a]	0.35 ± 0.11
	2	1.3 ± 0.2[a]	34.3 ± 2.4	0.33 ± 0.05	10.0 ± 1.8	0.52 ± 0.12
	4	2.2 ± 2.4	32.2 ± 1.7[a]	0.26 ± 0.02[a]	7.2 ± 0.4[a]	0.55 ± 0.04
Clozapine (33-37)	1	2.7 ± 0.2	24.4 ± 1.4	0.19 ± 0.02	12.8 ± 1.8	0.72 ± 0.15
	2	3.0 ± 0.4	30.2 ± 2.5	0.28 ± 0.03	11.4 ± 1.8	0.56 ± 0.12
	4	3.5 ± 0.2	26.0 ± 0.8	0.10 ± 0.01	7.3 ± 0.3[a]	0.58 ± 0.01[a]

[a] $p<0.05$ compared with control animals.
Source: Ref. 294.

TABLE 4.31 The Effect of Repeated Administration of Haloperidol or Sulpiride for 17 Days, and Subsequent Drug Withdrawal for 3 Days, on Striatal Dopamine Function in Sham-Operated and Hypophysectomized Rats

	Prolactin (ng/ml)		Stereotypy score	
Drug treatment (dose)	Sham-operated	Hypophysectomy	Sham-operated	Hypophysectomy
Saline	26.6 ± 8.6	N.D.	3.0 ± 0.4	2.5 ± 0.3
Haloperidol (0.75 mg/day)	65.0 ± 14.6[b]	N.D.	4.0 ± 0[a]	3.9 ± 0.2[a]
Sulpiride (2 × 15 mg/day)	22.3 ± 7.1	<7.5	4.0 ± 0[a]	3.7 ± 0.2[a]

[a] $p<0.05$ compared with saline-treated animals.
N.D.; not detectable.
Source: Ref. 297.

haloperidol administration caused an enhancement of apomorphine-induced stereotyped behavior and an increase in the number of [^{3}H]-spiperone binding sites in striatum. If the pituitary does play a role in the modulation of dopamine receptor supersensitivity, prolactin may not be the factor responsible.

E. Chronic Continuous Neuroleptic Administration

The data presented in the previous sections demonstrate that brief periods of repeated neuroleptic administration may cause the emergence of an underlying dopaminergic supersensitivity in the brain, at least in the striatal area. However, most dopamine-mediated behavioral effects continue to be suppressed by such short-term treatments if the drug is not withdrawn, presumably because sufficient neuroleptic is present in brain to continue to antagonize emerging supersensitive dopamine receptors. These experiments, however, last only a matter of days or at the most a few weeks. In contrast, chronic neuroleptic therapy to prevent relapse of schizophrenia is continued for many years while the abnormal movements characterizing tardive dyskinesia only occur after months or years of neuroleptic treatment. Recent interest has centered on effects of treating

[^{3}H]Spiperone			
B_{max} (pmoles/g tissue)		K_D (nM)	
Sham-operated	Hypo-physectomy	Sham-operated	Hypo-physectomy
30.9 ± 2.8	29.6 ± 1.0	0.23 ± 0.02	0.23 ± 0.02
49.3 ± 5.4[a]	40.3 ± 1.0[a]	0.35 ± 0.11	0.25 ± 0.04
39.5 ± 2.0[a]	37.5 ± 1.3[a]	0.27 ± 0.03	0.23 ± 0.02

rodents with neurloeptics for a prolonged period and examining changes in dopamine function without neuroleptic withdrawal so as to mimic what occurs in man.

1. Reversal of Acute Dopamine Receptor Blockade

In a series of studies involving a variety of neuroleptic drugs (Table 4.33), a pattern of change in brain dopamine function has become apparent on continuous chronic drug administration (Fig. 4.10). Initial dopamine receptor blockade was evidenced behaviorally by (1) the induction of catalepsy during the first few weeks of drug intake and (2) by the inhibition of apomorphine-induced stereotyped behavior, and biochemically by (1) a compensatory increase in dopamine release as witnessed by elevation in the dopamine metabolites homovanillic acid and 3,4-dihydroxyphenylacetic acid while normal dopamine levels were maintained, (2) a reduction in the ability of dopamine to stimulate cyclic AMP formation in striatal tissue in vitro during the first few weeks of drug administration, (3) in vitro identification of striatal dopamine receptors labeled by ligands such as [^{3}H]-spiperone which showed a reduction in total binding compared with tissue from control animals; this appeared to be due to a large

TABLE 4.32 The Effect of Repeated Administration of Haloperidol, Doperidone or Sulpride for 21 Days, Followed by 3 Days Drug Withdrawal on Striatal Dopamine Function

Drug treatment (mg/kg)	Prolactin (ng/ml)	Stereotypy score	B_{max} (pmoles/g)	K_D (nM)
Saline	31.7 ± 5.6	3.2 ± 0.2	17.9 ± 1.2	0.4 ± 0.01
Haloperidol (5 mg/kg)	364.0 ± 51.5[a]	4.1 ± 0[a]	26.5 ± 1.4[a]	0.23 ± 0.02
Sulpiride (5 mg/kg)	191.9 ± 26.4[a]	3.3 ± 0.2	18.0 ± 1.5	0.23 ± 0.01
Domperidone (5 mg/kg)	432.1 ± 45.7[a]	3.3 ± 0.2	19.0 ± 0.9	0.24 ± 0.03

Source: Ref. 299.

TABLE 4.33 Summary of Chronic Neuroleptic Studies

	Dose (mg/kg·day)	Period of administration (months)	Effect on apomorphine-induced stereotypy	Effect on B_{max} for striatal [^{3}H]Spiperone binding	Reference
Trifluoperazine	2.5-3.5	12	↓(0.125 mg/kg) ↑(0.5-1.0 mg/kg)	↑	[300]
Trifluoperazine	4.4-4.9	12	↓(0.125 mg/kg) ↑(0.5-1.0 mg/kg)	↑	[301]
Trifluoperazine	0.7-0.9	6-8	↑(0.5-2.0 mg/kg)	N.D.	[302]
Thioridazine	30-40	12	↑(0.125 mg/kg) ↑(0.5-1.0 mg/kg)	↑	[300]
Haloperidol	1.5	9	↓(0.15 mg/kg)	↑	[303]
Haloperidol	1.4-1.6	12	↓(0.125 mg/kg) ↑(0.5-1.0 mg/kg)	N.D.	[301]
cis-Flupenthixol	1.4-3.0	6	↓(0.15 mg/kg)	↑	[304]
cis-Flupenthixol	0.8-1.2	18	↑(0.125-2.0 mg/kg)	↑	[305]
Piflutixol	0.4	6	↓(0.15 mg/kg)	↑	[306]
Sulpiride	102-109	12	No change	No change	[301]
Metoclopramide	17	6	↑(0.15 mg/kg)	↑	[306]
Clozapine	24-27	12	No change	No change	[301]

N.D., not determined.

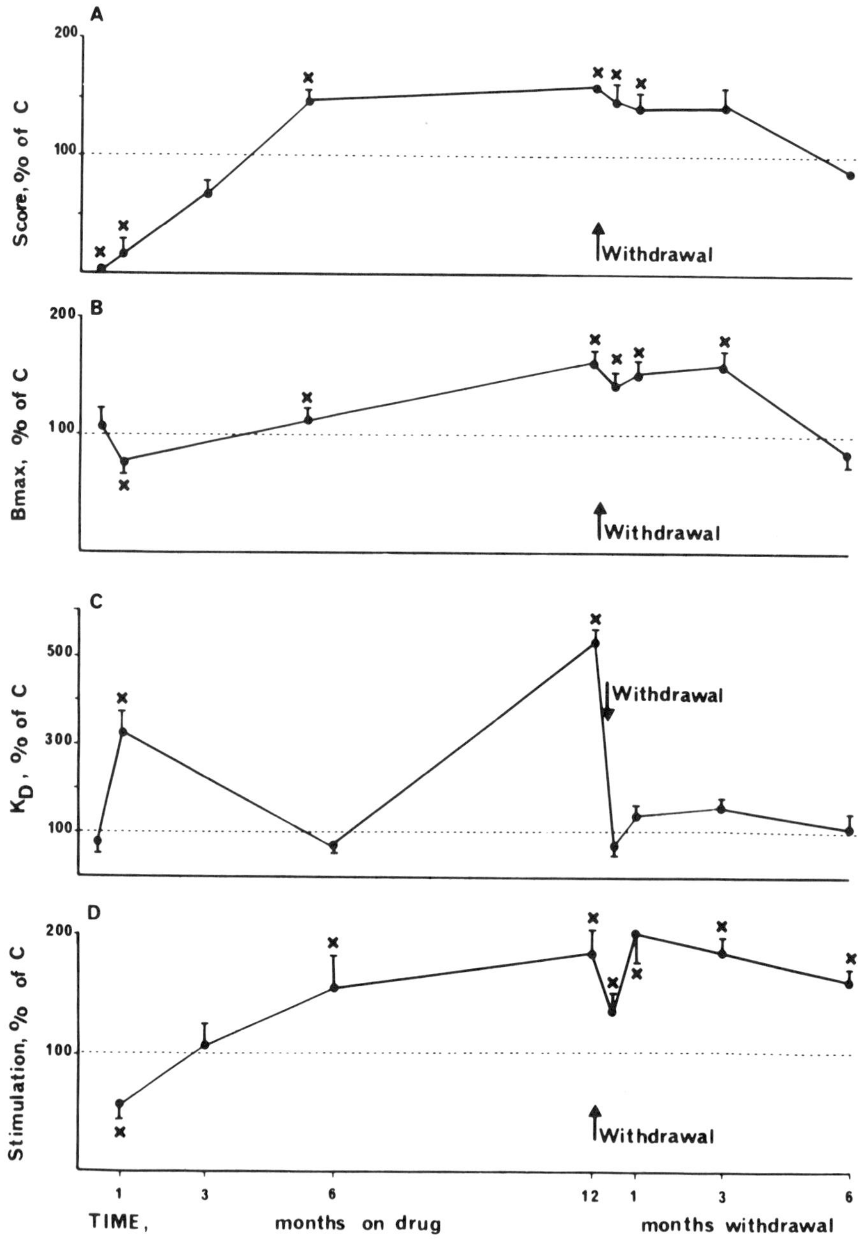

FIG. 4.10 The effect of continuous administration of trifluoperazine dihydrochloride (2.5–3.5 mg/kg/day p.o) to rats and its subsequent withdrawal for 6 months on apomorphine (0.5 mg/kg s.c.)-induced stereotyped behavior (A); specific striatal [^{3}H]spiperone

increase in the dissociation constant (K_D) rather than to change in receptor site numbers, an effect attributed to the presence of drug in the tissue preparations.

After 6 or 12 months drug intake, changes occurred in the characteristics of striatal dopamine receptors suggesting that acute dopamine receptor blockade was reversed and that striatal dopamine receptor supersensitivity had developed despite continued drug intake. Animals treated in this manner exhibited (1) an enhanced stereotyped response to high doses of apomorphine, although low-dose stereotypy may remain inhibited, (2) an increased ability of dopamine to stimulate striatal adenylate cyclase in vitro, and (3) an increased number of dopamine receptor binding sites as labeled by ligands such as [^{3}H]spiperone.

2. The Development of Functional Dopamine Receptor Supersensitivity

A critical question is whether the changes in dopamine receptor function induced by chronic neuroleptic treatment are operative in the intact, unprobed animal. It is not known what proportion of dopamine receptors labeled by [^{3}H]spiperone are required to produce a maximal pharmacological response. Any increase in the number of dopamine receptors also may be ineffective if they remain blocked in the intact animal by continued neuroleptic intake. Similarly, there is controversy over whether the enhancement of stereotyped behavior seen following administration of apomorphine reflects free and available receptors or the displacement of neuroleptic drug from receptors adequately blocked in vivo.

One way of deciding whether such changes are of functional significance in the intact animal is to measure some consequence of dopamine receptor occupation. In an area such as the striatum, dopamine receptors lie on the cell bodies of cholinergic interneurons and on the terminals of cortico-striate glutamate fibers. The action of dopamine at these sites is to inhibit release of acetylcholine or glutamate [152, 178]. It is therefore possibly by measuring changes in the release of these neurotransmitters to decide what alterations in dopamine receptor function have occurred in the presence of continued neuroleptic intake.

Activation of those receptors lying on the cell bodies of cholinergic interneurons by the administration of dopamine agonists causes an

---

binding sites (B_{max}) (B); the dissociation constant (K_D) for specific striatal [^{3}H]spiperone binding (C); and dopamine (50 μM) stimulation of striatal adenylate cyclase (D). All values are expressed as a percentage of values obtained for age-matched controls animals; * $p<0.05$.

increase in striatal acetylcholine content which is interpreted as being due to decreased cholinergic transmission [152]. If long-term continuous administration of neuroleptic drugs causes a functional increase in dopamine receptor activity in the intact animal this should be reflected by increased striatal acetylcholine content. Recently [307], we have found that treatment of rats for 14 months with *cis*-flupenthixol (0.8–1.2 mg/kg/day) induces enhanced apomorphine-induced stereotyped behavior and caused a twofold increase in basal striatal acetylcholine levels (Table 4.34).

In a recent series of experiments we have extended these findings [308]. While the acute administration of neuroleptic drugs led to an increase in [^{3}H]acetylcholine release from striatal slices this effect was abolished in those animals receiving chronic neuroleptic intake (Fig. 4.11). Also, while acute neuroleptic administration did not alter the release of [^{3}H]glutamate from striatal slices, in animals receiving neuroleptic intake for 12 months [^{3}H]glutamate release was markedly decreased compared with that occurring in age-matched control animals. Both these changes are consistent with the development of functional dopamine receptor supersensitivity as a result of chronic neuroleptic intake.

3. Alterations in the Nature of the Dopamine Receptor Population

If dopamine receptors are functionally active in rats receiving chronic neuroleptic intake, then why are such receptors not adequately blocked by the high concentration of neuroleptic drug present in the tissues of these animals? If these receptors were identical to the endogenous dopamine receptor population, then blockade by the neuroleptic administered would seem inevitable. The obvious explanation would seem to be that the nature of the dopamine receptor population is altered by chronic neuroleptic intake such that the new receptors are no longer adequately blocked by neuroleptic administration.

There is some evidence to support this hypothesis from a comparison of catalepsy and high-grade stereotypy induced by a range of neuroleptic drugs and dopamine agonists, respectively. Chronic neuroleptic-treated rats developed a gross exaggeration of stereotyped behavior but a marked reduction in the cataleptic response compared with the control animals (Fig. 4.12). The striatal dopamine receptor population appears to be altered by chronic neuroleptic intake in such a manner as to be agonist supersensitive but antagonist subsensitive.

Further evidence of alteration in the nature of the dopamine receptor population comes from the measurement of the number of [^{3}H]-spiperone binding sites (B_{max}) and the dissociation constant (K_D) in striatal preparations. In each of the long-term neuroleptic experiments that we have carried out, we have observed a series of changes in

TABLE 4.34 The Effect of Continuous Administration of *cis*- or *trans*-Flupenthixol for 14 Months on Striatal Dopamine Function and Striatal Acetylcholine Concentrations

Drug treatment (dose mg/kg/day)	Stereotypy score	Striatal acetylcholine (ng/g)
Controls (distilled water alone)	2.0 ± 0	4.1 ± 0.3
cis-Flupenthixol (0.8-1.2)	3.9 ± 0.1[a]	7.4 ± 0.7[a]
trans-Flupenthixol (0.9-1.2)	2.0 ± 0	3.9 ± 0.1

[a] $p<0.05$ compared with control animals.
Source: Ref. 304.

both B_{max} and K_D. As we have previously discussed, there was a progressive increase in B_{max} over the course of the neuroleptic intake. Usually by 6 and 12 months after starting administration, there was an enhanced number of [^{3}H]spiperone binding sites compared with the number observed in control animals. The changes in the dissociation constant K_D were more complex. In most experiments, after 1 month's neuroleptic intake, K_D was increased, and this was attributed to the presence of neuroleptic drug in tissue preparations (Fig. 4.13). By 3 months, however, K_D usually had decreased and by 6 months had returned to or towards normal. In some experiments, K_D remained at control values for 6 months, however, at 9 and 12 months after starting drug intake, K_D was increased in all experiments. We do not understand the underlying changes which cause this pattern of alteration in the dissociation constant during chronic drug intake, but it may indicate some subtle change in receptor affinity that is reflected in the dissociation constant. This may affect the whole receptor population since there was no evidence of more than one population of dopamine receptors at any stage during the course of these drug administration experiments.

4. Alterations in Different Dopamine Receptor Populations

Since dopamine receptors do not seem to be a single entity in the striatum, it is important to determine which of the various subgroups of receptors are altered by chronic neuroleptic intake. In animals treated chronically with *cis*- and *trans*-flupenthixol for 18 months [309],

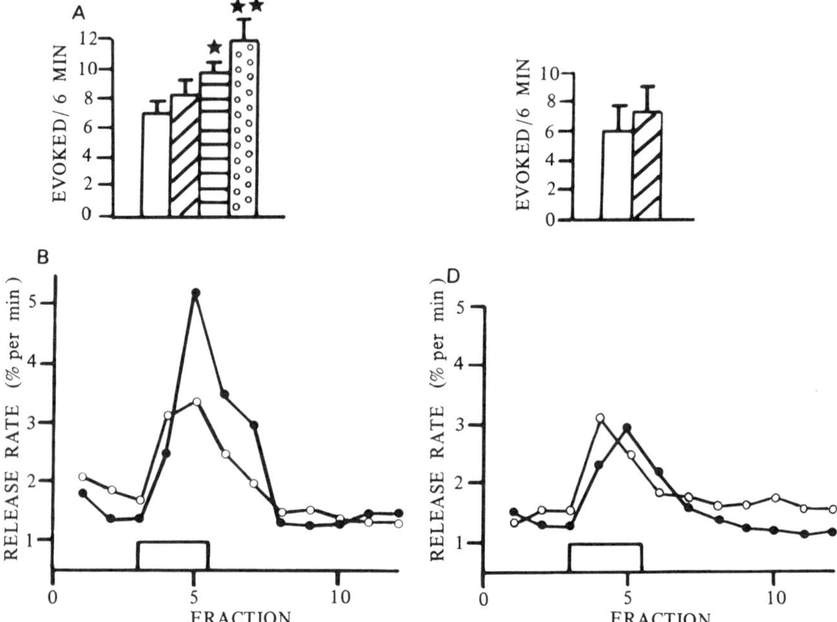

FIG. 4.11 Part i. Comparison of the effects of acute administration and chronic administration for 12 months of trifluoperazine to rats on [^{3}H]acetylcholine release from striatal slices. A. Amount of radioactivity released over the baseline during a 6-min period following K^+ stimulation in striatal slices from vehicle injected animals (□) and animals receiving 2.5 (▨), 5 (▤) and 10 (⚃) mg/kg trifluoperazine intraperitoneally 90 min before sacrifice, n = 8 and represents nonpooled tissue from individual animals. $^{**}p < 0.01$; $^{*}p < 0.05$ (Student's t-test). B. Individual curves showing the efflux of [^{3}H]acetylcholine from striatal slices from vehicle injected animals (○) and animals receiving 10 mg/kg trifluoperazine (●) 90 min previously. The addition of 25 mM KCl is indicated by the bar. Each point represents four animals. Standard errors are omitted for clarity but were in the range of 5–15%. C. Evoked release of [^{3}H] acetylcholine in striatal slices from control animals (□) and animals receiving continuous trifluoperazine for 1 year (▨; 4.5–5.1 mg/kg daily). Results are expressed as described for A above. n = 4 individual rats. D. Individual curves for the efflux of [^{3}H]acetylcholine from striatal slices of control (○) and from animals receiving trifluoperazine for 1 year (4.5–5.1 mg/kg·day) (●). For further explanation see B above.

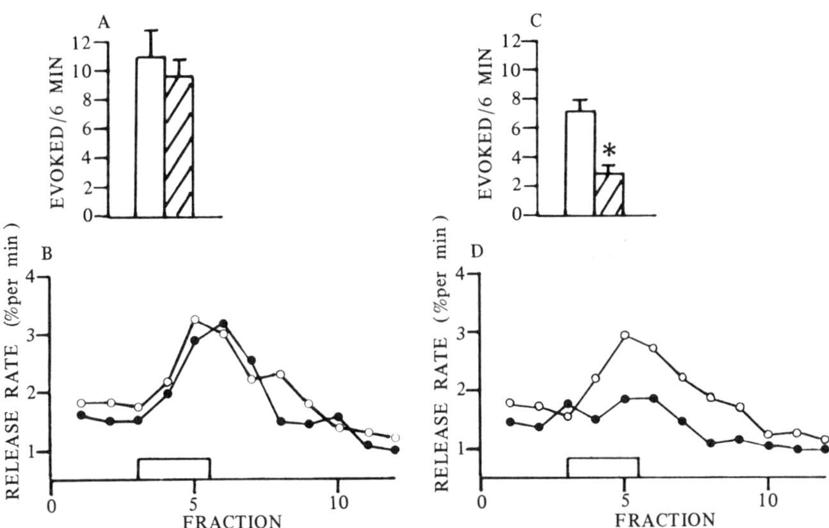

Part ii. Comparison of the effects of acute administration and chronic administration for 1 year of trifluoperazine on [^{3}H]glutamate release from striatal slices. A. Evoked release of [^{3}H]glutamate in striatal slices from vehicle-injected animals (□), and from animals receiving 10 mg/kg trifluoperazine (▨) 90 min prior to sacrifice. For further details see part i above. Trifluoperazine in doses of 2.5 and 5 mg (not shown) were without effect. n = 8 individual rats. B. Individual curves for efflux of [^{3}H]glutamate from striatal slices of control (○) and animals receiving 10 mg/kg trifluoperazine 90 min prior to sacrifice (●). For further details see part i above. C. Evoked release of [^{3}H]glutamate release in striatal slices from control animals (□) and animals receiving trifluoperazine for 1 year 4.5–5.1 mg/kg/day (▨). For further details see legent part i above. $^*p < 0.01$ (Student's t-test). D. Individual curves for efflux of [^{3}H]glutamate in striatal slices from control (○) and animals receiving trifluoperazine for 1 year (●). For further details see part i above.

we found a disparity between the changes of binding of [^{3}H]spiperone and [^{3}H]NPA to antagonist and agonist D-2 sites, respectively, and the binding of [^{3}H] piflutixol to D-1 sites (Table 4.35).

The number of [^{3}H]spiperone-binding sites was increased and there was a corresponding increase in the dissociation constant (K_D). There were a larger number of D-2 receptors of apparently lower affinity. In contrast, the number of [^{3}H]NPA-binding sites was decreased, but there was a corresponding decrease in K_D. This suggested that

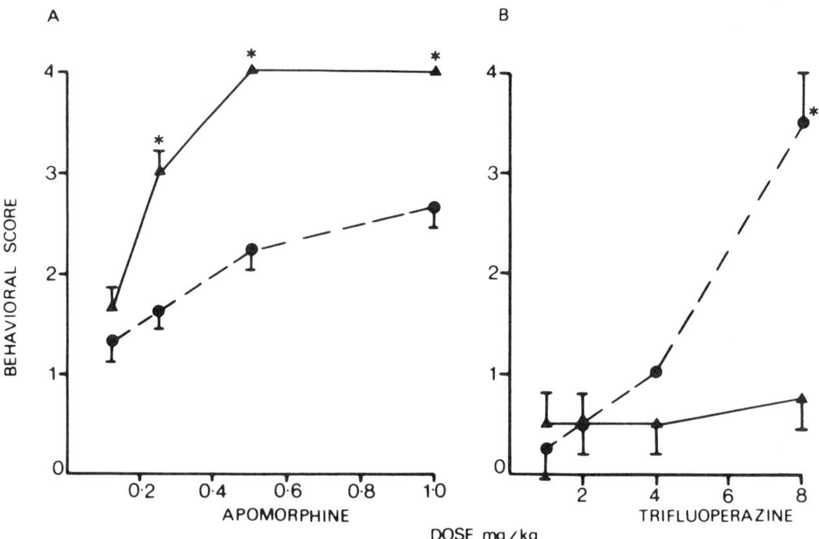

FIG. 4.12 Dose-response curves for induction of apomorphine (0.125–1.0 mg/kg s.c. 15 min previously)-induced stereotypy (A) and trifluoperazine (1–8 mg/kg 3 hr previously) catalepsy (B) in rats receiving *cis*-flupenthixol (0.8–1.2 mg/kg•day) for 18 months (▲) compared with age-matched control rats (●). $*p < 0.05$.

neuroleptic treatment produced a smaller number of higher affinity agonist binding sites. This finding might explain the apparent agonist supersensitivity and antagonist subsensitivity that was exhibited behaviorally by these animals. Only a fraction of the total receptor population needs to be occupied to obtain a maximum pharmacological response. Drug action at antagonist sites involved a larger number of lower affinity receptors, which might result in a small behavioral response. Action on agonist sites would have been associated with a smaller number of receptors with a higher affinity, which might result in enhanced behavioral response. These data also would provide some evidence to suggest that perhaps agonist and antagonist binding sites respond differently to neuroleptic drug treatment and that they, perhaps, are not identical entities. However, the reciprocal changes that occur suggest they do not act independently of each other.

Specific [^{3}H]piflutixol binding to D-1 sites in striatal preparations was not altered by the drug administration and there was no change in either the B_{max} or K_D for the interaction of this ligand with striatal tissue. So D-1 receptors do not appear to be altered by the administration of *cis*-flupenthixol, a drug known to act with more or less equal affinity on both D-1 and D-2 sites. This failure to alter [^{3}H]piflutixol

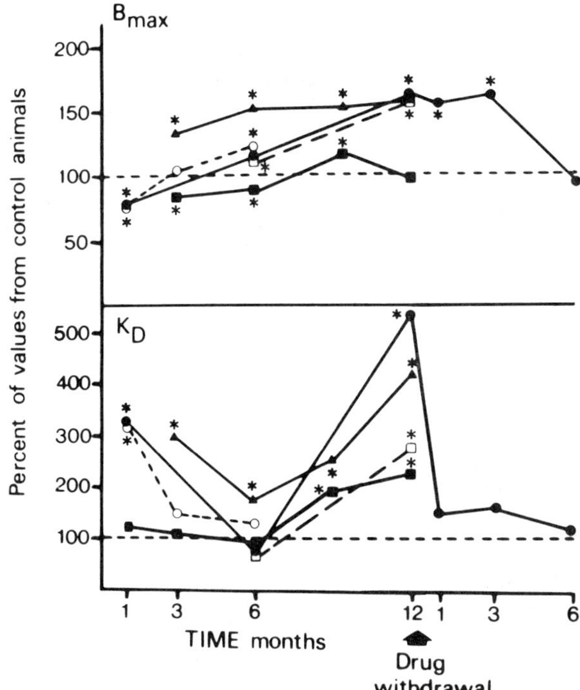

Fig. 4.13 Comparison of alteration in the number of binding sites (B_{max}) and the dissociation constant (K_D) for dopamine (10^{-4} M)-specific [^{3}H]spiperone (0.125–4.0 nM) binding to rat striatal preparations produced by the continuous administration of trifluoperazine or *cis*-flupethixol for up to 12 months in four distinct studies. Experiment 1: Trifluoperazine dihydrochloride, 2.5–3.5 mg/kg/day (●); thioridazine dihydrochloride, 30–40 mg/kg/day (□). Experiment 2: Trifluoperazine dihydrochloride, 2.8–4.9 mg/kg/day (○). Experiment 3: Trifluoperazine dihydrochloride, 4.5–5.6 mg/kg/day (▲). Experiment 4: *cis*-Flupenthxol hydrochloride, 0.8–1.2 mg/kg/day (■). $*p < 0.05$ compared with appropriate age-matched control animals.

TABLE 4.35 The Effect of Administration of *cis*-Flupenthixol (0.8–1.2 mg/kg/day) or *trans*-Flupenthixol (0.9–1.2 mg/kg/day) to rats for 18 months on Specific Striatal Binding of [^{3}H]Spiperone, [^{3}H]*N*,*n*-propylnorapomorphine, or [^{3}H]Piflutixol and Dopamine-Stimulated Adenylate Cyclase Activity

	[^{3}H]Spiperone (dopamine 10^{-4} M)		[^{3}H]*N*,*n*-propylnor-apomorphine [(±)-butaclamol 10^{-6} M]	
Drug treatment	B_{max} (pmoles/g tissue)	K_D (nM)	B_{max} (pmoles/g tissue)	K_D (nM)
Control	10.2 ± 0.8	0.14 ± 0.02	—	—
cis-Flupenthixol	14.0 ± 0.8[a]	0.88 ± 0.10[a]	2.4 ± 0.4[a]	0.52 ± 0.15[a]
trans-Flupenthixol	9.2 ± 0.8	0.25 ± 0.06	7.5 ± 1.7	1.29 ± 0.46

[a]$p<0.05$ compared with control or animals receiving *trans*-flupenthixol.
Source: Ref. 309.

binding occurs, however, in the presence of increased dopamine stimulation of striatal adenylate cyclase activity. It would appear that either the change in adenylate cyclase activity occurs at some site beyond the recognition site for dopamine, or that some change in receptor occupancy occurs to cause enhanced cyclic AMP formation.

The conclusion from these studies must be that only the D-2 adenylate cyclase-independent dopamine recognition sites are altered by chronic neuroleptic intake. Changes in adenylate cyclase activity appear to occur without a direct effect on D-1 recognition sites.

We would not wish to give the impression that changes in dopamine receptors occurring in response to chronic neuroleptic intake represent a static phenomenon. Receptors protein components of membranes exist in a dynamic state. The expectation, therefore, is that the relationship between various dopamine receptor populations might change with time of drug intake. Indeed, as illustrated in Fig. 4.14, the relationship between [^{3}H]spiperone binding and [^{3}H]NPA binding in animals receiving chronic haloperidol treatment varies according to the time period of study. It cannot be presumed that different research workers will obtain identical results if different time points are employed. Indeed, as we will see later, the effect observed also will vary according to the neuroleptic drug employed.

$[^3H]$Piflutixol (*cis*-flupenthixol 10^{-6} M)		$[^3H]$Piflutixol (plus sulpiride 3×10^{-5} M)		Adenylate cyclase (dopamine 50 μM)
B_{max} (pmol/g tissue)	K_D (nM)	B_{max} (pmol/g tissue)	K_D (nM)	(pmoles/2.5 min 2 mg tissue)
84.6 ± 3.3	0.29 ± 0.02	59.7 ± 4.5	0.53 ± 0.04	12.8 ± 4.2
89.4 ± 4.0	0.40 ± 0.02	53.6 ± 6.5	0.47 ± 0.08	31.8 ± 2.9
71.6 ± 3.2	0.26 ± 0.02	72.8 ± 8.8	0.57 ± 0.20	—

5. Alterations in Mesolimbic and Mesocortical Dopamine Receptors

So far we have concerned ourselves with the adaptive responses of striatal dopamine receptors to chronic continuous neuroleptic intake. Evidence of the effects of chronic neuroleptic treatment on mesolimbic and cortical dopamine function is sparse. Our own studies [310] have suggested that increased numbers of $[^3H]$spiperone binding sites and increased adenylate cyclase activity can be demonstrated in mesolimbic tissue. But this does mean that these receptors are no longer blocked by the neuroleptic drug. We have neither evidence from behavioral experiments to support such an assertion, nor a biochemical correlate of enhanced mesolimbic dopamine receptor activation. Until such evidence is available, no firm conclusion can be reached as to the functional status of mesolimbic dopamine receptors during chronic neuroleptic administration.

It has not been possible to establish whether dopamine receptor blockade in the mesocortical system is maintained during chronic neuroleptic therapy. No easily measurable behavioral correlate of cortical dopamine receptor function has been available and ligand-binding procedures in this region are not adequately established. It is possible to measure dopamine-sensitive adenylate cyclase in cortical areas [311],

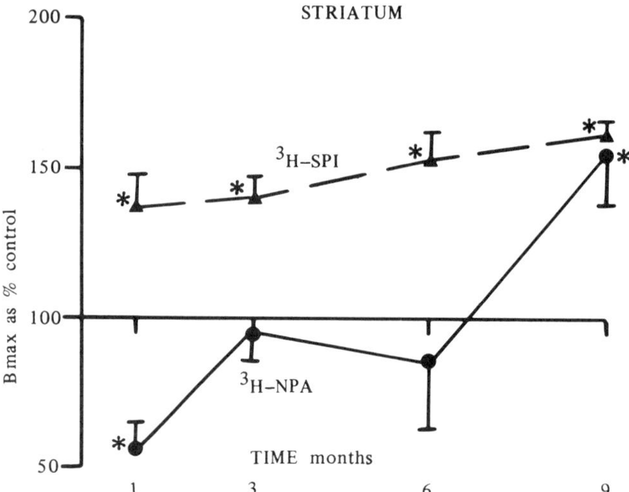

Fig. 4.14 The effects of continuous administration of haloperidol (1.6–1.7 mg/kg/day) for up to 9 months on specific [^{3}H]spiperone (0.1–4.0 nM) and [^{3}H]*N*,*n*-propylnorapomorphine (0.05–2.0 nM) binding to striatal tissue. Data are the values for B_{max} in drug-treated animals (± 1 SEM) expressed as a percentage of those values for age-matched control animals. Duration of treatment is indicated as time in months. Specific binding of [^{3}H]spiperone was defined using (−)-sulpiride (10^{-5} M) and that of [^{3}H]*N*,*n*-propylnorapomorphine defined using (±)-ADTN (10^{-6} M).

so some study of the effect of long-term neuroleptic administration on dopamine receptors in this area may be possible. At present no one can say what happens to cortical dopamine receptors during chronic neuroleptic intake.

6. The Effect of Neuroleptic Withdrawal

Withdrawal of rats from chronic neuroleptic intake leads to no further increase in those indices of striatal dopamine function that are enhanced during drug administration [312]. In general, the behavioral and biochemical indices of dopamine receptor supersensitivity induced by chronic neuroleptic administration to animals did not persist. Enhancement of apomorphine-induced stereotypy and the elevation in specific [^{3}H]spiperone binding produced by chronic neuroleptic treatment disappear by 3 months following drug withdrawal. However, the enhanced stimulation of adenylate cyclase by dopamine in vitro remained unchanged for between 6–12 months after drug withdrawal [313]. At present, there is no known function for the dopamine receptor linked to adenylate cyclase in the brain or for the cyclic AMP so formed. These observations might suggest an involvement in long-term adaptive phenomena.

7. Peri-Oral Movements

When animals receiving chronic neuroleptic intake were examined for behavioral manifestations related to tardive dyskinesia, it was found that they exhibited an exaggerated incidence of purposeless chewing movements [314,315] (Table 4.36). However, administration of cholinergic agonists enhanced the number of spontaneous peri-oral jaw movements, whereas anticholinergic drugs inhibited manifestations of this phenomenon. This suggests that these movements do not resemble tardive dyskinesia as it occurs in man. Cholinergic drugs decrease tardive dyskinesia, but anticholinergic drugs make it worse. Furthermore, if such movements did resemble tardive dyskinesia, then it might be expected that they would persist following neuroleptic withdrawal. However, we found that on removal of neuroleptic intake from animals treated for 1 year, a dramatic decrease in the number of spontaneous mouthing movements occurred, such that there was no difference from control animals 2 weeks following drug withdrawal [312].

8. Changes in Nondopamine Neuronal Systems

As discussed above, neuroleptic drugs can interact with a variety of neurotransmitter systems in brain. So are the changes in dopamine receptor function during chronic neuroleptic treatment specific, or do they reflect a general change in neurotransmitter systems?

In animals receiving 6-months' continuous trifluoperazine intake the change in dopamine receptors appeared to be selective (Table 4.37). There was an increase in the number of striatal dopamine receptors labeled by [^{3}H]spiperone, but the number and binding affinity of muscarinic receptors in the striatum, mesolimbic area, and cerebral cortex as identified by [^{3}H]dexetimide were unchanged; this was also the case for the H-1 receptors identified by [^{3}H]mepyramine, for α-noradrenergic receptors identified by [^{3}H]WB 4101 in cerebral cortex, and for GABA receptors in the cerebellum identified by [^{3}H]muscimol. Identification of 5-HT receptors in frontal cortex using [^{3}H]spiperone indicated no apparent change in receptor numbers, but a slight increase in K_D.

This study suffered from the deficit that many of the determinations were made outside the basal ganglia, in areas where dopamine-active drugs might not have influenced the activity of other neuronal systems.

TABLE 4.36 The Effect of Cholinergic and Anticholinergic Agents on Spontaneous Perioral Behavior in Control Rats and in Rats Treated with Haloperidol (1.4-1.6 mg/kg/day) for 4 months

Drug treatment	Incidence in 5-min test period		
	Chewing	Tongue protrusion	Gaping
Cholinergic drugs			
Control	22 ± 3	1.0 ± 0.6	0
Haloperidol	52 ± 6[a]	4.3 ± 1.6	0.1 ± 0.1
Pilocarpine (4 mg/kg i.p.)	145 ± 12[a]	9.7 ± 2.4[a]	5.8 ± 2.2[a]
Pilocarpine plus haloperidol	171 ± 13[a]	8.6 ± 2.1[a]	12.1 ± 4.0[a]
Physostigmine (0.2 mg/kg i.p.)	65 ± 11[a]	6.8 ± 3.1[a]	5.9 ± 2.3[a]
Physostigmine plus haloperidol	88 ± 8[a]	16.0 ± 2.8[a]	22.0 ± 3.8[a]
Anticholinergic drugs			
Control	21 ± 3	4.1 ± 0.6	0
Haloperidol	45 ± 5	4.3 ± 1.4	0
Atropine (25 mg/kg i.p.)	4 ± 1[a]	0[a]	0
Atropine plus haloperidol	14 ± 3[a]	0[a]	0
Scopolamine (0.5 mg/kg i.p.)	13 ± 1[a]	0.9 ± 0.4[a]	0
Scopolamine plus haloperidol	14 ± 2[a]	0.9 ± 0.4[a]	0

[a] $p < 0.05$ compared with control animals.
Source: Ref. 315.

TABLE 4.37 The Effect of Continuous Administration of Trifluoperazine (2.8-4.0 mg/kg/day) for 6 Months on Neurotransmitter Receptors in Rat Brain

Receptor	Ligand	Area	Direction of change
Dopamine	[^{3}H]Spiperone	Striatum	Increase
		Mesolimbic	Increase
	[^{3}H]Apomorphine	Striatum	?
		Mesolimbic	?
5-HT-2	[^{3}H]Spiperone	Frontal cortex	No change
Acetylcholine	[^{3}H]Dexetimide	Striatum	No change
		Mesolimbic	No change
		Cortex	No change
H_1-histamine	[^{3}H]Mepyramine	Cortex	No change
α_1-Adrenergic	[^{3}H]WB 4101	Cortex	No change
GABA	[^{3}H]Muscimol	Cerebellum	No change

Source: Ref. 316.

This is highlighted by the recent finding of Dawbarn and colleagues [317] that chronic trifluoperazine administration increased [^{3}H]5-HT binding in the striatum, and enhanced 5-HT mediated behaviors. The difference between this study and our own on 5-HT receptors in striatum and cerebral cortex might have been due to the different brain areas studied but also could have reflected the different 5-HT receptor populations labeled by these ligands [318]. [^{3}H]Spiperone selectively labels 5-HT-2 receptors, whereas [^{3}H]5-HT label 5-HT-1 receptors. Another change specific to the basal ganglia is the finding of Gale [319] of increased [^{3}H]GABA binding in substantia nigra following chronic neuroleptic treatment; this too may be of consequence of the change induced in striatal dopamine function.

Despite the fact that most neuroleptic drugs can act on a range of neurotransmitter systems in brain, it appears that the increase in receptor numbers produced by chronic neuroleptic intake may primarily affect dopamine systems. However, changes in brain dopaminergic mechanisms may cause secondary alterations in other neuronal systems with which dopamine interacts.

In addition to monoamine pathways, the striatum contains a number of peptide transmitter substances that also are altered by chronic neuroleptic administration. Hong and colleagues [182] showed haloperidol, pimozide, and chlorpromazine, but not clozapine, administration for 3 weeks to increase *met*-enkephalin levels selectively in dopamine-containing brain regions. For alterations in the rate of decline of *met*-enkephalin levels, following inhibition of synthesis using cycloheximide, they concluded the increase to be due to an increased rate of synthesis, presumably in response to continuing dopamine receptor blockade. We have examined striatal *met*-enkephalin concentrations after 14 months administration of *cis*-flupenthixol (unpublished observations) (Table 4.38). In contrast to the increase observed by Hong and colleagues [162], we find an approximate 50% decrease in striatal *met*-enkephalin concentration in drug-treated animals compared with age-matched controls. By analogy to the work of Hong et al. this can be tentatively ascribed to a decrease in peptide synthesis occuring in response to the development of dopamine receptor supersensitivity. At this time we observed also a rise in striatal cholecystokinin-8 concentration.

9. The Effects of Chronic Administration of Sulpiride or Clozapine

It is of particular interest to determine the effects of the atypical neuroleptics sulpiride and clozapine in such long-term experiments. If the ability of neuroleptic drugs to produce extrapyramidal disturbances is related to their actions in altering cerebral dopamine function, then it might be expected that sulpiride and clozapine would have different effects from typical neuroleptic compounds.

In animals that have received either haloperidol, clozapine, or sulpiride for 1 year [301], only haloperidol treatment caused enhancement of apomorphine-induced stereotyped behavior (Table 4.39). The effect of haloperidol was accompanied by an increase in the specific binding of [^{3}H]spiperone in striatal tissue preparations, whereas clozapine and sulpiride were without effect. The functional significance of the changes induced by haloperidol were shown by a corresponding increase in striatal acetylcholine content. Sulpiride was without effect on striatal acetylcholine but, interestingly, clozapine also increased acetylcholine content even though it had no effect on dopamine parameters. This probably reflects the high inherent anticholinergic activity of this compound, causing compensatory changes in striatal cholinergic function.

From this data it would seem that sulpiride and clozapine may well produce different effects on striatal dopamine function from those observed following administration of a typical neuroleptic such as haloperidol. Interestingly, sulpiride and clozapine, but not haloperidol, increased dopamine stimulation of striatal adenylate cyclase. Again, we do not know the meaning of this change, but, since it was caused by both of the atypical antipsychotic compounds, its relevance should not be overlooked.

TABLE 4.38 Peptide Concentrations in Basal Ganglia following 18 Months *cis*- or *trans*-Flupenthixol Administration

Dose treatment (dose mg/kg/day)	met-enkephalin[a]		Substance P	CCK-8[a]	
	ST	SN	SN	ST	GP
Controls (distilled water alone)	633 ± 59	65 ± 3	741 ± 72	41 ± 5	39 ± 3
cis-Flupenthixol (0.8-1.2)	443 ± 22[b]	61 ± 4	707 ± 74	58 ± 6[b]	39 ± 5
trans-Flupenthixol (0.9-1.2)	830 ± 80	87 ± 39	797 ± 39	46 ± 5	38 ± 5

[a] pmoles/g tissue.
[b] $p < 0.05$ compared with control animals.
Source: Ref. 320.

TABLE 4.39 The Effect of Continuous Chronic Administration for 12 Months of Haloperidol, Clozapine or Sulpride on Striatal Dopamine Function

Drug treatment (dose mg/kg/day)	Apomorphine-induced (0.5 mg/kg/sc) stereotypy score	$[^3H]$Spiperone		Striatal acetylcholine content (nmoles/g tissue)
		B_{max} (pmoles/g)	K_D (nM)	
Controls (distilled water alone)	3.09 ± 0.21	13.8 ± 1.0	0.13 ± 0.03	19.85 ± 2.08
Haloperidol (1.6-1.7)	3.91 ± 0.09[a]	26.4 ± 2.2[a]	0.20 ± 0.04	35.65 ± 3.33[a]
Sulpiride (102-109)	3.50 ± 0.22	17.2 ± 1.4	0.13 ± 0.02	26.54 ± 2.57
Clozapine (25-27)	3.16 ± 0.16	15.3 ± 0.9	0.15 ± 0.02	29.52 ± 3.36[a]

[a] $p<0.05$ compared with age-matched control animals; two-tailed Student's t-test for parametric data, Mann-Whitney U-test for nonparametric stereotypy scores.
Source: Ref. 301.

VII. DISCUSSION

Neuroleptic drugs exert a common action in blocking brain dopamine receptors following their acute administration. All such drugs have actions on other neuronal systems within brain, but there is no other consistent pattern of effect that would explain their actions. Extrapolating this data to man, it is evident that the antipsychotic activity of neuroleptic compounds also is directly correlated with the ability of neuroleptic drugs to interact with brain dopamine receptors. There is a linear relationship between the ability of drugs to displace ligands such as [^{3}H]spiperone or [^{3}H]haloperidol from their specific binding sites on rat striatal membranes and the average daily dose of such compounds used to control schizophrenia (Fig. 4.15) [195]. The correlation between antipsychotic activity and [^{3}H]spiperone binding also implies that the action of neuroleptic drugs in producing antipsychotic activity is related to their ability to interact with the D-2 dopamine receptor population. No such correlation exists with their ability to inhibit dopamine-sensitive adenylate cyclase, reflecting their actions at D-1 receptors.

Because of this close correlation between the interaction at dopamine receptors and the production of antipsychotic activity, all neuroleptic drugs produced in the past 30 years have been developed through animal screening models designed to detect their interaction with brain dopamine systems. It is unfortunate that this approach has also led to the selection of those drug molecules that are able to block dopamine-mediated motor behaviors, so ensuring that extrapyramidal motor disorders will also be an almost inevitable part of the profile of compounds developed in this manner.

Although neuroleptic drugs may act to block dopamine receptors on acute administration, it is apparent from the evidence that we have presented that this may not continue on repeated or chronic neuroleptic intake. It is necessary to relate the ability of brain dopamine systems to adapt to the presence of neuroleptic agents to their continuing antipsychotic activity and to the development of long-term motor disorders such as tardive dyskinesia. In so doing, it is necessary to look critically at the basic hypotheses on which neuroleptic drugs are used to treat schizophrenia.

A. What Is the Present Status of the Dopamine Hypothesis of Schizophrenia?

The dopamine hypothesis of schizophrenia has dominated biochemical concepts of schizophrenia for over a decade. However, the data we have discussed suggest that at least some of its foundations are open to criticism.

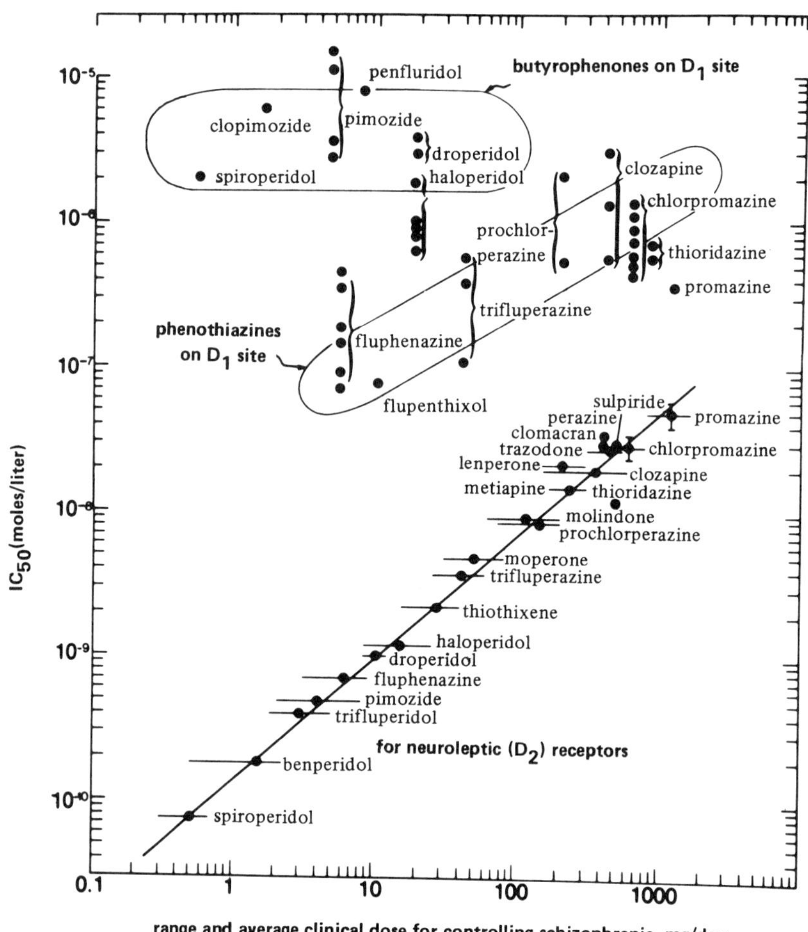

FIG. 4.15 Correlation between the ability of neuroleptic drugs to inhibit specific binding of [^{3}H]haloperidol to D-2 receptors on calf striatal preparations (IC_{50}) with the average daily dose used to control subacute schizophrenia [145]. Note again the lack of correlation with activity on the D-1 adenylate cyclase-linked site.

A major premise of the dopamine hypothesis of schizophrenia is that amphetamine induces psychotic states resembling paranoid schizophrenia, but this observation is not conclusive. Many patients who receive high-dose continuous amphetamine treatment for prolonged periods do not develop any psychiatric symptomatology and, in those who do, amphetamine is more likely to induce acute toxic confusional states than a schizophreniform illness. Increased dopamine release alone may not be sufficient to produce a schizophreniform psychosis. Indeed, there is controversy as to the effect of administering dopamine agonists such as *L*-dopa to schizophrenics not receiving neuroleptic treatment [321,322]. Whereas such treatment causes symptomatic deterioration, this may be due to nonspecific toxic confusion rather than to an exacerbation of schizophrenic symptoms such as thought disorder and hallucinations. Paradoxically, chronic schizophrenics maintained on neuroleptics also may show additional improvement if *L*-dopa is administered concurrently [323]. Although failure to deteriorate under these conditions might be expected from the continued presence of a neuroleptic, a positive response to *L*-dopa appears inconsistent with the dopamine hypothesis of schizophrenia.

The data reviewed in preceding sections strongly suggest that dopamine receptor blockade in the forebrain produced by acute neuroleptic administration is not maintained on chronic drug therapy, at least in striatal and mesolimbic areas. This raises doubt about the belief that benefical actions of neuroleptic agents on chronic administration to man are maintained by this mechanism. Our animal experiments show chronic neuroleptic treatment to lead to a reversal of receptor blockade such that rats have functionally supersensitive dopamine receptors at least in striatum and, at least initially, in the mesolimbic area. If the dopamine hypothesis of schizophrenia were correct, then theory would predict that chronic neuroleptic-induced cerebral dopamine receptor supersensitivity should exacerbate primary symptoms of schizophrenia. In contrast, the antipsychotic potency of neuroleptics is maintained during chronic neuroleptic therapy despite the manifestation of tardive dyskinesias associated with striatal dopaminergic overactivity. Moreover, in schizophrenics treated with *cis*-flupenthixol, therapeutic benefit emerges only after several weeks of treatment at a dosage effective in causing initial dopamine receptor blockade as judged by increased serum prolactin levels [324]. This corresponds to the time course for the development of tolerance to initial blockade and the presence of underlying dopamine receptor supersensitivity and might be taken to indicate that the antipsychotic effects of *cis*-flupenthixol and of neuroleptics in general are related to some change secondary to dopamine receptor blockade.

To date, postmortem studies of brain tissue from schizophrenic patients have failed to provide convincing data to verify the hypothesis of cerebral dopaminergic overactivity. There is no evidence for enhanced dopamine turnover in brain tissue from schizophrenics. If anything, the information presently available would suggest a compensatory decrease in dopamine function as a result of drug therapy. In drug-treated schizophrenics, there is little doubt that the increased numbers of dopamine receptors demonstrated in brain are not a true reflection of the disease process but are a consequence of chronic drug therapy. The study of tissue from untreated or drug-free schizophrenics so far has failed to resolve the issue since there is no clear agreement on changes in receptor numbers in such patients.

Antipsychotic drugs are used not only in schizophrenia but are also widely used to control acute psychotic episodes, whatever their cause. Physicians use neuroleptics to control acute toxic confusional states due to systemic illness while neurologists use the same drugs to control the acute behavioral disturbance of those with brain injury whether it be due to trauma, encephalitis, or stroke. Neuroleptics are employed successfully to control the psychotic and behavioral disburbances provoked by dopamine replacement therapy in Parkinson's disease, in which such dopamine agonists much more commonly cause acute toxic confusional states and depression rather than the rare schizophreniform psychosis. If dopamine overactivity does exist in schizophrenia, then it cannot be regarded as symptomatic of that disorder alone. These observations would support the concept of a dopamine hypothesis of acute psychotic disturbance, whatever its cause, rather than a restricted hypothesis relating to schizophrenia.

B. How Do the Actions of Neuroleptic Drugs Relate to the Emergence of Tardive Dyskinesia?

There are a few clues as to factors predisposing to the development of tardive dyskinesia. Postmortem studies have so far not been employed to detect underlying receptor changes. The pathophysiology of tardive dyskinesia is not established for certain, but most available clinical evidence supports the notion that it is due to cerebral dopamine overactivity. The animal studies we have described support the concept that chronic administration of neuroleptic drugs reverses the acute dopamine receptor blockade cuased by such compounds so as to produce functional dopamine receptor supersensitivity in striatum, even while neuroleptic intake continues. However, chronic neuroleptic drug adminstration does not simply alter dopamine receptors. It may also cause a change in the nature of the receptor. It may be the production of these abnormal dopamine receptors that leads to the appearance of tardive dyskinesia in man.

Despite producing the changes in striatal dopamine function that might be expected in tardive dyskinesia, no abnormal movements appeared in animals exposed to long-term neuroleptic intake that could be likened to tardive dyskinesia. However, it is not known how such a disorder would be manifest in rodents or, indeed, whether the same deficits that characterize tardive dyskinesia in man would produce behavioral change in the rat. It must also be remembered that all the animals treated in the studies described developed signs of dopamine receptor supersensitivity. However, only a proportion of those patients treated with neuroleptic drugs develop tardive dyskinesia. It may be that some other underlying, as yet undetected, factor predispose some individuals to the development of tardive dyskinesia and that this is not apparent in our rodent colonies. This might also explain why tardive dyskinesias are so difficult to treat. They may be suppressed by further neuroleptic treatment, but their reversal by drug treatment is difficult.

Although the emergence of cerebral dopamine receptor overactivity may be the primary change responsible for tardive dyskinesia, it may not be the sole cause. The alteration of striatal dopamine receptor function resulting from chronic neuroleptic exposure appears to lead to a series of changes in other basal ganglia neuronal systems including cholinergic activity, differences in 5-HT and GABA receptors, as well as altered peptide levels. It may be the balance or sum of these changes that causes tardive dyskinesia.

The data we have presented strongly support the proposal based on clinical experience that neuroleptic-induced dopaminergic supersensitivity arising in the basal ganglia is responsible for the emergence of tardive dyskinesia. It is an almost inevitable consequence that neuroleptic drugs should induce unwanted extrapyramidal side effects since they are often selected on the basis of their antidopamine motor properties. Screening tests for neuroleptics, such as the inhibition of apomorphine-induced stereotypy or the induction of catalepsy, have been argued to be more predictive of a neuroleptic's propensity to induce extrapyramidal side effects rather than to predict clinical antipsychotic activity. It is to be hoped that in future antidopamine properties will not continue to dominate screening procedures of potential new antipsychotic drugs.

REFERENCES

1. J. Delay, P. Deniker, and J. M. Harl, *Ann. Med.-Psychol.*, 110, 112 (1951).
2. H. H. Meyer, *L'Encephale*, 45:524 (1956).
3. National Institute of Mental Health, *Arch. Gen. Psychiat.*, 20:246 (1964).
4. B. Pollack, *Am. J. Psychiat.*, 112:937 (1956).
5. B. Pollack, *Am. J. Psychiat.*, 114:749 (1958).
6. J. P. Leff and J. K. Wing, *Br. Med. J.*, 2:599 (1971).

7. S. R. Hirsch, R. Gaind, P. D. Rohde, B. C. Stevens, and J. K. Wing, *Br. Med. J.*, 1:633 (1973).
8. T. J. Crow, *Br. Med. J.*, 280: 66 (1980).
9. C. D. Marsden, D. Tarsy, and R. J. Baldessarini, in *Psychiatric Aspects of Neurologic Disease* (D. F. Benson and D. Blumer, Eds.), Grune & Stratton, New York, 1875, p. 219.
10. C. D. Marsden and P. Jenner, *Psychol. Med.*, 10: 55 (1980).
11. J. Delay and P. Deniker, in *Psychotropic Drugs* (S. Garrattini and V. Ghetti, Eds.), Elsevier, Amsterdam, 1957, p. 485.
12. H. Steck, *Ann. Med. Psychol.*, 112: 373 (1954).
13. J. Sigwald, D. Bouttier, C. Raymondeaud, and C. Piot, *Rev. Neurol.*, 100:751 (1959).
14. L. Uhrbrand and A. Faurbye, *Psychopharmacologia (Berl.)*, 1:408 (1960).
15. M. P. Bishop, D. M. Gallant, and T. F. Sykes, *Arch. Gen. Psychiat.*, 3:155 (1965).
16. P. H. Connell, *Maudsley Monograph*, 6, Oxford, London, (1958).
17. A. Carlsson and M. Lindqvist, *Acta Pharmacol. Toxicol.*, 20:140 (1963).
18. N. E. Anden, S. G. Butcher, and H. Corrodi, *Eur. J. Pharmacol.*, 11:303 (1970).
19. P. Seeman, M. Chau-Wong, J. Tedesco, and K. Wong, *Proc. Natl. Acad. Sci. (USA)*, 72: 4376 (1975).
20. T. Lee, P. Seeman, W. W. Tourtellotte, I. J. Farley, and O. Hornykiewica, *Nature*, 274:897 (1968).
21. F. Owen, A. J. Cross, T. J. Crow, A. Longden, M. Poulter, and G. J. Riley, *Lancet*, 2: 233 (1978).
22. A. V. P. MacKay, E. D. Bird, E. G. Spokes, M. Rossor, and L. L. Iversen, *Lancet*, 2: 915 (1980).
23. T. Lee and P. Seeman, *Am. J. Psychiat.*, 137:191 (1980).
24. T. J. Crow, J. F. W. Deakin, and A. Longden, *Psychol. Med.*, 7:213 (1977).
25. G. E. Crane, *Br. J. Psychiat.*, 122:395 (1973).
26. D. Tarsy and R. J. Baldessarini, in *Clinical Neuropharmacology 1*, (H. L. Klawans, Ed.), Raven, New York, 1976, p. 29.
27. D. V. Jeste and R. J. Wyatt, *Arch. Gen. Psychiatry*, 39:803 (1982).
28. P. Jenner and C. D. Marsden, in *Neuroleptics and Tardive Dyskinesia* (S. J. Enna and J. Coyle, Eds.) Raven, New York, 1983 (in press).
29. H. L. Klawans, *Am. J. Psychiat.*, 130:82 (1973).
30. A. E. Caldwell, in *Principles of Psychopharmacology*, 2nd ed. (W. G. Clark and J. del Guidice, Eds.), Academic, New York, 1978, p. 9.
31. H. Laborit, P. Huguenard, and R. Alluaume, *Press Med.*, 60: 206 (1952).

32. P. Charpentier, *U. S. Patent 2*, 519:886 (1950).
33. A. V. P. MacKay, in *Drugs in Psychiatric Practice*, (P. J. Tyrer, Ed.), Buttersworths, London, 1982, p. 42.
34. T. van Putten, *Arch. Gen. Psychiat.*, 31:67 (1974).
35. P. A. J. Janssen, *Int. Rev. Neurobiol.*, 8:221 (1965).
36. J. M. Davis, *Arch. Gen. Psychiat.*, 13:552 (1965).
37. R. Deberdt, P. Elens, W. Berghmans, J. Heykants, R. Woestenborghs, F. Driesens, A. Reyntjens, and L. van Wijngaarden, *Acta Psychiat. Scand.*, 62:356 (1980).
38. I. Faloon, D. C. Watt, and M. A. Shepherd, *Psychol. Med.*, 8:59 (1978).
39. P. V. Petersen, N. Lassen, T. Holm, R. Kopf, and I. Moller-Nielsen, *Arz. Forsch*, 8:395 (1958).
40. A. Knights, M. S. Okasha, M. A. Salih, and S. R. Hirsch, *Br. J. Psychiat.*, 135:515 (1979).
41. J. Schmutz, F. Hunziker, G. Stille, and H. Lauener, *Bull. Chim. Ther.*, 6:424 (1967).
42. G. M. Simpson and E. Varga, *Curr. Ther. Res.*, 16:679 (1974).
43. B. M. Angrist, in *The Benzamides: Pharmacology, Neurobiology and Clinical Aspects* (J. Rotrosen and M. Stanley, Eds.), Raven, New York, 1982, p. 1.
44. M. Stanley, A. Lautin, J. Rotrosen, S. Gershon, and D. Kleinberg, *Psychopharmacology*, 71:219 (1980).
45. L. Justin-Besancon, C. Laville, and M. Thominet, *C. R. Acad. Sci.*, 258:4384 (1964).
46. L. Justin-Besancon, M. Thominet, and C. Laville, *C. R. Acad. Sci.*, 265:1253 (1967).
47. L. Justin-Besancon, C. Laville, J. Margarit, and M. Thominet, *C. R. Acad. Sci.*, 279:375 (1974).
48. R. Ropert, F. Caillard, and F. Petitjean, presented at *Joint Meeting of the American Psychiatric Association of the Societe Medico-Psychologique*, Atlants (1978).
49. P. Price, J. D. Parkes, and C. D. Marsden, *Lancet*, 2:1106 (1978).
50. U. Ungerstedt, *Acta Physiol. Scand.*, Suppl. 367: 1 (1971).
51. O. Lindvall and A. Bjorklund, in *Dopamine* (P. J. Roberts, G. N. Woodruff and L. L. Iversen, Eds.), Raven, New York, 1978, p. 1.
52. A. M. Thierry, J. P. Tassin, G. Blanc, and J. Glowinski, in *Dopamine* (P. J. Roberts, G. N. Woodruff, and L. L. Iversen, Eds.), Raven, New York, 1978, p. 205.
53. P. A. J. Janssen, C. J. E. Niemeggers, and K. H. L. Schellekens, *Arz.-Forsch.*, 15:504 (1965).
54. E. M. Boyd and J. K. Miller, *Fed. Proc.*, 13:338 (1954).
55. J. M. van Rossum, *Arch. Int. Pharmacodyn. Ther.*, 160:492 (1966).
56. A. Randrup, I. Munkvad, and P. Udsen, *Acta Pharmacol. Toxicol.*, 20:145 (1964).

57. P. Protais, J. Constantin, and J. C. Schwartz, *Psychopharmacology*, 50:1 (1976).
58. C. Pycock, D. Tarsy, and C. D. Marsden, *Psychopharmacologia (Berl.)*, 45:211 (1975).
59. B. Costall and R. J. Naylor, *Eur. J. Pharmacol.*, 35:161 (1976).
60. K. P. Bharvaga and O. Chandra, *Br. J. Pharmacol.*, 21:436 (1963).
61. J. W. Kebabian, G. L. Petzgold, and P. Greengard, *Proc. Nat. Acad. Sci. USA*, 69:2145 (1971).
62. D. R. Burt, I. Creese, and S. H. Snyder, *Molec. Pharmacol.*, 12:800 (1976).
63. K. H. Lu, Y. Amenomori, C. L. Chen, and J. Meites, *Endocrinology*, 87:667 (1970).
64. G. K. Aghajanian and B. S. Bunney, *Naunyn-Schmied. Arch. Pharmakol.*, 297:1 (1977).
65. B. S. Bunney, J. R. Walters, R. H. Roth, and G. K. Ahajanian, *J. Pharmacol. Exp. Ther.*, 185:560 (1973).
66. G. Di Chiara, M. L. Porceddu, L. Vargiu, A. Argiolas, and G. L. Gessa, *Nature*, 264:564 (1976).
67. B. Costall and R. J. Naylor, *Eur. J. Pharmacol.*, 40:9 (1976).
68. C. J. Carter and C. J. Pycock, *Br. J. Pharmacol.*, 42:402P (1978).
69. B. Costall, R. J. Naylor, and R. M. Pinder, *Eur. J. Pharmacol.*, 31:94 (1973).
70. B. Costall and R. J. Naylor, *Eur. J. Pharmacol.*, 33:301 (1975).
71. T. J. Crow and C. Gilbe, *Nature*, 245:27 (1973).
72. P. Muller and P. Seeman, *J. Pharmac. Pharmacol.*, 26:981 (1974).
73. P. H. Kelly and K. E. Moore, *Nature*, 263:695 (1976).
74. C. J. Pycock and C. D. Marsden, *Eur. J. Pharmacol.*, 47:167 (1978).
75. Y. C. Clement-Cormier, J. W. Kebabian, G. L. Petzgold, and P. Greengard, *Proc. Natl. Acad. Sci. USA*, 71:1113 (1974).
76. P. Seeman, *Biochem. Pharmacol.*, 26:1741 (1977).
77. P. Jenner, P. N. C. Elliott, A. Clow, C. Reavill, and C. D. Marsden, *J. Pharm. Pharmacol.*, 30:46 (1978).
78. B. D. Roufogalis, M. Thornton, and D. N. Wade, *Life Sci.*, 19:927 (1976).
79. W. C. Prozialeck and B. Weiss, *J. Pharmacol. Exp. Ther.*, 222:509 (1982).
80. W. C. Prozialeck, M. Cimino, and B. Weiss, *Molec. Pharmacol.*, 19:264 (1981).
81. M. E. Gnegy and Y. S. Lau, in *Ling-term Effects of Neuroleptics*, (F. Cattabeni, G. Racagni, P. F. Spano, and E. Costa, Eds.), Raven, New York, 1980, p. 147.
82. R. M. Levin and B. Weiss, *Molec. Pharmacol.*, 13:690 (1977).
83. R. M. Levin and B. Weiss, *J. Pharmacol. Exp. Ther.*, 208:454 (1979).

84. B. D. Roufogalis, *Biochem. Biophys. Res. Comm.*, 98:607 (1981).
85. R. W. Wrenn, N. Katoh, R. C. Schatzman, and J. F. Kuo, *Life Sci.*, 29:725 (1981).
86. D. R. Burt, I. Creese, and S. H. Snyder, *Molec. Pharmacol.*, 12:800 (1976).
87. D. R. Howlett, H. Morris, and S. R. Nahorski, *Molec. Pharmacol.*, 15:506 (1979).
88. J. E. Leysen, C. J. E. Niemegeers, J. P. Tollenaere, and P. M. Laduron, *Nature*, 272:163 (1978).
89. C. Kohler, S.-O. Ogren, L. Haglund, and T. Angeby, *Neurosci. Lett.*, 13:51 (1979).
90. C. Kohler, L. Haglund, S.-O. Ogren, and T. Angeby, *J. Neural. Trans.*, 52:163 (1981).
91. N. Klemm, C. Murrin, and M. J. Kuhar, *Brain Res.*, 169:1 (1979).
92. J. M. Palacios, D. L. Niehoff, and M. J. Kuhar, *Brain Res.*, 213:277 (1981).
93. J. G. Edwards. J. R. Alexander, M. S. Alexander, A. Gordon, and T. Zuchti, *Br. J. Psychiat.*, 137:522 (1980).
94. B. Costall, R. J. Naylor, and V. Nohria, *Eur. J. Pharmacol.*, 50:39 (1978).
95. A. J. Puech, P. Simon, and J.-R. Boissier, *Eur. J. Pharmacol.*, 36:349 (1976).
96. P. N. C. Elliott, P. Jenner, G. Huizing, C. D. Marsden, and R. Miller, *Neuropharmacology*, 16:333 (1977).
97. G. Bartholini, *J. Pharm. Pharmacol.*, 28:429 (1976).
98. A. Restelli, D. Lucchini, and A. Glasser, *Pharmacol. Res. Commun.*, 7:409 (1975).
99. B. Scatton, S. Bischoff, J. Dedek, and J. Korf, *Eur. J. Pharmacol.*, 44:287 (1977).
100. A. Tagliamonte, G. De Montis, M. Olianas, L. Vargiu, G. U. Corsini, and G. L. Gessa, *J. Neurochem.*, 24:707 (1975).
101. R. D. Pinnock, G. N. Woodruff, and M. J. Turnbull, *Eur. J. Pharmacol.*, 56:413 (1979).
102. B. Costall and R. J. Naylor, *Psychopharmacology*, 43:69 (1975).
103. F. Honda. Y. Satoh, K. Shimamura, H. Satoh, H. Noguchi, S. Uchida, and R. Kato, *Jpn. J. Pharmacol.*, 27:397 (1977).
104. H.-R. Olpe, *Eur. J. Pharmacol.*, 51:441 (1978).
105. P. Jenner, A. Clow, C. Reavill, A. Theodorou, and C. D. Marsden, *J. Pharm. Pharmacol.*, 32:39 (1980).
106. R. M. Ridley, P. R. Scraggs, and H. F. Baker, *Biol. Psychiat.* 15:165 (1980).
107. G. U. Corsini, M. Del Zompo, C. Cianchetti, A. Mangoni, and G. L. Gessa, *Psychopharmacology*, 47:169 (1976).
108. Delagrange Laborabories; personal communication.
109. A. M. Mancini, A. Guitelman, C. A. Vargas, L. Debelyjuk, and W. J. Aparicio, *J. Clin. Endocr. Metab.*, 42:181 (1976).

110. E. E. Muller, E. Stefanini, F. Camanni, V. Locatelli, F. Massara, P. F. Spano, and D. Cocchi, *J. Neural Trans.*, 46:205 (1979).
111. L. Bjerkenstedt, C. Harnryd, and G. Sedvall, *Psychopharmacology*, 64:135 (1979).
112. P. Borenstein, C. Champion, P. Cujo, P. Gekiers, C. Olivenstein, and P. Kramarz, *Sem. Hop. Paris*, 45:1301 (1969).
113. M. Trabucchi, R. Longoni, P. Fresia, and P. F. Spano, *Life Sci.*, 17:1551 (1975).
114. S. Fleminger, P. Jenner, and C. D. Marsden, unpublished observation.
115. A. Theodorou, M. Crockett, P. Jenner, and C. D. Marsden, *J. Pharmac. Pharmacol.*, 31:424 (1979).
116. G. N. Woodruff and J. B. Freedman, *Neuroscience*, 6:407 (1981).
117. P. Jenner, A. Theodorou and C. D. Marsden, in *The Benzamides Pharmacology, Neurobiology and Clinical Aspects* (M. Stanley and J. Rotrosen, Eds.), Raven, New York, 1982, p. 109.
118. A. Theodorou, M. D. Hall, P. Jenner, and C. D. Marsden, *J. Pharmac. Pharmacol.*, 32:441 (1980).
119. A. Theodorou, P. Jenner, and C. D. Marsden, *Life Sci.*, in press (1982).
120. E. Stefanini, A. M. Marchiso, P. Devoto, F. Vernaleone, R. Collu, and P. F. Spano, *Brain Res.*, 198:229 (1980).
121. B. Costall, D. H. Fortune, and R. J. Naylor, *J. Pharmac. Pharmacol.*, 30:796 (1978).
122. H. R. Burki, A. C. Sayers, W. Ruch, and H. Asper, *Arzneim-Forsch.*, 17:1561 (1977).
123. J. Buus Lassen, *Acta Pharmacol. (Kbh.), 35/Suppl.*, 1:39 (1974).
124. P. Worms and K. G. Lloyd, *Pharmacol. Ther.*, 5:443 (1979).
125. C. J. Pycock, D. Tarsy, and C. D. Marsden, *J. Pharmac. Pharmacol.*, 27:445 (1975).
126. S. Wilk and M. Stanley, *Eur. J. Pharmacol.*, 51:101 (1978).
127. P. Seeman, T. Lu, M. Chan-Wong, and K. Wong, *Nature*, 261:717 (1976).
128. G. Bartholini, W. Haefely, M. Jalfre, A. H. Keller, and A. Pletscher, *Br. J. Pharmacol.*, 46:736 (1972).
129. G. Stille, H. Lauener, and E. Eichenberger, *Il Farmaco*, 26:603 (1971).
130. B. S. Bunney and G. K. Aghajanian, in *Anti-psychotic Drugs: Pharmacodynamics and Pharmacokinetics* (G. Sedvall and B. Urnas, Eds.) Pergamon, Oxford, 1976, p. 305.
131. B. Fjalland, A. V. Christensen, and J. Hyttel, *Naunyn-Schmied. Arch. Pharmakol.*, 301:5 (1977).
132. J. Gerlach, P. Koppelhus, E. Helweg, and A. Monrad, *Acta Psychiat.*, 50:410 (1974).
133. R. Matz, W. Rick, D. Oh, H. Thompson, and S. Gershon, *Curr. Ther. Res.*, 16:687 (1974).

134. H. Y. Meltzer, D. J. Goode, P. M. Schyve, M. Young, and V. S. Fang, *Am. J. Psychiat.*, 136:1550 (1979).
135. D. C. U'Prichard, D. A. Greenberg, and S. H. Snyder, *Molec. Pharmacol.*, 13:454 (1977).
136. D.B. Bylund and S. H. Synder, *Molec. Pharmacol.*, 12:568 (1976).
137. F. Sulser and S. E. Robinson, in *Psychopharmacology: A Generation of Progress* (M. A. Lipton, A. Di Mascio, and K. F. Killam, Eds.), Raven, New York, 1978, p. 943.
138. J. B. Blumberg, R. E. Tyler, and F. Sulser, *J. Pharmac. Pharmacol.*, 27:125 (1975).
139. R. Freedman and B. J. Hoffer, *J. Neurobiol.*, 6:277 (1975).
140. D. L. Nelson, A. Herbet, A. Enjalbert, J. Bockaert, and M. Hamon, *Biochem. Pharmacol.*, 29:2445 (1980).
141. K. von Hungen, S. Roberts, and D. F. Hill, *Brain Res.*, 85:257 (1975).
142. N. G. Bacopoulos, *J. Pharmacol. Exp. Ther.*, 219:708 (1981).
143. M. Grabowska, *Pol. J. Pharmacol. Pharmac.*, 28:253 (1976).
144. R. B. Rastogi, R. L. Singhal, and Y. D. Lapierre, *Life Sci.*, 29:735 (1981).
145. D. A. Bender and P. M. Cockfort, *Biochem. Sco. Trans.* 5:155 (1977).
146. A. Carlsson, in *Psychopharmacology; A Generation of Progress*, (M. A. Lipton, A. Di Mascio, and K. F. Killma, Eds.), Raven, New York, 1978, p. 1057.
147. D. Chadwick, M. Hallett, P. Jenner, and C. D. Marsden, *J. Neurol. Sci.* 35:157 (1978).
148. S. J. Hill and M. Young, Eur. J. Pharmac., 52:397 (1978).
149. M. D. Spiker, G. C. Palmer, and A. A. Marian, *Brain Res.*, 104:401 (1976).
150. J. Coupet and V. A. Szuchs-Myers, *Eur. J. Pharmacol.*, 74:149 (1981).
151. C. R. Calcutt, *Gen. Pharmacol.*, 7:15 (1976).
152. V. H. Sethy and M. H. Van Woert, *Res. Commun. Chem. Path. Pharmacol.*, 8:13 (1974).
153. H. Stadler, K. G. Lloyd, M. Gadea-Ciria, and G. Bartholini, *Brain Res.* 55:476 (1973).
154. P. L. McGeer, D. S. Grewaal, and E. G. McGeer, *Brain Res.*, 80:211 (1974).
155. P. G. Guyenet, Y. Agid, F. Javoy, J. C. Beaujouan, J. Roissier, and J. Glowinski, *Brain Res.*, 84:227 (1975).
156. B. Scatton, *J. Pharmacol. Exp. Ther.*, 220:197 (1982).
157. E. Marco, C. C. Mao, A. Revuelta, E. Peralta, and E. Costa, *Neuropharmacology*, 17:589 (1978).
158. E. Marco. C. C. Mao, D. L. Cheney, A. Revuelta, and E. Costa, *Nature*, 264:263 (1976).
159. J. S. Hong, H. -Y. T. Yang, and E. Costa, *Neuropharmacology*, 17:83 (1978).

160. D. J. Pettibone and R. J. Wurtman, *Brain Res.*, 86:409 (1980).
161. G. R. Hanson, L. Alphs, W. Wolf, R. Levine, and W. Lovenberg, *J. Pharmacol. Exp. Ther.*, 218:568 (1981).
162. J. S. Hong, H.-Y. T. Yang, W. Fratta, and E. Costa, *J. Pharmacol. Exp. Ther.* 205:141 (1978).
163. J. S. Hong, H.-Y. T. Yang, J. C. Gillen, and E. Costa, in *Long-Term Effects of Neuroleptics* (F. Cattabeni, G. Racagni, P. F. Spano, and E. Costa, Eds.), Raven, New York, 1980, p. 223.
164. J. E. Leysen, in *Clinical Pharmacology in Psychiatry: Neuroleptic and Antidepressant Research* (E. Usdin, S. Dahl, L. F. Gram, and O. Lingjaerde, Eds.), MacMillan, Basingstoke, Hants, 1982, p. 35.
165. D. Hauser and A. Closse, *Life Sci.*, 23:557 (1978).
166. B. M. Cohen, M. Herschel, and A. Aoba, *Psychiatry Res.*, 1:199 (1979).
167. D. B. Bylund, *J. Pharmacol. Exp. Ther.*, 217:81 (1981).
168. D. H. York, *Brain Res.*, 20:233 (1970).
169. I. Creese, D. R. Burt, and S. H. Snyder, *Science*, 197:596 (1977).
170. J.-P. Schwarcz, I. Creese, J. T. Coyle, and S. H. Snyder, *Nature*, 271:766 (1978).
171. M. Garcia-Munoz, N. Nicolaou, I. F. Tulloch, A. K. Wright, and G. W. Arbuthnott, *Nature*, 265:363 (1977).
172. G. Di Chiara, M. L. Porceddu, W. Fratta, and G. L. Gessa, *Nature*, 267:270 (1977).
173. A. Carlsson, J. N. Davis, W. Kehr, M. Lindqvist, and C. V. Atack, *Naunyn-Schmied. Arch. Pharmakol.*, 275:153 (1972).
174. A. Handforth and T. L. Sourkes, *Eur. J. Pharmacol.*, 34:311 (1975).
175. P. Seeman and T. Lee, *J. Pharmacol. Exp. Ther.*, 190:131 (1974).
176. L.-O. Farnebo and B. Hamberger, *Acta Physiol. Scand.., Suppl.* 371:35 (1971).
177. L. L. Iversen, M. A. Rogawski, and R. J. Miller, *Molec. Pharmacol.*, 12:251 (1976).
178. P. R. Mitchell and N. S. Doggett, *Life Sci.*, 26:2073 (1980).
179. L. B. Geffen, T. M. Jessell, A. C. Cuello, and L. L. Iversen, *Nature*, 260:258 (1976).
180. G. K. Aghajanian and B. S. Bunney, in *Frontiers of Neurology and Neuroscience Research* (P. Seeman and G. M. Brown, Eds.), University of Toronto Press, Toronto, 1974, p. 4.
181. P. M. Groves, C. Wilson, S. Young, and G. Rebec, *Science*, 190: 522 (1975).
182. T. D. Reisine, J. I. Nagy, H. C. Fibiger, and H. I. Yamamura, *Brain Res.*, 169:209 (1979).
183. M. C. Olianas, G. M. De Montis, A. Concu, A. Tagliamonte, and G. Di Chiara, *Eur. J. Pharmacol.*, 49:223 (1978).

184. P. F. Spano, M. Trabucchi, and G. Di Chiara, *Science*, 196: 1343 (1977).
185. B. Costall, D. H. Fortune, S.-C. G. Hui, and R. J. Naylor, *Eur. J. Pharmacol.*, 63:347 (1980).
186. T. Alander, N.-E. Aden, and M. Grabowska-Anden, *Naunyn-Schmied. Arch. Pharmakol.*, 312:145 (1980).
187. F. Cerrito, G. Maura, and M. Raiteri, in *Apomorphine and Other Dopaminomimetics*, (G. L. Gessa and G. U. Corsini, Eds.), Raven, New York, 1981, p. 123.
188. A. Ruffieux and W. Schultz, *Nature*, 285:240 (1980).
189. J. W. Kebabian and D. B. Calne, *Nature*, 277:93 (1979).
190. I. Creese, D. R. Burt, and S. H. Snyder, *Life Sci.*, 17:993 (1975).
191. M. Titeler, P. Weinreich, D. Sinclair, and P. Seeman, *Proc. Nat. Acad. Sci. USA*, 75:1153 (1978).
192. I. Creese, Presented at Third World Congress of Biological Psychiatry (Stockholm), 1981.
193. I. Creese, T. Usdin, and S. H. Snyder, *Nature*, 278:577 (1979).
194. P. Sokoloff, M.-P. Martres, and J.-P. Schwartz, *Naunyn-Schmied. Arch. Pharmakol.*, 315:89 (1980).
195. P. Seeman, *Pharmacol. Rev.*, 32:229 (1980).
196. J. W. Kebabian and T. E. Cole, *Trends Pharmacol. Sci.*, 2:69 (1981).
197. R. Markstein, P. L. Herrling, H. R. Burki, H. Asper, and W. Ruch, *J. Neurochem.*, 31:1163 (1978).
198. J. Hyttel, *Progr. Neuro-Psychopharmacol.*, 3:329 (1978).
199. J. Hyttel, *Life. Sci.*, 23:551 (1978).
200. J. Hyttel, *Psychopharmacology*, 75:217 (1981).
201. K. Tsuruta, E. A. Frey, C. W. Grewe, T. E. Cote, R. J. Eskay, and J. W. Kebabian, *Nature*, 292:463 (1981).
202. D. R. Sibley, S. E. Leff, and I. Creese, *Life Sci.*, 31:637 (1982).
203. G. N. Woodruff, S. B. Freedman, and J. A. Poat, *J. Pharm. Pharmacol.*., 32:802 (1980).
204. M. Rodbell, *Nature*, 284:17 (1980).
205. S. Fleminger, H. van de Waterbeemd, N. M. J. Rupniak, C. Reavill, B. Testa, P. Jenner, and C. D. Marsden, *J. Pharm. Pharmac.* in press (1983).
206. J. C. Stoff and J. W. Kebabian, *Nature*, 294:366 (1981).
207. M. Munemura, R. Eskay, and J. W. Kebabian, *Endocrinology*, 106:1795 (1980).
208. P. Seeman, *Biochem. Pharmacol.*, 31:2563 (1982).
209. I. Creese and D. R. Sibley, *Biochem. Pharmacol.*, 31:2568 (1982).
210. M. Titeler, S. List, and P. Seeman, *Commun. Psychopharmacol.*, 3:411 (1979).
211. J. E. Leysen, in *Long-Term Effects of Neuroleptics* (E. Cattabeni, G. Racagni, P. F. Spano, and E. Costa, Eds.), Raven, New York, 1980, p. 123.

212. J. E. Leysen, *Commun. Psychopharmacol.*, 3:397 (1979).
213. V. Nomura, K. Oki, and T. Segawa, presented at the 8th International Congress of Pharmacology, Tokyo, 1981.
214. M. Memo, L. Lucchi, P. F. Spano, and M. Trabucchi, *Brain Res.* 202:488 (1980).
215. M. H. Makman, B. Dvorkin, and P. N. Klein, *Proc. Natl. Acad. Sci. USA*, 79:4212 (1982).
216. S. Leff, L. Adams, J. Hyttel, and I. Creese, *Eur. J. Pharmacol.*, 70:71 (1981).
217. P. Weinreich and P. Seeman, *Brain Res.*, 198:491 (1980).
218. T. D. Reisine, J. I. Nagy, H. C. Fibiger, and H. J. Yamamura, *Brain Res.*, 169:209 (1979).
219. J. L. Nagy, T. Lee, P. Seeman, and H. C. Fibiger, *Nature*, 274:278 (1978).
220. J. E. Leysen, W. Gommeren, and P. M. Laduron, *Arch. Int. Pharmacodyn. Ther.*, 249:312 (1979).
221. M. D. Hall, P. Jenner, and C. D. Marsden, *Neurosci. Lett.*, *Suppl.* 7:S363 (1981).
222. M. D. Hall, P. Jenner, E. Kelly, and C. D. Marsden, *Br. J. Pharmacol.*, in press (1983).
223. M. Quik, P. C. Emson, and E. Joyce, *Brain Res.*, 167:355 (1979).
224. T. D. Reisine, J. I. Nagy, H. C. Fibiger, and H. I. Yamamura, *Brain Res.*, 169:209 (1979).
225. T. Hattori and H. C. Fibiger, *Brain Res.*, 238:245 (1981).
226. M. Schachter, P. Bedard, A. G. Debono, P. Jenner, C. D. Marsden, P. Price, J. D. Parkes, J. Keenan, B. Smith, J. Rosenthaler, R. Horowski, and R. Dorow, *Nature*, 286:157 (1980).
227. B. Costall and R. J. Naylor, *Neuropharmacology*, 13:353 (1974).
228. C. J. Carter and C. J. Pycock, *Br. J. Pharmacol.*, 62:402p (1978).
229. P. R. Sanberg, M. Pisa, and H. C. Fibiger, *Eur. J. Pharmacol.*, 74:347 (1981).
230. P. R. Sanberg, *Nature*, 284:472 (1980).
231. G. Bartholini, K. G. Lloyd, B. Scatton, and P. Worms, *Br. J. Pharmacol.*, 72:128p (1980).
232. A. M. Zarkovsky, A. M. Nurk, L. K. Rago, and L. H. Allikmets, *Neuropharmacology*, 21:155 (1982).
233. P. Sokoloff, M.-P. Martres, and J.-C. Schwarts, presented at 8th International Congress of Pharmacology, Tokyo, 1982.
234. P. Sokoloff, Presented at Symposium on Special Aspects of Psychopharmacology, St. Maxime, France, 1982.
235. H. Asper, M. Baggiolini, H. R. Burki, H. Lauener, W. Ruch, and G. Stille, *Eur. J. Pharmacol.*, 22:287 (1973).
236. I. Moller Nielsen, B. Fjalland, V. Pedersen, and M. Nymberg, *Psychopharmacologia (Berl.)*, 34:95 (1974).
237. E. M. Boyd, *J. Pharmacol. Exp. Ther.*, 128:75 (1960).

238. N. M. J. Rupniak, P. Jenner, and C. D. Marsden, unpublished observation.
239. A. C. Sayers, H. R. Burki, W. Ruch, and H. Asper, *Psychopharmacologia (Berl.)*, 41:97 (1975).
240. B. Scatton, *Eur. J. Pharmacol.*, 46:363 (1977).
241. M. B. Bowers, Jr. and A. Rozitis, *J. Pharmac. Pharmacol.*, 26: 743 (1974).
242. Y. Clement-Cormier, in *Long-Term Effects of Neuroleptics* (F. Cattabeni, G. Racagni, P. F. Spano, and E. Costa, Eds.), Raven, New York, 1980, p. 103.
243. B. S. Bunney and A. A. Grace, *Life Sci.*, 23:1715 (1978).
244. N. G. Bacopoulos, *Eur. J. Pharmacol.*, 70:585 (1981).
245. I. Moller-Nielsen and A. V. Christensen, *J. Pharmacol (Paris)*, 6:277 (1975).
246. J. C. Schwartz, J. Constentin, M. P. Martes, P. Protais, and M. Baudry, *Neuropharmacology*, 17:665 (1978).
247. H. Kolbe, A. Clow, P. Jenner, and C. D. Marsden, *Neurology (NY)*, 31:434 (1981).
248. M. Valchar, J. Metysova, J. Chelbounova, and A. Dlabac, *Psychopharmacology*, 76:381 (1982).
249. A. V. Christensen and I. Moller-Nielsen, in *Tardive Dyskinesia* (W. E. Fann, R. C. Smith, J. M. Davis, and E. F. Domino, Eds.), Spectrum, New York 1980, p. 35.
250. J. Hyttel, *Psychopharmacology*, 59:211 (1978).
251. H. Kolbe, N. M. J. Rupniak, E. Kelly, D. Cooper, C. Reavill, P. Jenner, and C. D. Marsden, unpublished data.
252. J. C. Schwartz, presented at 7th International Congress of Pharmacology, Paris, 1976.
253. B. H. C. Westerink and A. S. Horn, *Eur. J. Pharmacol.*, 58:39 (1979).
254. P. Muller and P. Seeman, *Psychopharmacology*, 60:1 (1978).
255. D. Tarsy and R. J. Baldessarini, *Nature*, 245:262 (1973).
256. G. Gianutsos and K. E. Moore, *Life. Sci.*, 20:1585 (1977).
257. P. F. Von Voigtlander, E. G. Losey, and H. J. Triezenberg, *J. Pharmacol. Exp. Ther.*, 193:88 (1975).
258. K. Fuxe, S.-E. Ogren, H. Hall, L. F. Agnati, K. Andersson, C. Kohler, and R. Schwarca, in *Advances in Biochemical Psychopharmacology*, Raven, New York, 1980, p. 193.
259. R. C. Smith, W. Narasimhachari, and J. M. Davis, *J. Neural. Trans.*, 42:159 (1978).
260. D. R. Burt, I. Creese, and S. H. Snyder, *Science*, 196:326 (1977).
261. D. J. Heal, A. R. Green, D. J. Boullin, and D. G. Grahame-Smith, *Psychopharmacology*, 49:287 (1976).
262. J. Rotrosen, E. Friedman, and S. Gershon, *Life Sci.*, 17:563 (1975).

263. G. Yarborough, *Eur. J. Pharmacol.*, 21:367 (1975).
264. A. M. Zarkovsky, A. M. Nurk, L. K. Rago, and L. H. Allikmets, *Neuropharmacology*, 21:155 (1982).
265. D. M. Jackson, N.-E. Anden, J. Engel, and S. Liljequist, *Psychopharmacology*, 45:151 (1975).
266. K. L. Davis, L. E. Hollister, and W. C. Fritz, *Life Sci.*, 23: 1543 (1978).
267. I. Moller-Nielsen, A. V. Christensen, and J. Hyttel, in *Dopamine* (P. J. Roberts, G. N. Woodruff, and L. L. Ivesen, Eds.), Raven, New York, 1978, p. 267.
268. R. P. Ebstein, D. Pickhclz, and R. H. Belmaker, *J. Pharmac. Pharmacol.*, 31:558 (1979).
269. S. List and P. Seeman, *Life Sci.*, 24:1447 (1979).
270. J.-C. Schwartz, M. Baudry, M.-P. Martres, J. Costentin, and P. Protais, *Life. Sci..*, 23:1785 (1978).
271. A. M. Marshall and R. K. Mishra, in *Long-Term Effects of Neuroleptics* (F. Cattabeni, P. F. Spano, G. Racagni, and E. Costa, Eds.), Raven, New York, 1980, p. 153.
272. R. M. Kobayashi, J. Z. Fields, R. E. Hruska, K. Beaumont, and H. I. Yamamura, in *Animal Models in Psychiatry and Neurology* (I. Hanin and E. Usdin, Eds.), Pergamon, New York, 1977, p. 405.
273. P. Muller and P. Seeman, *Life Sci.*,21:1751 (1977).
274. E. Meller, K. Bohmaker, H. Rosengarten, and A. J. Friedhoff, *Res. Commun. Chem. Path. Pharmacol.*, 37:323 (1982).
275. J. W. Schweitzer, R. Schwarts, and A. J. Friedhoff, *Res. Commun. Chem. Pathol. Pharmacol.*, 38:21 (1982).
276. S. Fleminger, N. M. J. Rupniak, M. D. Hall, P. Jenner, and C. D. Marsden, *Biochem. Pharmacol.*, in press (1983).
277. M. Gnegy, P. Uzunov, and E. Costa, *J. Pharmacol. Exp. Ther.*, 202:558 (1977).
278. M. Goldstein, J. Y. Lew, T. Asano, and K. Ueta, *Commun. Psychopharmacol.* 4:21 (1980).
279. M. D. Hall, N. M. J. Rupniak, P. Jenner, and C. D. Marsden, *Psychopharmacology*, in press (1983).
280. J. E. Rosenblatt, D. Shore. L. M. Neckers, M. J. Perlow, W. J. Feed, and R. J. Wyatt, *Eur. J. Pharmacol.*, 60:387 (1979).
281. W. C. Friend, G. M. Gregory, G. Jawahir, T. L. Lee, and P. Seeman, *Am. J. Psychiat.*, 135:839 (1978).
282. O. Svendsen, *Eur. J. Pharmacol.*, 53:387 (1979).
283. P. Jenner, M. D. Hall, K. Murugaiah, N. Rupniak, A. Theodorou, and C. D. Marsden, *Biochem. Pharmacol.*, 31:325 (1982).
284. K. Fuxe, S.-O. Ogren, H. Hall, L. F. Agnati, K. Anderson, C. Kohler, and R. Schwarcz, in *Long-Term Effects of Neuroleptics* (F. Cattabeni, G. Racagni, P. S. Spano, and E. Costa, Eds.), Raven, New York, 1980, p. 193.

285. M. Trabucchi, M. Memo, F. Battaini, A. Reggiani, and P. F. Spano, in *Long-Term Effects of Neuroleptics* (F. Cattabeni, G. Racagni, P. F. Spano, and E. Costa, Eds.), Raven, New York, 1980, p. 275.
286. J. Bannet, S. Gillis, R. P. Ebstein, and R. H. Belmaker, *Int. Pharmacopsychiat.*, 15:334 (1980).
287. N. Montanara, R. Dall'Olio, O. Gandolfi, and A. Vaccheri, presented at International Workshop on Application of Behavioral Pharmacology in Toxicolory, Capri.
288. M. Gnegy, P. Uzunov, and E. Costa, *J. Pharmacol. Exp. Ther.*, 202:558 (1977).
289. R. M. Kobayashi, J. Z. Fields, R. E. Hurska, K. Beaumont, and H. I. Yamamura, in *Animal Models in Psychiatry* (E. Usdin, Ed.), Pergamon, New York, 1978, p. 405.
209. G. Racagni, F. Bruno, A. Bugatti, M. Parenti, J. A. Apud, V. Sankin, A. Carenz, A. Groppetti, and F. Cattabeni, in *Long-Term Effects of Neuroleptics* (F. Cattabeni, G. Racagni, P. F. Spano, and E. Costa, Eds.), Raven, New York, 1980, p. 45.
291. I. Creese and S. H. Snyder, in *Long-Term Effects of Neuroleptics* (F. Cattabeni, G. Racagni, P. F. Spano, and E. Costa, Eds.), Raven, New York, 1980, p. 89.
292. R. C. Smith and J. M. Davis, *Life Sci.*, 19:725 (2976).
293. T. F. Seeger, L. Thal, and E. L. Gardner, *Psychopharmacology*, 76:182 (1982).
294. N. M. J. Rupniak, M. Hall, P. Jenner, and C. D. Marsden, unpublished observations.
295. R. E. Hruska, L. Ludmer, and E. K. Silbergeld, *Eur. J. Pharmacol.*, 65:455 (1980).
296. R. E. Hruska, K. Pitman, E. K. Silbergeld, and L. M. Ludmer, *Life Sci.*, 30:547 (1982).
297. P. Jenner, N. M. J. Rupniak, M. D. Hall, R. Dyer, N. Eight, and C. D. Marsden, *Eur. J. Pharmacol.*, 76:31 (1981).
298. R. E. Hruska and E. K. Pitman, *Eur. J. Pharmacol.*, 85:201 (1982).
299. N. M. J. Rupniak, M. Hong, S. Mansfield, S. Fleminger, R. Dyer, P. Jenner, and C. D. Marsden, *Eur. J. Pharmac.*, in press (1983).
300. A. Clow, A. Theodorou, P. Jenner, and C. D. Marsden, *Eur. J. Pharmacol.*, 63:135 (1980).
301. N. M. J. Rupniak, M. D. Hall, S. Fleminger, P. Jenner, and C. D. Marsden, unpublished observations.
302. D. Dawbarn and C. Pycock, *Eur. J. Pharmacol.*, 71:233 (1981).
303. J. L. Waddington and S. J. Gamble, *Eur. J. Pharmacol.*, 67:363 (1980).
304. J. L. Waddington, S. J. Gamble, and R. C. Bourne, *Eur. J. Pharmacol.*, 69:511 (1981).

305. K. Murugaiah, A. Theodorou, P. Jenner, and C. D. Marsden, *Neuroscience*, in press (1983).
306. R. C. Bourne, S. J. Gamble, and J. L. Waddington, *Br. J. Pharmacol.* 76:232P (1982).
307. K. Murugaiah, A. Theodorou, P. Jenner, and C. D. Marsden, *Life Sci.*, 21:181 (1982).
308. R. W. Kerwin, N. M. J. Rupniak, P. Jenner, and C. D. Marsden, *Neuroscience*, in press (1983).
309. K. Murugaiah, S. Fleminger, M. D. Hall, A. Theodorou, P. Jenner, and C. D. Marsden, *Neuropharmacology*, in press (1983).
310. A. Clow, A. Theodorou, P. Jenner, and C. D. Marsden, *Psychopharmacology*, 69:227 (1980).
311. J. P. Tassin, H. Simon, D. Herve, G. Blanc, M. Le Moal, J. Glowinski, and J. Bockaert, *Nature*, 295:696 (1982).
312. A. Clow, A. Theodorou, P. Jenner, and C. D. Marsden, *Eur. J. Pharmacol.*, 63:145 (1980).
313. K. Murugaiah, S. Fleminger, A. Theodorou, P. Jenner, and C. D. Marsden, *Biochem. Pharmacol.*, in press (1983).
314. B. J. Sahakian, T. W. Robbins, and S. D. Iversen, *Eur. J. Pharmacol.*, 37:169 (1976).
315. N. M. J. Rupniak, P. Jenner, and C. D. Marsden, *Psychopharmacology*, 79:226 (1983).
316. A. Theodorou, W. Gommeren, A. Clow, J. Leysen, P. Jenner, and C. D. Marsden, *Life. Sci.*, 28:1621 (1981).
317. D. Dawbarn, S. K. Long, and C. J. Pycock, *Br. J. Pharmacol.*, 73:149 (1981).
318. S. J. Peroutka and S. H. Snyder, *Molec. Pharmacol.*, 16:687 (1979).
319. K. Gale, *Brain Res. Bull,*, 5:897 (1980).
320. K. Murugaiah, P. D. Marley, P. Emson, P. Jenner, and C. D. Marsden, unpublished data.
321. M. Alpert, A. J. Friedhoff, L. R. Marcos, and F. Diamond, *Am. J. Psychiatry*, 135:1329 (1978).
322. M. Alpert and A. J. Friedhoff, *Schizophrenia Bull.*, 6:387 (1980).
323. P. Fleming, H. Makar, and K. R. Hunter, *Lancet*, 2:1186 (1970).
324. E. C. Johnstone, T. J. Crow, C. D. Frith, M. W. P. Carney, and J. S. Price, *Lancet, 1:848 (1978).*

5
Drugs Used in the Regulation of Endocrine and Motor Activity

JAMES A. CLEMENS *Central Nervous System and Endocrine Research, The Lilly Research Laboratories, A Division of Eli Lilly and Company, Indianapolis, Indiana*

I. INTRODUCTION

The purpose of this chapter is to describe the drugs and the biological rationale for using the drugs in treating various endocrine and CNS motor disturbances. The application of the various drugs in treating the diseases will be viewed in the light of what is known about the etiology of the disease. Most of the endocrine diseases mentioned herein result from disturbances of the hypothalamus–pituitary axis. The CNS disorders of motor activity are those that are related to malfunctions within the extrapyramidal system.

II. DRUGS USED TO TREAT ENDOCRINE DISTURBANCES

A. Hyperprolactinemia

The term "hyperprolactinemia" is used to refer to the condition where serum prolactin levels are elevated beyond the normal range. Other conditions are produced by hyperprolactinemia, and in most instances it is the discovery of the secondary condition that finally leads to the measurement of serum prolactin levels. Since the measurement of serum prolactin levels is not a part of routine physical examinations, the true incidence of hyperprolactinemia is not known. In the female, one of the most common disturbances resulting from high serum prolactin levels is amenorrhea and/or galactorrhea. In the male, unlike the female, there are few symptoms other than sexual impotence that signal the presence of hyperprolactinemia.

Many causes of hyperprolactinemia exist. In patients with serum prolactin levels consistently >50 ng/ml, the presence of a pituitary tumor needs to be ruled in or out, as well as possible. In many instances, small, hard-to-detect microadenomas exist that are difficult to find in routine skull X-rays.

The causative factors in the production of prolactin-secreting tumors are unknown. In animals, the most efficient way of causing prolactin-secreting pituitary tumors is to administer estrogens [1]. Estradiol or an estradiol metabolite may be the carcinogen, or perhaps an eventual reduction of the dopamine inhibitory influence on the mammotroph (as has been reported for estradiol [2]) is the cause of the tumor. When the influence of dopamine on the pituitary is removed, prolactin release continues unabated [3,4]. The possibility exists that, in the human, the continuous action of estradiol or a defective tuberoinfundibular dopaminergic system allows the pituitary to escape from the inhibitory influence of dopamine and leads to the formation of an adenoma or a tumor.

Hyperprolactinemia can also be drug induced. All of the currently marketed neuroleptic drugs are potent stimulators of prolactin release [5]. Clozapine, which had been withdrawn from the market, was the only neuroleptic drug that did not stimulate prolactin release. Two of the commonly used antihypertensive drugs, reserpine and α-methyldopa, stimulate prolactin release [6,7].

Neuroleptic drugs block the interaction of dopamine with its receptor at the level of the pituitary, whereas reserpine depletes hypothalamic dopamine levels and α-methyldopa inhibits dopamine synthesis. The net effect of all of the drugs is to make dopamine functionally unavailable to the pituitary gland. Other substances including morphine, methadone, β-endorphin and other opioids, thyrotropin-releasing factor (TRH), and estrogens have been shown to elevate prolactin release.

The most effective drug therapy for hyperprolactinemia is the administration of dopamine agonists. The first treatment utilized along this line was the dopamine precursor, L-dopa. L-dopa was found to be of little value, because prolactin suppression was transient [7–9] and side effects, particularly nausea, were prominent and forced discontinuation in several cases. For hyperprolactinemia, the greatest advance in drug therapy to date has been the development of bromocriptine. Bromocriptine lowers serum prolactin levels, and in many instances restores menses to amenorrhea-galactorrhea patients [10–18]. In some patients with prolactin-secreting pituitary tumors, bromocriptine has been found to shrink the size of the tumor [19–21], and in most patients with prolactin-secreting tumors it substantially lowers serum prolactin levels. Side effects include nausea, postural hypotension, and mental changes. Two potential drugs, pergolide [21–24] and lisuride [25,26] are still in the clinical trial stage, and it is too early to tell if one of these or possibly both will have a better therapeutic ratio than bromocriptine.

Both agents have shown good efficacy in treating prolactin-dependent disorders. The side effects of both potential drugs appear to be qualitatively similar to those of bromocriptine. Of the three agents, pergolide appears to be the most potent and longest acting.

B. Amenorrhea-Galactorrhea

In patients with high serum prolactin levels, amenorrhea and galactorrhea may both present. However, many of the women with galactorrhea have normal levels of serum prolactin and regular menses. Cyclic estrogen-progesterone therapy has been tried, but this often diminishes galactorrhea without eliminating it; and the condition resumes on cessation of therapy. Bromocriptine has been shown to be a much more effective therapy for galactorrhea [10–18]. Amenorrhea without galactorrhea also occurs, and drugs to treat this condition will be mentioned in the section on infertility.

C. Benign Breast Disease

Benign fibrocystic disease of the breast is the most common breast disorder in women. The disease can occur at any age, but the incidence is higher in women 30–50 years old. Most of the breast surgery (about 74%) is performed on women to remove lumps that appear in the breast as a result of this disease [27]. The reason for the surgery is that it has been difficult to distinguish a benign lump or nodule from a cancer, and because the fear of cancer is so great. Recent advances in diagnostic procedures, however, are making it easier to distinguish a benign lesion from a malignant one.

Diagnostic procedures will not be covered here, but for an excellent review, consult the work of Greenblatt, *et al.* [27].

In many instances, little effort is made to treat this disease except for surgical removal of suspicious nodules or lumps. More effort needs to be focused on treating and finding a cure for this disease, because women with benign breast disease have a three times greater risk of developing a breast cancer than normal women [28,29]. Since breast cancer is the most frequent cancer in women, it may be possible to reduce significantly the number of deaths by effectively treating benign breast disease.

The cause of fibrocystic disease is unknown. It is believed that this condition results from a hormonal imbalance [30–32]. The nature of the hormonal imbalance has not been clearly established [27,33]. Prolactin may play a permissive role in the development of the disease, but most studies report no significant correlation with serum prolactin levels [30,33]. The role of ovarian steroids is also unclear, because in most cases the administration of oral contraceptives and other estrogenic preparations does not result in an increased incidence of benign breast disease [34]. Perhaps one of the clues that provides us with a better understanding of the actual etiology of the disease is the finding that estrogen and progesterone receptor levels parallel the degree of mammary dysplasia [35]. Thus, the increased receptor levels may induce a hypersensitivity of epithelial elements to steroid hormones.

Fibrocystic disease has been treated with oral estrogens and/or oral progestins, as well as androgens [36,37] for many years. These treatments were effective to a limited degree. However, prolonged exposure to estrogens appears to increase the risk of uterine cancer. The antiestrogen, tamoxifen, has been used to treat figrocystic disease and appears to be useful [38].

Danazol, a new impeded androgen with fewer masculinizing side effects than prior forms of androgen therapy, has been used by several investigators who have reported elimination or partial resolution of nodosities plus relief from pain and tenderness in a high percentage of women [39–42]. Danazol suppresses ovarian function by blocking the luteinizing hormone (LH) surge and interferes with ovarian steroidogenesis [43,44]. This action diminishes ovarian hormone secretion, which is believed to be a causative factor in the disease.

Side effects that have been reported for Danazol include nausea, hot flushes, nervousness, depression, weight gain, mild hirsutism, and muscle cramps. In addition, amenorrhea or menstrual irregularities can be expected. Danazol is not recommended for nursing mothers, pregnant women, or patients with liver, kidney, or heart disease.

Nonsteroidal therapy has also been used in the treatment of fibrocystic disease. Mastalgia, or pain in the breast, is a common symptom of fibrocystic disease. It may occur on a cyclical basis. In one double-blind study [45] and three open studies [30,46,47], bromocriptine was reported to be effective in relieving the pain. In an additional open study [33], 192 patients were given 3 × 2.5 mg p.o. bromocriptine continuously for 3 months. In about 75% of the cases, there was improvement or complete recovery. Thus, dopamine agonists may prove to be a useful new form of therapy for benign fibrocystic breast disease.

D. Acromegaly

Acromegaly is a relatively rare disease. It is almost always associated with a growth hormone-secreting pituitary tumor. The preferred treatment for this disorder is hypophysectomy. In cases of large tumors, many times hypophysectomy does not result in a permanent lowering of serum growth hormone levels. The only form of drug therapy that has been documented to be of benefit in acromegaly is the use of dopamine agonists. Bromocriptine [48–52] has been used over the last 7 years with varying degrees of success. In the acromegalic patient, the side effects of bromocriptine therapy include hypotension, headache, nasal stuffiness, nausea, and dyspepsia. The newer ergolines, lisuride, pergolide, and CU32-085 may also be of value in treating acromegaly. Although dopamine agonist therapy does not appear to cure this disease, it appears to be of benefit in slowing the progression.

E. Cushing's Disease

Cushing's disease, or pituitary-dependent Cushing's syndrome, is another relatively rare condition and is characterized by excessive ACTH secretion from the pituitary. ACTH secretion is controlled by corticotropin-releasing factor (CRF), which is produced by the hypothalamus. Whether the disease is primarily pituitary or hypothalamic in origin is not clear. In most patients, the disease is associated with a pituitary tumor that can be surgically removed to cure the condition [43,54].

In a small number of patients, hyperplasia of the adrenocorticotropin (ACTH)-secreting cells in the pituitary is found, with no distinct adenoma [53]. In these patients, the disease may be hypothalamic in origin and result from excessive CRF secretion.

The optimal therapy for Cushing's disease has not yet been agreed upon. Different methods of treatment have been developed. Nondrug therapy includes selective pituitary adenoma removal and pituitary irradiation with or without bilateral adrenalectomy. In drug therapy, treatment with enzyme blockers such as metyrapone to inhibit steroid synthesis [55] has been used. Krieger and co-workers [56] have pioneered the treatment of Cushing's disease with cyproheptadine, a serotonin antagonist. The drug lowered cortisol levels, a desired effect, but it did not restore the circadian rhythm of ACTH.

In a small number of patients, bromocriptine has proven to be of benefit in lowering ACTH levels in patients with Cushing's disease [57,58]. A central depletion of dopamine stores has been suggested to be implicated in the pathophysiology of the disease [59]; however, only a small number of patients have shown a response to bromocriptine.

Aminoglutethimide is an adrenal inhibitor that has been used in Cushing's disease for several years. It lowers serum cortisol levels and has been used as a substitute for surgical adrenalectomy [60–62]. The reputed sites of action of aminoglutethimide include inhibition of conversion of cholesterol to pregnenolone and blockade of the C11, C18, and C20 steroid hydroxylations [63–65]. Thus, this drug not only inhibits adrenal steroid formation, but it interferes with placental, ovarian, and testicular steroidogenesis [66].

Unfortunately, none of the drugs that are used to treat this condition result in a cure, but only alleviate the symptoms. The underlying disease process continues. A more effective treatment for this disease may be arrived at when it is determined if the disease is of hypothalamic or of pituitary origin.

F. Infertility

Most of the attention here is devoted to treatment of polycistic ovarian (PCO) syndrome, because it is one of the most common causes of infertility in women. Several possible causes of this disease exist. A defect in the hypothalamus–pituitary axis may cause the disease, or there may be an inappropriate pituitary feedback caused by abnormal steroidogenesis in the polycystic ovary. Another possibility is that the follicle may not mature properly because of an abnormal response to follicle-stimulating hormone (FSH). Regardless of the exact cause of the PCO syndrome, or even if a single cause exists, it is well known that the CNS-hypothalamic complex, the pituitary, and the ovary must interact in a highly integrated manner to achieve normal ovarian cyclicity.

Sclerocystic changes in the human ovary that were associated with a clinical syndrome of amenorrhea, hirsutism, and obesity were reported by Stein and Leventhal [67] in 1935 and became known as the Stein-Leventhal syndrome. Patients were usually treated by bilateral ovarian wedge resection, and this resulted in a high percentage (80–95%) reversal to normal menstrual cycles [68].

Subsequent endocrinological investigations of the subject revealed that the combination of bilateral ovarian failure, hirsutism, obesity, and the presence of polycystic ovaries was associated with several endocrine disorders of diverse etiology. Thus, amenorrhea, hirsutism, and obesity together with polycystic ovaries, although necessary, are not sufficient for the diagnosis of polycystic ovarian syndrome.

Some additional biochemical and endocrinological abnormalities characteristic of the PCO syndrome include androgen excess, lower levels of steroid hormone-binding globulin, elevated DHEA levels [69], erratic and inappropriately elevated blood LH levels with relatively constant and low FSH levels [70] and chronic anovulation. Whereas most of the studies indicate the existence of multiple hormonal abnormalities in the PCO syndrome, the cause does not appear to reside in an inherent defect in the hypothalamic–pituitary axis, but rather resides in an abnormality in steroid metabolism by the ovaries and adrenal glands. For two excellent reviews on the PCO syndrome, consult the work of Yen [71] and Goldzieher [72].

The aims in the treatment of the PCO syndrome are to establish fertility by the production of ovulatory menstrual cycles, reduce the probability of endometrial cancer, and reverse the hirsutism. The treatment may differ somethat depending on whether the patient wants to become pregnant.

The ovulation-inducing properties of clomiphene, an antiestrogen, are well established. The administration of clomiphene is considered to be an effective therapy for patients who are interested in conception, but it is not advised as a method merely to produce menstrual cycles. The success rate in patients with PCO syndrome is very high [73,74]. Clomiphene appears to increase FSH secretion, which results in an increase in estradiol production by the follicle. The positive feedback by estradiol on the hypothalamus results in an ovulatory surge of LH and FSH.

Gonadotropin-releasing hormone (GN-RH, LH-RH) has been used to treat the PCO syndrome [75]. The results with this therapy have been rather disappointing, however, possibly because of its short half-life. Synthetic analogs with greater potency and longer duration of activity are being tested, but these may be of limited value because of the peripheral antigonadotropic effects of potent LH-RH analogs [76].

Gonadotropin preparations have been used to treat cases of infertility where clomiphene did not work. In cases of a "luteal phase defect," LH (as HCG) has been given to patients where clomiphene was unsuccessful. Properly timed administration of preparations relatively high in FSH, such as Pergonal, is also used. A recent summary [77] of the use of gonadotropin preparations in clomiphene-resistant patients indicates that about two-thirds of the patients became pregnant. However, there was a 24% abortion rate, 36% multiple pregnancies, and three cases of severe hyperstimulation syndrome.

For women who do not wish to become pregnant immediately, oral contraceptives have been used. It appears desirable to use an oral contraceptive preparation containing 80 μg or more of ethynyl estrogen for several cycles. Many clear-cut benefits of contraceptive steroid treatment have been enumerated [72].

In some cases of PCO syndrome, hyperprolactinemia has been reported [78,79]. Therapy with the dopamine agonist, bromocriptine, was found to be of benefit in lowering serum prolactin levels and restoring menstrual cycles. Dopamine and dopamine agonists have been shown to have an inhibitory effect on LH release in humans [80,81]. In the PCO syndrome where estrogens are chronically elevated, the LH sensitivity to dopaminergic inhibition is enhanced [82]. Thus, the beneficial effect of dopamine agonist therapy in PCO syndrome may be due to an effect on both prolactin and LH release.

III. DRUGS USED IN THE CNS REGULATION OF MOTOR ACTIVITY

A. Parkinson's Disease

Parkinson's disease is a disease of motor function. To be more precise, it is a disease of the basal ganglia. The basal ganglia are responsible for the automatic execution of learned motor plans [83]. Unlike many of the other diseases of motor activity, Parkinson's disease appears to result primarily from the loss of dopaminergic input to the basal ganglia. In Parkinson's disease, the dopaminergic nigro-striatal neurons are virtually destroyed, which leads to gross disruption of the activity of the basal ganglia.

Tremor is associated with Parkinson's disease, and resting tremor characteristic of the disease. Resting tremor is tremor that is present while the patient's hands are folded in the lap or placed on the knees. The tremor tends to be less pronounced when the patient holds the hands outstretched to the front and tends to disappear with intentional movement. Patients with Parkinson's disease sit rigidly in one position with a set facial expression and stooped posture. Overall, there is a marked lack of spontaneous movement.

Initial drug therapy of Parkinson's disease included anticholinergic drugs resembling the belladonna alkaloids as well as the antihistamines which possessed anticholinergic activity. The commonly used drugs are listed in Table 5.1.

Anticholinergic drugs are used because dopamine acts in the corpus striatum to inhibit the release of acetylcholine from cholinergic neurons. The anticholinergic drugs offer a mild benefit, at best, in the treatment regimen. The side effects are dry mouth, blurred vision, urinary retention in males, and disturbed mentation.

Table 5.1 Anticholinergic Drugs Used in the Treatment of Parkinson's Disease

Drug	Dose range (mg/day)
Benztropine mesylate (Cogentin*®)	1–5
Biperiden (Akineton*®)	1–10
Chlorophenoxamine (Phenoxene*®)	50–100
Cycrimine (Pagitane*®)	1–10
Diphenhydramine (Benadryl*®)	25–200
Procyclidine (Kemadrin*®)	1–10
Trihexyphenidyl (Artane*®)	1–10

*® Trademark.

L-Dopa is used to increase dopaminergic activity. Treatment with L-dopa is effective in improving all of the signs and symptoms of Parkinson's disease in about 85% of treated individuals. Tremor is the sign least improved. The response is seen within 2 weeks of drug therapy. L-dopa can be used in combination with a decarboxylase inhibitor, carbidopa [carbidopa/levodopa (Sinemet*®)]. The addition of the carbidopa allows reduction in the dose of L-dopa and a corresponding reduction in some of the side effects. L-dopa is decarboxylated to dopamine, and the carbidopa prevents the peripheral decarboxylation of L-dopa, thereby making more L-dopa available for decarboxylation to dopamine by brain tissue. Carbidopa does not appreciably cross the blood brain barrier.

Even during L-dopa therapy, the disease appears to progress relentlessly. After about 5 years only about one-third of the patients retain the initial degree of improvement. One-third lose certain abilities and the other third deteriorate to the extent that they are worse off than they were at the onset of treatment.

Side effects of L-dopa therapy are nausea and vomiting, cardiac dysrhythmias, hypotension, and mental changes; with continued use, dyskinesias becomes apparent. Patients can experience unusual vacillations from brief period of improvement, followed by dyskinesia and then reemergence of Parkinsonian signs. Additionally, periodically during the day the patient can suddenly freeze in place and be unable to move for varying periods of time. These fluctuations are variations of the "on-off" phenomenon.

Amantadine hydrochloride (Symmetrel*®), a dopamine releaser, was found to be of benefit in the treatment of Parkinson's disease. It was initially used in patients intolerant or refractory to L-dopa as an adjunctive drug but has not provided much added benefit.

Monoamine oxidase (MAO) inhibitors have been used in Parkinson's disease. The type-B MAO inhibitor, L-deprenil, was reported to offer some benefit to Parkinson's patients concomitantly treated with L-dopa without the risk of hypertension seen with other MAO inhibitors [84].

One of the new approaches for the drug therapy of Parkinson's disease is the use of postsynaptic dopamine receptor agonists. One of the oldest recognized dopamine agonists is apomorphine. Apomorphine administration to patients with Parkinson's disease induced dose-dependent improvement of tremor, rigidity, and akinesia beginning at 160–600 mg/p.o. but had to be discontinued because of the production of azotemia [85]. An analog of apomorphine, *N*-propylnorapomorphine, produced improvement in Parkinson's disease with oral doses of 10–15 mg, although it had to be given six times a day [85]. Attempts to induce further improvement by increasing the dose produced azotemia.

---

*® Trademark.

The maximal improvement was sustained for about 3 weeks, after which a gradual diminution of symptomatic control developed. The tachyphylaxis could be abolished by coadministration of Sinemet®. Patients treated with *N*-propylnorapormophine showed "on-off" similar to when taking L-dopa, and other side effects were similar.

The ergot alkaloid dopamine agonist, bromocriptine, was the first agent in this series to be tested against Parkinson's disease [86,87], and a large number of studies with bromocriptine in Parkinson's disease have been reported. These have been summarized by Hoen [88]. Bromocriptine appeared to offer some promise to patients who suffer "on-off" phenomena. By titrating the dose of bromocriptine and L-dopa a more sustained degree of improvement was reported. High doses result in mental changes and a risk of hypotension. Bromocriptine alone can effect an improvement; however, a greater beneficial effect is obtained when it is combined with L-dopa.

Because of variations in individual response, bromocriptine can ameliorate some of the problems of prolonged L-dopa therapy; i.e., declining efficacy, fluctuations in response, and the development of abnormal involuntary movements. Thus, the consensus appears that bromocriptine is a valuable adjunct in the treatment of Parkinson's disease.

A novel idea to reduce the side effects of bromocriptine therapy was to add a peripheral dopamine antagonist to the treatment. In patients treated with the peripheral dopamine antagonist, domperidone, at a dose of 50 mg three times a day, the dose of bromocriptine could be increased rapidly to a mean dose of 148 mg/day. The side effects of nausea and vomiting were virtually eliminated [89]. A significant clinical improvement over baseline score was obtained.

Lisuride and pergolide are not ergot alkaloids, but synthetic ergoline derivatives that have been found to possess potent dopamine agonist activity. Both agents are currently in clinical trials for the treatment of Parkinson's disease.

Lisuride was found to be active against Parkinson's disease and was fairly well tolerated [90–93]. The optimal dose of lisuride was about 4.5 mg/day but the dose needed to be individualized. Most patients experienced a dose-related improvement of the full range of symptoms. The degree of improvement was similar to that obtained with bromocriptine [93]. Side effects include mental changes, sedation, lightheadedness, postural hypotension, vestibular impairment, hallucinations, and nausea. The side effects of lisuride are similar to those of bromocriptine.

Pergolide mesylate has been shown to be a potent, long-acting dopamine agonist in animals [96] and in man [22,24]. Many of the beneficial effects of pergolide in the treatment of Parkinson's disease are similar to those produced by lisuride and bromocriptine [95]. Early side effects of pergolide—nausea, orthostatic hypotension, nasal stuffiness, sweating, and alterations in liver function tests—were usually transient. In a study where pergolide was compared with lisuride in treatment of Parkinson's disease [96], it was reported that pergolide was more effective and was of longer duration (4–8 hr compared with 1–3 hr for lisuride) in smoothing out the L-dopa oscillations.

One of the most promising aspects of pergolide therapy is the finding that it is particularly useful in patients with "on-off" phenomena [97–100]. For the most part, pergolide has only been used in patients also receiving L-dopa, and in most studies the dose of L-dopa could be substantially reduced.

In an attempt to find useful drugs to treat the "on-off" syndrome, naloxone was used and found to be of some benefit [101]. Although naloxone did not change the cardinal symptoms of Parkinson's disease, the opiate antagonist did modify the "on-off" syndrome. The switch from the rigid to the mobile phase and from the mobile to rigid phase became more gradual, and thereby increased the total duration of the "on" phases. Naloxone also reduced the L-dopa-induced dyskinesia. Thus, opiate receptors may be important in the control of abnormal involuntary movements.

In conclusion, none of the drugs mentioned above are able to cure Parkinson's disease, but can only improve the symptoms. It would seem to be of value to try to find drugs that can prevent the insidious destruction of the nigro-striatal dopaminergic system that occurs in this disease.

B. Tardive Dyskinesia

Tardive dyskinesia may be defined as a choreic movement disorder, characterized by involuntary movements of the tongue, lips, and jaw. Tardive dyskinesia appears in a significant number of patients after continuous prolonged treatment with neuroleptic drugs. Tardive dyskinesia usually occurs late in neuroleptic treatment and often appears when neuroleptic medication is discontinued.

The exact mechanism of tardive dyskinesia is unknown, but currently the favored hypothesis is the denervation supersensitivity hypothesis. Some investigators have suggested that chronic neuroleptic administration induces a postsynaptic dopamine receptor supersensitivity that can lead to the development of tardive dyskinesia [101,102].

Drug treatment of tardive dyskinesia is a very challenging problem, because there is no consensus on the most effective treatment. An amazing number of drugs have been tested as treatments for tardive dyskinesia. Many of the drugs have been shown to be of some benefit. The drugs reported to be effective in treating tardive dyskinesia are listed in Table 5.2.

TABLE 5.2 Drugs Reported to Be of Benefit in the Treatment of Tardive Dyskinesia

Dopamine antagonists	GABAeric agents
phenothiazines	Valproate
butyrophenones	baclofen
clozapine	Serotonin antagonists
pimozide	cyproheptadine
sulpride	Cholinergic agents
oxiperomide	deanol
papaverine	physostigmine
metoclopramide	choline and lecithin
Dopamine agonists	Catecholamine-depleting agents
apomorphine	reserpine
bromocriptine	tetrabenazine
lisuride	
Catecholamine synthesis inhibitors	
methyldopa	
α-methyltyrosine	
fusaric acid	
disulfiram	

In spite of the large number of drugs that appears in Table 5.2, a beneficial response to most of these agents is compatible with the dopamine receptor supersensitivity hypothesis. If a postsynaptic dopamine receptor supersensitivity occurs in tardive dyskinesia, then any treatment that decreases the amount of postsynaptic stimulation by dopamine may prove beneficial. Dopamine antagonists block the action of dopamine and at modest doses reduce the tardive dyskinesia symptoms [103]. Reserpine, which depletes dopamine stores, is beneficial [104, 105], and dopamine agonists are beneficial in doses that primarily stimulate presynaptic dopamine autoreceptors and thereby reduce dopaminergic neuronal activity [106,107]. Agents that enhance γ-aminobutyric acid (GABA) activity reduce dopaminergic neuronal activity. Agents that have cholinergic effects are beneficial [107,108] by reducing the dopaminergic influence in the striatum, because it is well recognized that dopamine inhibits acetylcholine release in the striatum.

Perhaps a highly effective drug for treating tardive dyskinesia would be a selective dopamine autoreceptor stimulant. A drug of this nature might shut down or attenuate dopaminergic neuronal function without influencing postsynaptic dopamine receptors. In addition, it could be used as a neuroleptic. An agent such as pergolide, which is long acting and has autoreceptor-stimulating properties at doses far below the doses where postsynaptic stimulation is seen [109], eventually may prove useful for this disease. At the present time, the best treatment for tardive dyskinesia appears to be to try to avoid it by decreasing the dose of neuroleptic medication as much as possible without losing control of the psychotic disorder.

C. Tourette Syndrome

Gilles de la Tourette syndrome is a familial neurological disorder characterized by a combination of chronic fluctuating motor tics usually involving the head and frequently other parts of the body, torso, and upper and lower limbs. Involuntary verbalizations are present and include various complicated sounds, words, or in some cases coprolalia. It may be associated with hyperactivity or minimal brain dysfunction. Some investigators believe that Tourette syndrome may result from a dopaminergic receptor supersensitivity [110].

The most widely used drug to treat the symptoms of Tourette syndrome is haloperidol [111–113]. The dosage has to be titrated for each patient to achieve optimum effectiveness. Benztropine is used in combination with haloperidol at the start of treatment. Side effects include Parkinson-like symptoms, akathisia, akinesia, acute dystonia, tardive dyskinesia, and cognitive impairment.

Other dopamine antagonists, pimozide [114] and fluphenazine [115], were reported to be effective in treating Tourette syndrome. Fluphenazine may have fewer side effects. Recently Tanner at al. [116] reported that scopolamine improved motor tics but exacerbated vocal tics in patients with Tourette syndrome. The reverse was seen with physostigmine.

D. Huntington's Disease

Huntington's disease is similar to tardive dyskinesia and L-dopa dyskinesias in that it is characterized by many hyperkinetic abnormal movements, but differs from these dyskinesias in that it is inherited as an autosomal dominant trait. It is characterized by progressive, involuntary movements and dementia, has an onset at about 36–37 years of age [117] and has defied all treatment.

Pathological changes in Huntington's disease include loss of neurons in the putamen and caudate nuclei and in the cerebral cortex and other sites [118]. Glutamate is believed to be involved in the degeneration of striatal (caudate, putamen) neurons in this disease [119]. Glutamate may be related to nerve cell death in the brains of patients with Huntington's disease [120]. An analog of glutamic acid, kainic acid, has been used to produce lesions in the striatum that are a model for the morphological and biochemical changes found in brains from Huntington's patients [121]. Biochemical studies of brains of patients with Huntington's disease indicated a loss of GABA, its synthesizing enzyme glutamic acid decarboxylase, and choline acetyltransferase [122,123]. Many investigators proposed that if brain GABA activity could be increased, Huntington's disease might be controlled.

Disappointing results have been obtained in clinical trials that had been built around the above pharmacological rationale. Neither inhibitors of GABA breakdown nor GABA agonists were shown to be of clear-cut benefit in treating Huntington's disease [124–127].

Some believe that Huntington's disease is related to a functional overactivity of dopaminergic influences relative to the cholinergic and GABA system in the striatum [128]. A dopaminergic supersensitivity may also be involved. The current mainstay of therapy is dopamine receptor antagonists and is in line with the above concept.

Phenothiazines and butyrophenones are the accepted mode of therapy in Huntington's disease [129]. Haloperidol and chlorpromazine are the two most widely used drugs. Selective presynaptic dopamine autoreceptor stimulants may eventually prove useful in treating this disease, because apomorphine has been found to be useful in reducing involuntary movements [130]; however, the usefulness of apomorphine is hampered by its short half-life.

Other forms of treatment have been tried with varying degrees of success. Increasing acetylcholine activity with physostigmine or deanol has produced inconsistent results. Choline administration was reported to improve the involuntary movements [131].

In conclusion, Huntington's disease is another of the CNS motor disorders that has no known cure. The most that can be done with drug treatment is an amelioration of the symptoms in the more fortunate patients.

ACKNOWLEDGMENTS

The author wishes to thank Lee Ann Bertram for excellent help in preparing the bibliography and Linda Johnson for her expert secretarial assistance.

REFERENCES

1. K. Nakagawa, T. Obaha, and K. Tashiro, *Endocrinology*, 106: 1033 (1980).
2. F. Casnueva, D. Cocchi, V. Locatelli, C. Flauto, F. Zambotti, G. Bestetti, G. Rossi, and E. Muller, *Endocrinology*, 110:590 (1982).

3. J. A. Clemens and J. Meites, in *Lactogenic Hormones: Fetal Nutrition and Lactation* (J. B. Josimovich, M. Reynolds, and E. Cobo, Eds.) Wiley, New York, 1974, p.111.
4. C. W. Welsch, M. D. Squires, E. Cassell, C. L. Chen, and J. Meites, *Am. J. Physiol.*, 221:1714 (1971).
5. J. A. Clemens, E. B. Smalstig, and B. D. Sawyer, *Psychopharmacologia*, 40:123 (1974).
6. A. G. Frantz and D. L. Kleinberg, *Science*, 170:745 (1970).
7. A. G. Frantz, in *Lactogenic Hormones: Fetal Nutrition and Lactation* (J. B. Josimovich, M. Reynolds, and E. Cobo, Eds.) Wiley, New York, 1974, p. 379.
8. M. Edmonda, R. Volpe, and H. Friesen, *Can Med. Assoc. J.*, 107:534 (1972).
9. W. B. Malarkey, L. S. Jacobs, and W. H. Daughaday, *New Engl. J. Med.*. 285:1160 (1971).
10. G. M. Besser and C. R. W. Edwards, *Br. Med. J.*, 2(5808):280 (1972).
11. L. Varga, P. M. Lutterbeck, J. S. Pryor, R. Wenner, and H. Erb, *Schweiz, Med. Wochenschr.*, 36:1284 (1972).
12. E. Fluckiger, K. Saameli, and W. H. Daughaday, *New Engl. J. Med.*, 286:547 (1972).
13. E. del Pozo, A. Audibert, and P. M. Lutterbeck, *New Engl. J. Med.*, 287:723 (1972).
14. R. del Re Brun, E. del Pozo, P. deGrandi, H. Friesen, M. Hinselmann, and H. Wyss, *Obstet. Gynecol.*, 41:884 (1973).
15. E. del Pozo, *J. Clin. Endocrinol. Metab.*, 39:18 (1974).
16. K. Schulz, W. Geiger, J. Kuenzig, and K. H. Lohse, *Acta Endocrinol.*, 78 (Suppl. 193):27 (1975).
17. E. S. Canales, G. Forsbach, J. Soria, and A. Zarate, *Fertil. Steril.*, 27:1335 (1976).
18. R. Rolland, L. A. Schellekens, and R. M. Lequin, *Clin. Endorinol.*, 3:155 (1974).
19. A. M. McGregor, M. F. Scanlon, K. Hall, D. B. Cook, and R. Hall, *N. Engl. J. Med.*, 300:291 (1979).
20. A. M. McGregor, M. F. Scanlon, R. Hall, and K. Hall, *Br. Med. J.*, 2:700 (1979).
21. D. Muhlenstedt, F. Osmers, and H. P. G. Schneider, *Arch. Gynecol.*, 226:341 (1978).
22. D. L. Kleinberg, A. Lieberman, J. Todd, J. Greisling, A. Neophyides, and M. Kupersmith, *J. Clin. Endorcinol. Metab.*, 51:152 (1980).
23. S. Franks, P. M. Horrocks, S. S. Lynch, W. R. Butt, and D. R. London, *Lancet*, :659 (1981).
24. L. Lemberger and R. E. Crabtree, *Science*, 205:1151 (1979).
25. A. Liuzzi, P. G. Chiodini, G. Oppizzi, L. Botalla, G. Verde, L. deStefano, G. Colussi, K. J. Graf, and R. Horowski, *J. Clin. Endocrinol. Metab.*, 46:196 (1978).

26. P. G. Chiodini, *Clin. Endocrinol.*, 12:47 (1980).
27. R. B. Greenblatt, J. Vaspuez, and C. Samaras, *Postgraduate Med.*, 71:159 (1982).
28. L. J. Coombs and A. Lilienfeld, *Prev. Med.*, 8:40 (1979).
29. C. D. Haagensen, N. Lane, and R. Lattes, *Cancer*, 42:737 (1978).
30. J. Martin-Comin, P. Pujol-Amat, V. Cararach, E. Davi, and C. Robyn, *Obstet. Gynecol.*, 48:703 (1976).
31. R. C. Golinger, *Surg. Gynecol. Obstet.*, 146:273 (1978).
32. P. H. Rolland, P. M. Martin, A. J. Rolland, M. Bourry, and H. Serment, *Obstet. Gynecol.*, 54:715 (1979).
33. C. Santoro, M. Cappa, C. Moretti, A. Fabbri, V. LaVecchia, L. R. Marcellino, and F. Fraioli, *Int. J. Clin. Pharmacol. Therapy Toxicol.*, 20:479 (1982).
34. H. Ory, P. Cole, B. MacMahon, and R. Hoover, *New Engl. J. Med.*, 294:419 (1976).
35. J. D. Jacquemier, P. H. Rolland, D. Vague, R. Lieutaud, J. M. Spitalier, and P. M. Martin, *Cancer*, 49:2534 (1982).
36. E. Novak, in *Gynecology and Female Endocrinology* (E. Novak, Ed.), Little Brown, Boston, 1941, p. 545.
37. S. Chinuki and M. Koyama, *Yonago Acta Med.*, 10:211 (1966).
38. I. Ricciardi and A. Ianniruberto, *Obstet. Gynecol.*, 54:80, (1979).
39. N. H. Lauersen and K. H. Wilson, *Obstet. Gynecol.*, 48:93 (1976).
40. L. J. Humphrey and L. C. Estes, *Postgrad. Med. J.*, 55:48 (1979).
41. H. W. Baker and P. A. Snedecor, *Am. Surg.*, 45:727 (1979).
42. C. Neghat, R. H. Asch, and R. B. Greenblatt, *Am. J. Obstet. Gynecol.* 137:604 (1980).
43. R. B. Greenblatt, W. P. Dmowski, V. B. Mahesh, and H. F. Scholer, *Fertil. Steril.*, 22:102 (1971).
44. R. L. Barbieri, J. A. Canic, A. Makris, R. Todd, I. Davies, and H. K. Ryan, *Fertil. Steril.*, 28:809 (1977).
45. M. Blichert-Toft, N. A. Andersen, O. B. Henriksen, and T. Mygind, *Br. Med. J.*, 1:237 (1979).
46. B. V. Palmer and J. C. M. P. Monteiro, *Br. Med. J.*, 1:1083 (1977).
47. K.-D. Schultz, E. Del Pozo, K. H. Lose, H. J. Kunzig, and W. Geiger, *Archiv. Gynakologie*, 220:83 (1975).
48. M. O. Thorner, A. Chait, M. Aitken, G. Benker, S. R. Bloom, C. H. Mortimer, P. Sanders, A. S. Mason, and G. M. Besser, *Br. Med. J.*, 1:299 (1975).
49. P. G. Chiodini, A. Luizzi, L. Botalla, E. Oppizzi, E. Muller, and F. Silvestrini, *J. Clin. Endocrinol. Metab.*, 40:705 (1975).
50. V. K. Summers, L. J. Hipkin, M. J. Diver, and J. C. Davis, *J. Clin. Endocrinol. Metab.*, 40:904 (1975).

51. G. Ueda, Y. Sato, M. Yamasaki, T. Shioji, T. Aono, and K. Kurachi, *Endocrinol. Japon.*, 22:265 (1975).
52. J. Kobberlins, H. C. Blossey, H. Dirks, and G. Mayer, *New Engl. J. Med.*, 306:748 (1982).
53. M. H. B. Carmalt, G. A. Dalton, R. F. Fletcher, and W. Smith, *Q. J. Med.*, 46:119 (1977).
54. R. M. Salassa, E. R. Laws, P. C. Carpenter, and R. C. Northcutt, *Mayo Clin. Proc.*, 53:24 (1978).
55. W. J. Jeffcoate, L. H. Rees, S. Tomlin, A. E. Jones, C. R. W. Edwards, and G. M. Besser, *Br. Med. J.*, 2:215 (1977).
56. D. T. Krieger, L. Amorosa, and F. Linick, *N. Engl. J. Med.*, 293:893 (1975).
57. G. Benker, K. Hackenberg, B. Hamburger, and D. Reinwein, *Clin. Endocrinol.*, 5:187 (1976).
58. S. W. J. Lamberts and J. C. Berkenhager, *J. Endocrinol.*, 70: 315 (1976).
59. S. W. J. Lamberts, H. A. T. Timmermans, F. H. DeJong, and J. C. Birkenhager, *Clin. Endocrinol.*, 7:185 (1977).
60. J. Givens, A. Cumacho, and P. Patterson, *Metabolism*, 19:808 (1970).
61. L. Fishman, G. Liddle, D. Island, N. Fleishman, and O. Kochel, *J. Clin. Endocrinol. Metab.*, 27:481 (1967).
62. R. Santen, A. Lipton, and J. Kendall, *J. Am. Med. Assoc.*, 230: 1661 (1974).
63. Y. Touitou, J. LeGrand, and P. Desgrez, *Biomedicine*, 18:185 (1973).
64. R. Dexter, L. Fishman, R. Ney, and G. Liddlel, *J. Clin. Endocrinol. Metab.*, 27:473 (1967).
65. E. Samojlik, R. Santen, and S. Wells, *J. Clin. Endocrinol. Metab.*, 45:480 (1977).
66. R. Santen, N. Cohen, R. Misbin, E. Sarmojlik, and E. Foltz, *J. Clin. Endocrinol. Metab.*, 49:631 (1979).
67. I. F. Stein and M. L. Leventhal, *J. Obstet. Gynecol.*, 29:181 (1935).
68. I. F. Stein, *West J. Surg.*, 72:237 (1964).
69. A. Kirschner and L. Jacobs, *J. Clin. Endocrinol. Metab.*, 33:199 (1971).
70. S. S. C. Yen, P. Vela and J. Rankin, *J. Clin. Endocrinol. Metab.*, 30:435 (1970).
71. S. S. C. Yen, *Clin. Endocrinol.*, 12:177 (1980).
72. J. W. Goldzieher, *Fertil. Steril.*, 35:371 (1981).
73. S. G. Raj, I. E. Thompson, M. J. Berger, and M. L. Taymor, *Obstet. Gynecol.*, 49:552 (1977).
74. S. S. C. Yen, P. Vela, and K. J. Ryan, *J. Clin. Endocrinol. Metab.*, 31:7 (1970).
75. C. B. Hammond, R. H. Wiebe, A. F. Haney, and S. G. Yancy, *Am. J. Obstet. Gynecol.*, 135:924 (1979).

76. C. Rivier, J. Rivier, and W. Vale, *Endocrinology*, 103:2299 (1979).
77. C. F. Wang and C. Gernzell, *Fertil. Steril.*, 33:479 (1979).
78. E. del Pozo and P. Falaschi, *Scott. Med. J.*, 25:S89 (1980).
79. M. Alger, L. Vazquez-Matute, M. Mason, E. Canales, and A. Zarate, *Fertil. Steril.*, 34:70 (1980).
80. G. C. L. Lachelin, H. Leblanc, and S. S. C. Yen, *J. Clin. Endocrinol. Metab.*, 44:728 (1977).
81. S. J. Judd, J. S. Rakoff, and S. S. C. Yen, *J. Clin. Endocrinol. Metab.*, 47:494 (1978).
82. M. E. Quigley, J. S. Rakoff, and S. S. C. Yen, *J. Clin. Endocrinol. Metab.*, 52:231 (1981).
83. C. D. Marsden, *Neurology*, 32:514 (1982).
84. W. Birkmayer, P. Riederer, and L. Ambrozi, *Lancet*, 1:439 (1977).
85. G. C. Cotzias, P. S. Papavasiliou, E. S. Tolosa, J. J. Mendez, and M. Bell-Midura, *N. Engl. J. Med.*, 294:567 (1976).
86. A. Lieberman, M. Kupersmith, and E. Estey, *N. Engl. J. Med.*, 295:1400 (1976).
87. C. S. Hutt, R. S. Snider, and S. Fahn, *Neurology*, 27:505 (1977).
88. M. M. Hoehn, *J. Amer. Geriat. Soc.*, 251 (1981).
89. N. Quinn, A. Illas, F. L'hermitte, and Y. Angrid, *Neurology*, 31:662 (1981).
90. A. Lieberman, A. Neophytides, and N. Leibowitz, *Neurology*. 30:366 (1980).
91. J. D. Parkes, N. Schachter, C. D. Marsden, B. Smith, and A. Wilson, *Ann. Neurol.*, 9:48 (1981).
92. G. Gopinathan, H. Teravainen, J. M. Dambrosia, and D. B. Calne, *Neurology*, 31:371 (1981).
93. P. A. LeWitt, G. Gopinathan, C. D. Ward, J. N. Sanes, J. M. Dambrasia, R. Durso, and D. B. Calne, *Neurology*, 32:69 (1982).
94. R. W. Fuller, J. A. Clemens, E. C. Kornfeld, H. D. Snoddy, E. B. Smalstig, and N. J. Bach, *Life Sci.*, 24:375 (1979).
95. C. M. Tanner and H. L. Klawans, *Ann. Intern. Med.*, 96:522 (1982).
96. A. J. Lees and G. M. Stern, *Lancet*, 2:577 (1981).
97. J. Ilson, S. Fahn, R. Mayeux, and L. Cote, *Neurology*, 32:A181 (1982).
98. J. Jankovic, *Neurology*, 32:A182 (1982).
99. A. Lieberman, M. Goldstein, G. Gopinathan, A. Neophytides, M. Liebowitz, R. Walker, and E. Hiesiger, *Neurology*, 32:A182 (1982).
100. A. Lieberman, M. Goldstein, M. Leibowitz, A. Neophytides, M. Kupersmith, V. Pact, and D. Kleinberg, *Neurology*, 31:675 (1981).
101. R. Rubovitz and H. Klawans, *Arch. Gen. Psychiat.*, 27:502 (1972).

102. A. V. Christensen and I. Nielsen, *Psychopharmacology*, 62:111 (1979).
103. H. Kazamatsuri, C. P. Chien, and J. O. Cole, *Am. J. Psychiat.*, 130: (1973).
104. D. V. Jeste, S. G. Potkin, S. Sinha, S. L. Feder, and R. J. Wyatt, *Arch. Gen. Psychiat.*, 36:585 (1979).
105. S. W. Asher and M. J. Aminoff, *Neurology*, 30:383 (1980).
106. R. C. Smith, C. A. Tamminga, J. Haraszti, J. Pandey, and J. Davis, *Am. J. Psychiat.* 134:763 (1977).
107. D. E. Casey, *Diseases of the Nervous System*, 38:7 (1977).
108. J. Growdon, A. Gelenberg, J. Doller, M. Hirsch, and R. Wurtman, *N. Engl. J. Med.*, 298:1029 (1978).
109. R. W. Fuller, J. A. Clemens, and M. D. Hynes III, *J. Clin. Psychopharmcol.*, 2:371 (1982).
110. H. S. Singer, I. J. Butler, L. E. Tune, W. E. Seifert, and J. Coyle, *Ann. Neurol.*, 12:361 (1982).
111. A. K. Shapiro, E. S. Shapiro, R. D. Bruun, and R. C. Sweet, *Gilles de la Tourette Syndrome*, Raven, New York, 1978.
112. L. E. Nee, E. Caine, R. Polinsky, R. Eldridge, and M. Ebert, *Ann. Neurol.*, 7:41 (1980).
113. F. Abuzzahab and R. Anderson, *Minn. Med.*, 56:492 (1973).
114. M. Ross and H. Moldofsky, *Lancet*, 1:103 (1977).
115. R. Borison, L. Ang. B. Diamond, and J. Davis, *Neurology*, 32:A114 (1982).
116. C. Tanner, C. Goetz and H. Klawans, *Neurology*, 32:1315 (1982).
117. H. Merrit, *A Textbook of Neurology*, 5th ed., Lea and Febiger, Philadelphia, 1973.
118. M. Dresse and M. Netsky, in *Pathology of the Nervous System* (J. Minkler, Ed.) McGraw-Hill, New York, 1968, p. 1186.
119. E. McGeer and P. McGeer, *Nature*, 236:517 (1976).
120. E. Kohler and R. Schwarcz, *Brain Res.*, 211:485 (1981).
121. J. Coyle and R. Schwarcz, *Nature*, 263:244 (1976).
122. T. L. Perry, S. Hansen, and M. Kolster, *N. Engl. J. Med.*, 288:337 (1973).
123. E. D. Bird and L. L. Iversen, *Brain*, 97:457 (1974).
124. G. Symington, D. Leonard, P. Shannon, and F. Vajda, *Am. J. Psychiatry*, 135:352 (1978).
125. R. Fisher, J. Norris, F. DeManuele, B. Ridgley, and C. Malyon, *Canad. Med. J.*, 15:605 (1982).
126. T. Perry, J. M. Wright, S. Hansen, S. Thomas, B. Allan, P. Baird, and P. Diewold, *Neurology*, 32:354 (1982).
127. G. Tell, P. Bohlen, P. Schechter, J. Koch-Weser, Y. Agid, A. Bonnet, G. Coquillat, G. Chazot, and C. Fischer, *Neurology*, 31:207 (1981).
128. H. Klawans, *Eur. Neurol.*, 4:148 (1970).

129. C. Goetz and W. Weiner, *J. Am. Geriat. Soc.*, 27:23 (1979).
130. E. Tolosa and S. Sparber, *Life Sci.*, 15:1371 (1974).
131. K. Davis, L. Hollister, and J. Barchas, *Life Sci.*, 1507 (1976).

6
Drugs of Ethno-Origin

PETER J. HOUGHTON and NORMAN G. BISSET *Department of Pharmacy, Chelsea College, University of London, London, England*

I. INTRODUCTION

Most cultures throughout the history of the world have used plants for medicinal purposes and these include the use of plants that affect the CNS. In some cultures this activity has been turned to account medicinally, but in many societies the use of CNS-active plants is also connected with a mixture of social and religious rites because of the euphoria or alteration in the conscious state often induced upon taking them. Several such plants have aroused interest and have been exploited in the leisure activities of hedonistic 20th-century Western culture. There are some plants whose psychoactivity has been observed not through sociomedicinal uses but rather through the effects of poisoning, e.g., the outbreaks of hallucinatory experiences recorded historically when populations were poisoned by eating ergot-infested rye bread.

The aim of this chapter is to present the ethnic uses of the more important plants with CNS activity and, where the requisite knowledge is available, to outline the chemical and pharmacological justification for these uses as revealed by modern scientific research. Where appropriate, some indication is given of any actual or potential clinical uses.

Over the last 20 years, much has been published concerning the ethnopharmacology, chemistry, and pharmacology of psychoactive plants and their constituents. These articles and reviews deal with the plants mentioned in this chapter in greater detail from the following points of view: (1) ethnology—Schultes and Hofmann [1], Efron [2], Schultes [3], Emboden [4], Hoffer and Osmond [5], Diaz [6], Watt [7]; (2) botany—Schultes and Hofmann [1], Efron [2], Emboden [4], Hoffer and Osmond [5], Diaz [6], Watt [7], Lewis and Lewis [8], Schultes [9], Schultes and Farnsworth [10]; (3) chemistry—Schultes and Hofmann [1],

Efron [2], Hoffer and Osman [5], Schultes [9], Schultes and Farnsworth [10], Tyler [11], Shulgin [12]; (4) pharmacology—Efron [2], Hoffer and Osmond [5], Diaz [6], Lewis and Lewis [8], Tyler [11], Shulgin [12], Hoffmeister and Stille [13].

Available information can be classified in a variety of ways, e.g., geographically, taxonomically, chemically, etc. However, the system used here, which is more in keeping with the subject matter of this book, is based on the overall effect of the drug on the CNS, i.e., on whether it is a stimulant, a depressant, or an agent that combines one or other of these effects with an alteration in the conscious state—perception of the self or of external stimuli.

It is important to realize that in most cases the substances used are not pure compounds but rather mixtures consisting of either the plant material or its crude extract or a complex mixture with other plants. Therefore, the overall effect observed will be the result of the pharmacological effects due to the individual components. In many cases, recent chemical research has led to the isolation and structure elucidation of the major active constituents and, to a lesser extent, to a study of their pharmacology. The pharmacological effects brought about by these constituents usually explain most of the effects of the drug itself. Nevertheless, the presence of minor substances may profoundly alter the action of the whole drug as compared with that shown by the major constituent(s). An example of this is the seeming lack of addiction connected with coca chewing but the addictive nature of cocaine, the major active constituent of coca leaves.

Although the observable effects of some of the drugs mentioned have been investigated thoroughly, there is little certain knowledge about the mechanisms at the cellular and molecular level underlying these effects. Many of the chemical substances are thought to inhibit or mimic neurotransmitters in the CNS, but since there is still much to learn about these, it is not surprising that our understanding of the reasons for the various kinds of psychoactivity is still in its infancy. For this reason, the information that follows consists largely of ethnological, chemical, and behavioral observations rather than a theoretical explanation of the types of CNS activity noted.

Some drugs have passed from folk use into medicine and their properties and modern clinical uses are well documented in other chapters of this book and in other established texts and reference sources. These drugs are: opium, rauwolfia, cocaine, scopolamine, caffeine, tobacco, cannabis, and alcohol. Only a brief summary of their current use and properties is given here; references to fuller treatments of these aspects are given elsewhere in the book.

A summary is given at the end of the chapter outlining those areas of current interest that have some therapeutic potential. This is not meant to be exhaustive but mainly to indicate that plants with CNS activity still have a contribution to make to modern medicine.

II. PSYCHOSTIMULANTS

These drugs stimulate the CNS, resulting in loss of fatigue and enabling work to be carried out more efficiently. Many of these drugs form an integral part of the cultures in most of the regions of the world, and psychological, but not physical, dependence on them is widespread.

A. Caffeine-Containing Drugs

Caffeine (1a), a xanthine alkaloid with a stimulating action, occurs in many higher plants and several of these are commonly used in one form or another as mild stimulants. Theobromine (1b), a less active compound, usually accompanies caffeine.

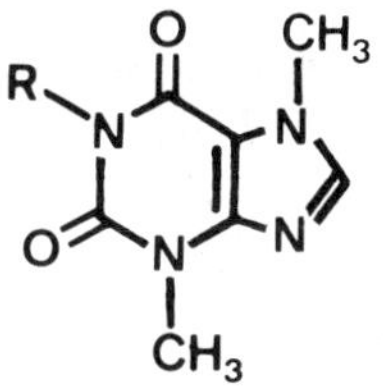

(1a) Caffeine R = CH_3
(1b) Theobromine R = H

1. Tea

Tea consists of a hot infusion of the prepared leaves of *Thea sinensis* L. (Theaceae) and is widely drunk in many parts of the world, although it originated in India and China. The leaves contain 1–4% caffeine.

2. Coffee

Coffee is prepared as a hot infusion from the ground roasted seeds of *Coffea arabica* and other *Coffea* species (Rubiaceae). The caffeine content of the seeds is about 1%. Coffee originated in Ethopia and was used extensively by the Arabs before its introduction into European culture in the 17th century. Like tea, its use as a mild stimulant has now spread throughout the world.

3. Cocoa

Cocoa and chocolate are obtained from the seeds of *Theobroma cacao* L. (Sterculiaceae), which is indigenous to the Amazon basin but is now cultivated throughout the tropics, particularly in West Africa. The Mexican Amerindians prepared a drink from the seeds. Commercial cocoa is made by roasting the fermented seed kernels and grinding them to a powder. The drink cocoa is made by mixing this powder with hot water or milk, whereas chocolate is prepared by mixing it with the fat found in the seeds, known as cocoa butter. Cocoa contains very little caffeine but 1.0–3.0% theobromine (1b), which, although a very weak stimulant, is a more powerful diuretic than caffeine.

4. Cola Nuts

Cola nuts are the dried cotyledons of *Cola nitida* L. and other *Cola* species (Sterculiaceae) found in West Africa. The cotyledons contain 1.0–2.5% caffeine and have been used as a masticatory stimulant throughout West Africa. Over the last century, an extract of cola has also become popular as the major ingredient of several well-known commercial soft drinks. These have about 0.3% w/v caffeine in them.

5. Maté

Maté is the best known example of a caffeine-containing infusion prepared from *Ilex* species (Aquifoliaceae). It is made from the dried and cured leaves of *Ilex paraguensis* L. and is a major drink in the Paraguay-Northern Argentina region of South America. Other species of *Ilex* have been used in North America by the indigenous and immigrant populations to produce drinks similar to maté, particularly in the absence of the imported beverages. Up to 2% caffeine is present in maté and it enjoys a reputation as a nutritive as well as a stimulant because of its vitamin C content.

6. Guarana

Guarana is another South American preparation which contains 2.5–5% caffeine. In Brazil, it is prepared by mixing the crushed seeds of *Paullinia cupana* L. (Sapindaceae) with cassave flour to give a paste that is formed into bars and dried. These bars are a convenient way in which to carry the stimulant, and it is drunk as an extract of scrapings from the bar as required. An intensely bitter drink is made in Colombia by using the bark of *P. yoco* L. which has about 2.8% caffeine.

The psychopharmacology of caffeine has been extensively reviewed [14–17] and is summarized briefly below. Although caffeine is the major substance responsible for the stimulant action of these various preparations, other substances present may affect its absorption into the bloodstream or may themselves affect the CNS.

Caffeine is a psychomotor stimulant. This has been demonstrated by many studies, although only a few have been designed to minimize bias due to habitual use, subjective observation, and variations in effect with dose administered.

Effects on mood are dose- and time-dependent and are also strongly influenced by individual habits. Thus, habitual users generally feel more alert and more physically active than casual users, but the contrary applies in regard to feelings of nervousness.

The results of research into the effects of caffeine on attention are more equivocal. Many studies have shown that caffeine reduces fatigue and delays the onset of sleep. Earlier investigations were subjective, but the more recent ones, making use of more objective criteria such as EEG, have revealed a decrease in the quality as well as quantity of sleep. And although this increase in alertness and release from fatigue usually means an increase in total work performed, it is offset to a certain extent by a decrease in motor performances and tremors induced by high doses of caffeine.

Many variables have to be considered when psychomotor activities such as calculation, typewriting, driving and learning are assessed. Although published work shows considerable variation in detail, it seems that moderate doses of caffeine improve performance in calculation, driving skills and learning, particularly in situations where control groups experience fatigue. On the other hand, there appears to be some impairment of comprehension and recall performance.

B. Khat

Khat, or chat, is a masticatory stimulant grown and used in Ethiopia and the Yemen. It is also exported to most of the surrounding countries. Khat consists of the fresh leafy twigs of *Catha edulis* Forsk. ex Scop. (Celastraceae), and its cultivation occupies a large amount of the time and space of farmers in certain parts of Ethiopia, particularly around Harar. A comprehensive account of its cultivation and distribution is given by Getahun and Krikorian [18,19]. Although first used by holy men to keep awake to pray, it is now in widespread use as a leisure activity amongst the student and unemployed populations in the towns. Unlike alcohol, the use of khat is not forbidden by Islam and in Ethiopia it is used more by Moslems than by Christians.

A typical farmer chews for 2 or 3 hr before work and consumes 250–750 g khat in that time. The drug causes thirst, so that a large amount of water is drunk. Until the khat has been chewed, regular users feel frustrated and unhappy, but after chewing it for 2–3 hr work is done without fatigue and this is sustained, after a short break for a meal and more khat, until nightfall. In the urban environment, khat is chewed as a pastime. Many reports speak of the euphoria it produces, as well as of the alertness, hyperactivity, and release from fatigue. Adverse effects include anorexia, gastric disturbances due to the high tannin content of the leaves, and some irrationality associated with the euphoria. Unsubstantiated folk beliefs among the local Christian population associate the use of khat with a high incidence of insanity and stomach and intestinal cancers. Other disadvantages of its widespread use are the inflammation and chlorophyll-staining of the mouths of khat chewers and the health hazards posed by the discarded chewed material on the floor and ground round the houses.

The most esteemed khat comes from the fresh leaves and twigs, but preparations such as pastes from dried leaves are available for use by old people.

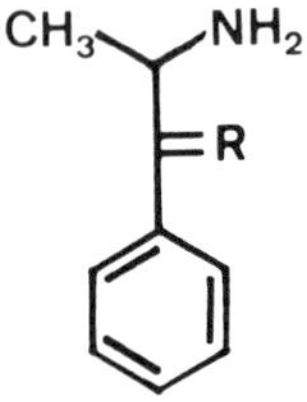

(2a) *d*-Nor-pseudoephedrine R = H, β-OH
(2b) Cathinone R = O

At one time, the stimulant activity of khat was thought to be due to the presence of caffeine. However, in 1930 Wolfes [20] isolated *d*-nor-pseudoephedrine (2a) from khat, together with minor amounts of related compounds. This was taken to be the compound responsible for the stimulation of the CNS, although insufficient amounts seemed to be present in the samples examined to account for the activity since Hofmann et al. [21] found that it had only one-sixth of the activity of methedrine. During the last decade, small amounts of a series of sesquiterpene alkaloids, called cathedulins, have been isolated [22–24]. Scharno and Steinegger [25] obtained 0.1% cathinone (2b) from young shoots of *Catha edulis*, which accounted for 70% of the total alkaloid. In the fully developed leaves, on the other hand, no cathinone was present. As khat chewers prefer fresh young twigs, it seemed then that it was the cathinone which was mainly responsible for the stimulant effect. This has been confirmed by Peterson et al. [26], who discovered that cathinone is at least seven times more potent than *d*-nor-pseudoephedrine and that its action has a more rapid onset but a shorter duration. The activity closely resembles that due to the amphetamines on the psychomotor centers of the CNS. Quedan [27] examined the volatile oil distilled from khat and found it to contain thujone, which is known to affect the CNS (see p. 323). However, the oil content is so small, 0.04% v/w, that it is unlikely to contribute much to the psychoactivity of khat.

A WHO report on the use of khat [28] noted the effects of habitual chewing of the drug, but concluded that there was no physical dependence but quite commonly psychic dependence.

C. Tobacco

Tobacco, originally in use for shamanistic purposes by the Maya [29] and many other groups of Amerindians, is now used worldwide in cigars and cigarettes for smoking and to a lesser extent as an inhaled snuff or as a masticatory. It consists of the dried leaves of *Nicotiana tabacum* L. (Solanaceae), the chief active component of which is nicotine (3).

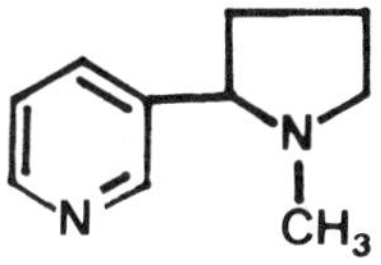

(3) Nicotine

The action of nicotine on the peripheral nervous system is well known, and it also affects the concentration of neurotransmitters in the cortex of the brain [30]. Many users of tobacco have it as a mild stimulant, but in South America it has been, and still is, used more specifically as a psychomimetic stimulant by the Huitoto and Bora Indians in Colombia, by the Warao Indians in Venezuela, and by the Creoles and Bush Negroes in French Guiana and Surinam. In these cultures the tobacco is mixed with the alkaline ashes of certain specific plants, moistened with water, and squeezed. The dark brown drops of liquid are taken as a liquid snuff to produce a short-lived intense ectasy [31,32].

The CNS action of tobacco depends on the way in which it is taken into the body, since pyrolysis products will be present in inhaled smoke but absent when the tobacco is taken as snuff or chewed. Nicotine increases the amount of acetylcholine in the brain, thus causing euphoria [33]. Tobacco has also been shown to contain the sedative psychoactive compounds β-carboline (nor-harman) (25a) and harman (25b) [34].

D. Betel

Betel is chewed in lands bordering the Indian Ocean and it is estimated that over 100,000 tons are produced annually to be used by more than

450 million people [3]. It brings about mild euphoria and stimulation. Although several substances may be added for flavoring, the basic ingredients are a mixture of lime and slices of the fruit of the palm *Areca catechu* L. (Palmae) enclosed in the leaves of *Piper betle* L. (Piperaceae). The quid is worked around the mouth and chewed. Salivation is increased and the saliva turns red and is spat out. Continued use leads to the formation on the teeth of a black deposit containing calcium carbonate.

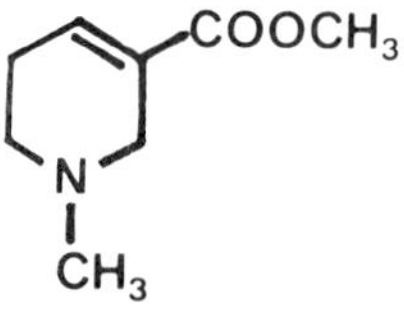

(4) Arecoline

The main stimulant is found in the *Areca* fruit and is an alkaloid arecoline (4), which is present to the extent of about 0.5% w/w. Related alkaloids are present in smaller amounts. The fruit also has large amounts of tannins, which counteract dysentery, and the lime is useful in the diet. Arecoline is employed in veterinary medicine as an anthelmintic and the habit of betel chewing helps to keep the intestines free of parasites in human users. Arecoline has long been known to have a cholinergic action and was formerly used as a pharmacological tool. Holmstedt [33] showed that arecoline increases the amount of acetylcholine present in the brain and activates waves shown on the EEG. This is presumably the basis of its stimulant action. The *Piper betle* leaves may also contribute to the overall activity, since they contain a phenolic volatile oil with a CNS-stimulant action and small traces of an alkaloid reputed to have cocaine-like properties [35].

E. Kratom

Kratom is the Thai name for the leaves of *Mitragyna speciosa* Korth. (Rubiaceae), a small tree indigenous to Southeast Asia and ranging from Thailand to Papua-New Guinea. In Thailand the leaves are chewed and smoked as a stimulant and have been used as a substitute for opium [36]. Because of the widespread abuse of *kratom* it was made illegal in Thailand in 1943, but it is still much used. A comprehensive study of *kratom* eaters has been carried out by Suwanlert [37]. More than 25 leaves are chewed daily to overcome a sense of weariness and to work more efficiently, as well as to produce a calm state of mind. Another effect is the desire of the *kratom* eater to be alone. Insomnia and anorexia leading to loss of weight are results of habitual use, and withdrawal symptoms occur if the chewer is deprived of the drug. A large number of indole alkaloids have been isolated from *Mitragyna speciosa* and related species [38]. The principal alkaloid in *kratom* is mitragynine (5).

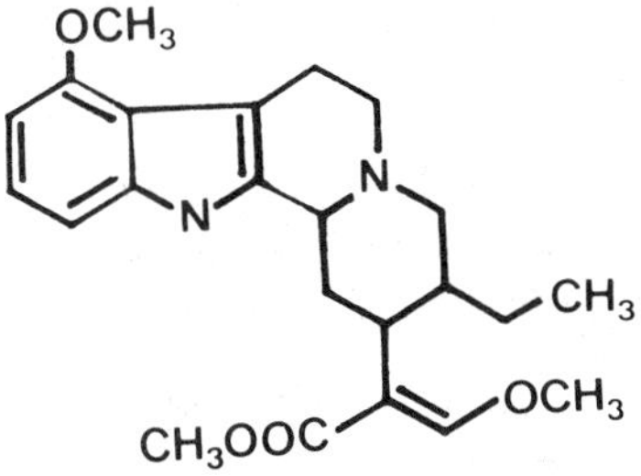

(5) Mitragynine

The pharmacology of mitragynine has been reported by Frewal [39] and Macko et al. [40]. It increases the excitability of the medulla and possibly also of the motor centers of the CNS; in addition, it elevates the pain threshold. Most of the other alkaloids present in *kratom* have not been investigated pharmacologically, but the related alkaloid rhynchophylline, which occurs in some other species of *Mitragyna* and in the nearby genus *Uncaria*, is used in China as a sedative [41].

F. Niando

Niando is the name given in parts of Zaire to the roots of the shrub *Alchornea floribunda* Muell.-Arg. (Euphorbiaceae). The powdered roots are added to food or palm wine and ingested to provide energy for fighting or festivities [11]. A state of intense excitement is followed by deep depression. An alkaloidal extract of the roots was found to possess sympathetic-excitant properties. At first it was thought that yohimbine was the major alkaloid present, although this has an opposite effect on the sympathetic nervous system. It was shown later [42] that yohimbine was not present and that the major alkaloid in the plant was an imidazopyrimidine, alchorneine (6), which exhibited sympathetic activity in accordance with the known excitatory properties of *niando*.

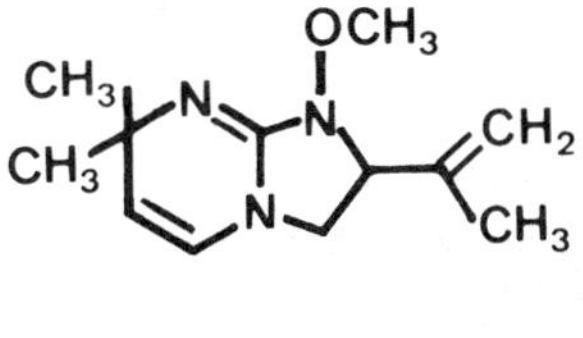

(6) Alchorneine

G. Ginseng and *Eleutherococcus*

Ginseng, the roots of *Panax ginseng* C. A. Mey. (Araliaceae), has been used in Chinese and Korean medicine for many centuries for a wide range of conditions, but chiefly as a tonic to maintain health and vigor. A North American species, *P. quinquefolium* L., has been used for the same purpose for the last 200 years. Other Far Eastern species such as *P. japonicum* C. A. Mey. and *P. notoginseng* (Burk.) F. H. Chen are also used.

Over the last 20 years there has been much commercial interest and consequent scientific interest in ginseng and its reputed properties of helping the body to withstand stress. The term "adaptogen" has been coined to describe the overall effect of drugs like ginseng. Several reviews dealing with ginseng and other adaptogens have been published [43–48] and they form the source of the information given below.

Although ginseng has been inherited from Chinese traditional medicine, a search for other plants with adaptogenic activity has resulted in the discovery and introduction into clinical use in the Soviet Union of a related plant *Acanthopanax senticosus* (Rupr. et Maxim.) Harms [= *Eleutherococcus senticosus* (Rupr. et Maxim.) Maxim.], known as *Eleutherococcus* or Siberian ginseng [49]. This plant and its extracts are said to have been used by Soviet astronauts and athletes to counteract fatigue and stress so that vigorous training programs can be carried out [50].

Ginseng and *Eleutherococcus* are related botanically but contain different types of glycosides. Ginseng has glycosides of the dammarane triterpenoids protopanaxadiol (7a) and protopanaxatriol (7b), whereas *Eleutherococcus* glycosides are based on phenylpropides such as eleutheroside B (8).

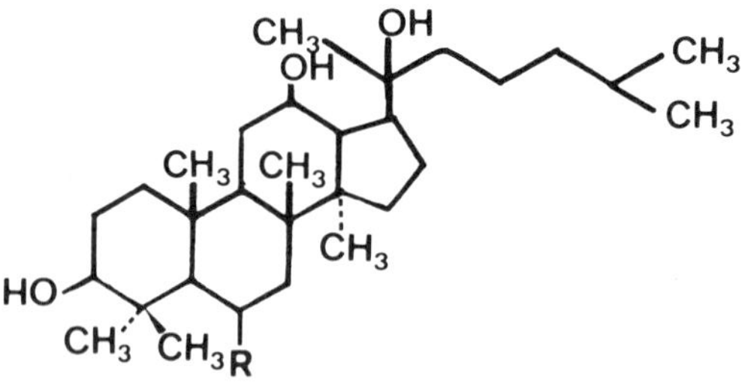

(7a) Protopanaxadiol R = H
(7b) Protopanaxatriol R = OH

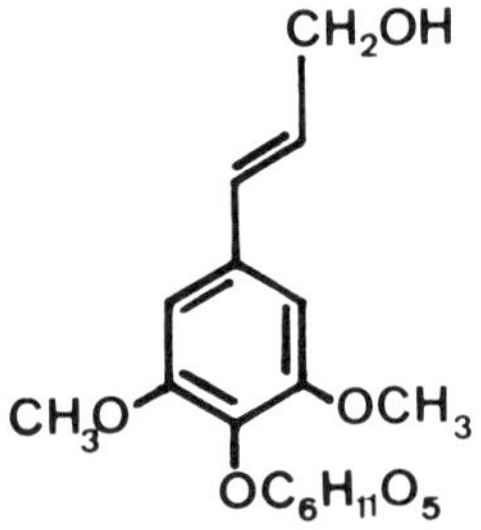

(8) Eleutheroside B

Considerable research has been conducted into the CNS activity of the ginseng glycosides but less into that of the *Eleutherococcus* compounds. The antifatigue activity of total extracts of the drugs has been demonstrated by animal experiments and is thought to be due to an increase in glycogen, lactic acid, and pyruvic acid metabolism.

More direct effects on the CNS are observed and can be summarized by stating that at low doses stimulation is observed while at high doses the overall effect is sedative. The stimulant action has been investigated by Petkov [51], who ascribed it to a cholinomimetic and antinarcotic effect in the cerebral cortex. However, there are differences in the reported effects and the somewhat confusing picture might well be due to the fact that most investigations have been carried out using crude extracts which probably have contained widely differing proportions of the glycosides and their genins. It has been shown that the individual glycosides have different activities. Thus, ginsenoside Rb_1 [(20*S*)-protopanaxadiol glycoside] is a CNS depressant and ginsenoside Rg_1 [(20*S*)-protopanaxatriol glycoside] is a stimulant. Consequently, it is easy to see how the observed activity of total extracts could vary considerably. Although they are being used increasingly for self-medication in the West, ginseng and *Eleutherococcus* have not yet been generally accepted by the medical establishment, even although there appears to be considerable experimental evidence for their usefulness.

H. Calamus

Calamus is the root of *Acorus calamus* L. (Araceae). The plant is widespread throughout the northern temperate zone, but its stimulating properties have been utilized only by the Cree Indians in Alberta, Canada. They used it as a stimulant and antifatigue substance. Higher doses are said to give experiences similar to those encountered with LSD-25 [5]. Calamus contains asarone (9) as its major active ingredient; and although structurally similar to mescaline and nutmeg constituents, its pharmacological properties tend to be opposite.

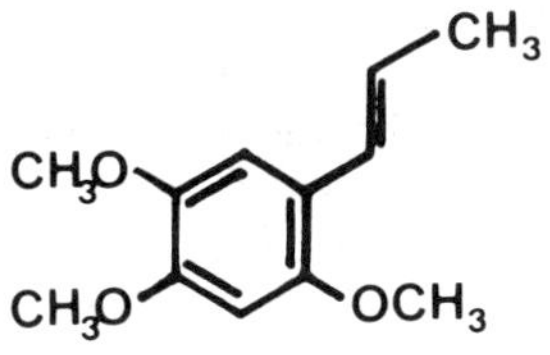

CH_3

CH_3O

CH_3O OCH_3

(9) Asarone

Asarone antagonizes the action of amphetamine and mescaline in rats [51,53] and, indeed, calamus is used as a sedative as well as a tonic in Ayurvedic medicine [35]. It seems thus that the active stimulant principle may not yet be known.

I. Coca

Coca consists of the leaves of *Erythroxylum coca* Lam., known as Bolivia coca, and *E. novogratense* (Morris) Heron and *E. novogratense* var. *truxillense* (Rusby) Plowman, known as Peruvian coca. The plants are not found in the wild state. Coca has been used in South America for many centuries, as testified by pottery figures showing it being chewed and by its presence in mummified bodies. Its use was originally restricted to the noble and priestly castes of the Inca civilization. However, its ability to enable hard work to be carried out resulted in its becoming available to the general population shortly before the Spanish Conquest. It has been available ever since. Its use is widespread among the Quechuas in the Andes of Peru and Bolivia. A different method of preparation is employed by various ethnic groups in the Amazon basin where the *ipadu* variety is used. The uses of coca have been reviewed by Martin [54], Ashley [55], Grinspoon and Bakalar [56], Holmstedt and Frega [57], Weil [58], and Andrews and Solomon [59].

In the highlands of the Andes, the midribs of the fresh leaves are removed and the leaves are then toasted or immediately chewed for a while and made into a ball called the *acullio*. Alkali in the form of lime or ashes from plants is then added and the mixture kept as a wad in the mouth, causing a bulge in one of the cheeks. The mass may be moved in the mouth from time to time but it is not actually chewed—the juice is allowed to trickle down the throat. New leaves are added from time to time and eventually the quid is ejected. About 50 g of coca leaves are commonly taken daily, and the practice enables the Indians to perform arduous work without food or drink for long periods, since hunger, thirst, and fatigue are suppressed. An infusion of the leaves is also taken, more as a medicine than masticatory, for the treatment of altitude sickness, toothache, and rheumatism.

In the Amazon basin, various groups of Indians use the *ipadu* variety of coca in a rather different way [60]. The leaves are toasted and powdered and mixed with the ashes of *Cecropia sciadophylla* Mart. (Moraceae). The mixture is sifted to form a fine powder which is put in the mouth and allowed to mix with the saliva and trickle down the throat. The mixture is easily taken on hunting expeditions and enables the Indians to go without food for several days. Some tribes in the northwestern Amazon basin take powdered coca as a snuff.

Even although coca is habitually chewed by many of the Indians in the regions mentioned above, there are several accounts that indicate that the habit is not addictive. Indeed, it has been shown that coca contains minerals and vitamins beneficial to the diet and its use does not cause long-term anorexia.

Cocaine (10) is the principal alkaloid among several found in coca. It was isolated in 1860 and caused an impact in medicine when its potent local anesthetic properties were discovered. Chemical modification of the cocaine molecule has led to the development of the modern local anesthetics such as lignocaine (11). The tingling sensation experienced when coca is chewed is due to the local anesthesia induced by the cocaine. At the same time, cocaine was used for its stimulating euphoric effect, and it was incorporated into several popular drinks. Its application in the treatment of opium addiction was recommended by Freud, but its addictive properties soon became evident and it rapidly fell out of use. The highly euphoric state it produces has meant a resurgence in the illegal use of cocaine, particularly as a snuff, in Western culture and especially in North America. In contrast to coca leaves, cocaine is addictive and only recently has there been interest in the therapeutic value of coca leaves in their own right [58]. Their use has in the past been ignored because it was thought that they also were addictive.

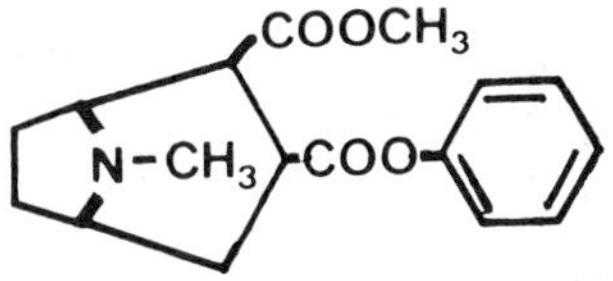

(10) Cocaine

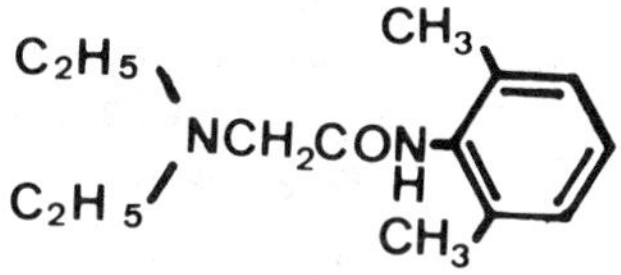

(11) Lignocaine

It is difficult to explain this contrast, but Weil [58] has pointed out that whereas a snuff or intravenous injection is a sudden infusion of cocaine into the body, the chewing of coca leads to a slow release of small quantities of cocaine that have to be absorbed from the gastrointestinal tract. Consequently, there is no "rush and crash" effect. Experimental evidence shows that the presence of lime increases the effect as compared with a corresponding dose of leaves taken as a hot-water infusion. Other components present in the leaves may counteract or modify the addictive mechanism that operates when cocaine is used on its own.

The euphoric activity is probably due to the fact that coca stimulates the nor-adrenergic pathways in the brain and possibly also the dopamine pathways, thus having an amphetamine-like action. Coca also restores tone to the gastrointestinal tract, which indirectly affects the mood of the user.

J. *Schizandra chinensis*

The fruits of *Schizandra chinensis* DC. (Magnoliaceae) have been used in the Far East to counteract fatigue, and the pharmacology of crude extracts and of the compound schizandrine (12), isolated from the plant, has been reported by Volicer et al. [61].

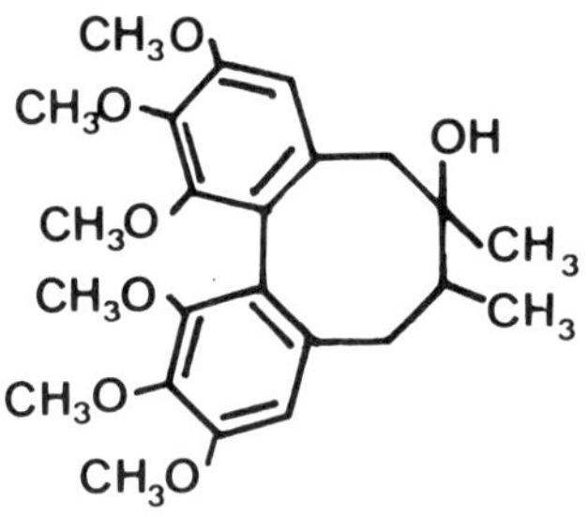

(12) Schizandrine

Potentiation of the central effects of reserpine was noted and also a dose-dependent response in the interaction of schizandrine with nicotine and cholinomimetic drugs. In small doses, the central effects of these drugs are potentiated, whereas with larger doses these effects are antagonized. Thus, in its action schizandrine resembles the CNS stimulant methylphenidate rather than the amphetamines.

III. PSYCHODEPRESSANTS

This group of drugs exerts an overall depressant effect on the CNS, leading to sedation and in many cases sleep. Drugs that also cause hallucinatory effects are included in the next section.

Some of the drugs mentioned here, notably opium and kava, also have a euphoric effect and because of this are widely used individually and socially.

A. Opium

Opium consists of the dried latex collected from the incised capsules of *Papaver somniferum* L. (Papaveraceae). It has been used as a medicine to induce narcosis for at least 3000 years and probably originated in the western part of the Mediterranean. Its cultivation and use has spread from there through India to Burma, Thailand, and China. Today, opium itself is little used in medicine but is the source of the analgesic alkaloids morphine (13a) and codeine (13b).

Morphine is found only in *P. somniferum* and is used for the relief of acute, severe pain. The annual world requirement is estimated to be 50 kg. Because of the labor-intensive methods used for opium production and the abuse of opium, the alkaloid is now produced in Turkey by extraction directly from the crushed capsules and no opium is produced legally. The demand for codeine, on the other hand, is much greater. Part of it is obtained from the capsules at the same time as the morphine. Nevertheless, there has been considerable research over the last few years directed toward finding a plant from which codeine but not morphine can be obtained. Some forms of *P. bracteatum* Lindl., in particular, produce thebaine, which can be easily converted to codeine but not to morphine.

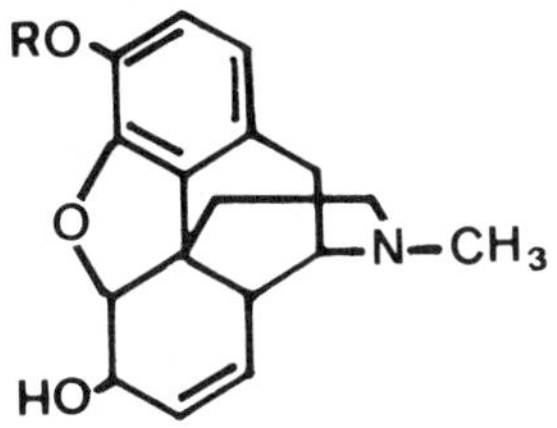

(13a) Morphine R=H
(13b) Codeine R=CH_3

From early times, opium has been taken by eating or drinking it, often in admixture, and for the last 500 years the smoking of opium in a pipe has been common. The tincture of opium is called laudanum and this also has been used.

Opium and its constituent alkaloids have a long history of abuse as well as valid medical use as narcotics and analgesics. Opium contains about 25% alkaloids; of this, 9–17% ought to be morphine, the alkaloid mainly responsible for the abuse. Nowadays, much opium is produced illegally as raw material for making the diacetyl derivative of morphine, heroin, which is one of the more serious drugs of abuse. The CNS effects of morphine and heroin are basically the same, and the reasons for the abuse are the euphoria experienced and the suppression of the natural drives of hunger, thirst, and aggression. Morphine stimulates the spinal cord, vagus, and vomiting centers and it depresses the thalamus and sensory cortex, thus causing diminution in awareness and response to disagreeable circumstances. Tolerance and dependence, which are regular features of the use of opium, morphine, and heroin, contribute to the moral and social degeneration arising from the illicit use of the drugs. Legal measures have been only partially successful in controlling their supply and the use. The use and abuse of opium and its alkaloids is covered more fully in Martindale [62] and Goodman and Gilman [63].

B. Kanna

Kanna is the present-day name given to certain species of South African *Mesembryanthemum* (or *Sceletium*) species (Aizoaceae). The roots and leaves of *M. expansum* L. and *M. tortuosum* L. are chewed and smoked by Hottentots [1]. The plants contain 1–1.5% alkaloids, the chief of which is mesembrine (14).

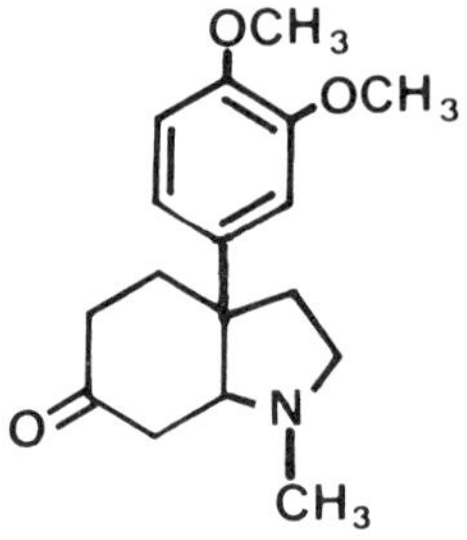

(14) Mesembrine

The alkaloid has been shown to possess sedative and cocaine-like properties and to produce torpor [11]. A hallucinogen "kanna" was reported over 200 years ago to be used by the Hottentots, but mesembrine has not been shown to have any hallucinogenic activity and the identity of the original "kanna" is not known. Other alkaloids have been isolated from other species of the plant family Aizoaceae, but no pharmacological work on them has been reported [64].

C. Kava

Kava is the name given to a drink made from the roots of *Piper methysticum* L. (Piperaceae). It is used extensively as a social drink in the islands of the South Pacific, particularly Fiji, Its use, chemistry, and pharmacology have been reviewed by Keller and Klohs [65], Holmes [66], Klohs [67], Meyer [68], Buckley et al. [69], and Shulgin [70], and the current state of knowledge is summarized below.

The use of kava was first brought to the attention of Europeans after Captain Cook's expedition to the Pacific islands in the late 18th century. The way in which it is used varies somewhat between different islands. In Fiji, the roots, which must be at least 4 years old, are cut, pounded or grated, and soaked in water; this is a tonic and stimulant only. In the Tonga region, the roots, after being cut up, are chewed and then spat out into water and allowed to ferment. A cloudy amber liquid results, which is taken during complicated ceremonial occasions, as an adjunct to social gatherings, and in daily life. It induces a trance-like state.

The drink prepared by chewing is said to bring about anesthesia of the tongue and lining of the mouth, loss of taste, visual and auditory changes, and particularly a euphoric state with improved appetite, loss of fatigue, and a benign social attitude. Sometimes, loquacity may be induced or, on the other hand, a dreamy state. Large doses cause muscular incoordination and ultimately stupor with no subsequent "hangover." It seems likely that digestive enzymes cause the compounds present to change into a more potent form.

Kava does not appear to contain alkaloids or glycosides as its active principles, but several aromatically substituted α-pyrones of the general structure (15) have been isolated.

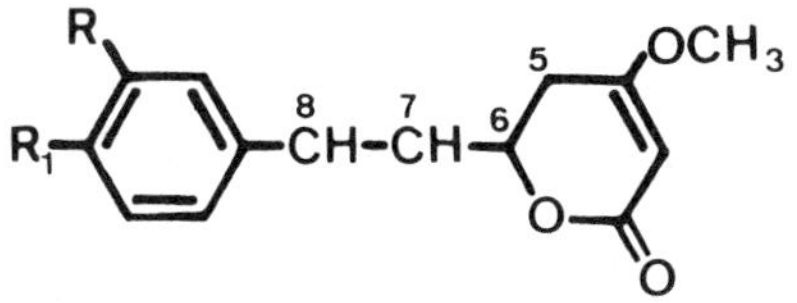

(15a) Kawain $R = R_1 = H, \Delta^7$
(15b) Dihydrokawain $R = R_1 = H$
(15c) Methysticin $R, R_1 = OCH_2O, \Delta^7$
(15d) Yangonin $R = H, R_1 = OCH_3, \Delta^5$

The major components present are kawain (15a), dihydrokawain (15b), and methysticin (15c). In some samples of kava, yangonin (15d) also occurs in reasonable amounts. Chalcones, called flavokuwins, are also present and on prolonged use of the drug they cause a yellow skin discoloration.

Experimental pharmacological studies on kava extracts and individual constituents have shown that they are more potent when given intravenously than orally. Some constituents, e.g., yangonin, are relatively ineffective when given by mouth but have activity comparable with that of the other components when injected parenterally. Those that are active orally are quickly absorbed and show activity after a few minutes. Certain components, e.g., methysticin, are effective in protecting against strychnine convulsions, whereas others, dihydromethysticin, increase the length of barbital-induced sleeping time [67]. A common effect is a general muscular relaxation. Meyer [68] has shown that synergism may occur; yangonin administered on its own has little effect, yet when given in conjunction with one of the pyrones it shows considerable activity. As well as the muscular relaxation noted above, the pyrones depress polysynaptic reflexes and reduce adema produced by irritants.

Interest was at one time shown in the use of these compounds and some semisynthetic derivatives as antiepileptic drugs, but trials were discontinued after test animals treated with kava extracts showed little change in their EEG patterns.

The activity mentioned above is connected with the lipophilic pyrones, but not all the observed effects of kava can be explained by the presence of these compounds, particularly since the drug is used as an aqueous infusion. Buckley et al. [69] investigated water-soluble components of kava. No compounds were isolated but administration of some fractions obtained led to a considerable reduction in the spontaneous motor activity of mice without impairing reflexes. The duration of the arousal response noted on the EEG of cats was markedly diminished and a slowing of cortical and skeletal-muscle relaxant activity was also seen.

It appears, therefore, that some of the active compounds still await characterization.

D. Valerian

Valerian is the dried root, rhizome, and stolon of *Valeriana officinalis* L. (Valerianaceae). The drug has been in use in European medicine since the early days of Greek civilization and it is still official in many pharmacopeias. Other species are used elsewhere in the world, e.g., *V. wallichii* DC. in India. The drug has been extensively employed in medical practice as a sedative and it has not been used socially in any way. It is commonly given orally as a tincture. Little was understood about the nature of the sedative compounds present until 1966 when Thies [71] reported the isolation of iridoid glycosides that were named valepotriates, e.g., valtrate (16), and which he stated were the active constituents. Some sedative activity resides in the volatile oil, and it

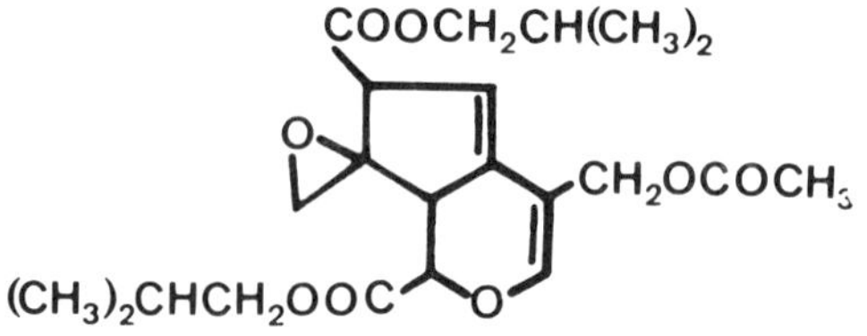

$COOCH_2CH(CH_3)_2$ CH_2OCOCH_3 $(CH_3)_2CHCH_2OOC$ O O

(16) Valtrate

CH_3 OH O CH_3 OH CH_3 CH_3

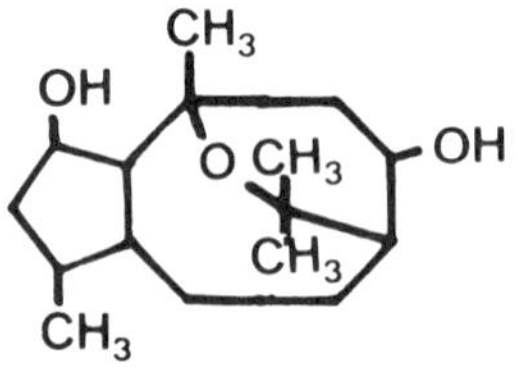

(17) Kessyl alcohol

was found by Hikino et al. [72] that valerian samples containing little valepotriate but much volatile oil had a more pronounced sedative activity, as measured by the increase in the barbital-induced sleeping time of rats, than samples having reasonable amounts of valepotriates. The sedative activity of the oil was ascribed to the kessyl alcohol (17) content. The constituents of Japanese valerian volatile oil, however, are substantially different from those of the European species.

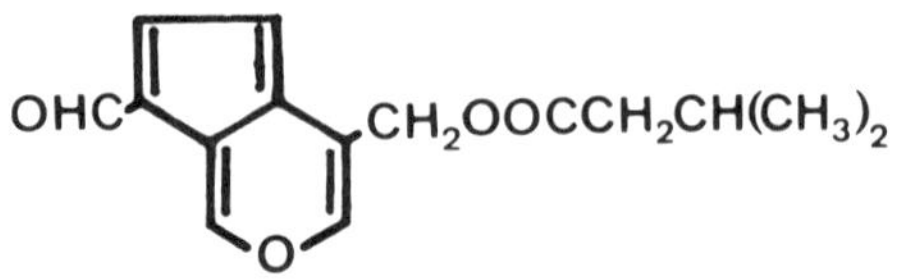

OHC $CH_2OOCCH_2CH(CH_3)_2$ O

(18) Homobaldrinal

Wagner et al. [73] showed that the valepotriate decomposition product homobaldrinal (18) from European valerian has a high sedative activity. Therefore, there is still some confusion as to which compounds present in valerian contribute most to its sedative action. The drug is still official in most European pharmacopeias, and extracts containing the valepotriates are marketed in some countries.

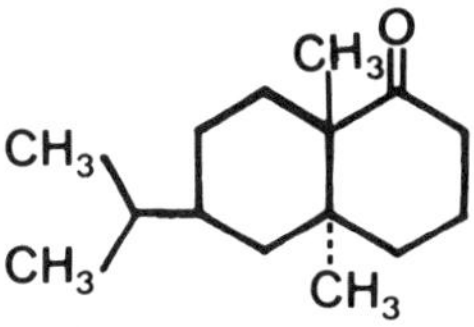

(19) Jatamansone

Jatamansone (19), synonymous with valeranone, another sesquiterpene with tranquilizing activity, has been isolated from the oil of a related plant, *Nardostachys jatamansii* DC. [74]. This drug has been used in Ayurvedic and Yunani medicine for a variety of disorders of the CNS such as hysteria and epilepsy [35, cf. 75]. It is thought to act by reducing the 5-hydroxytryptamine and epinephrine levels in the brain.

E. Rauwolfia*

The Indian snakeroot *Rauvolfia serpentina* (L.) Benth. ex Kurz (Apocynaceae) has long been used in Ayurvedic medicine as the drug *sarpagandha* for the treatment of snakebites and insanity, but it was not until 50 years ago that initial investigations led to the isolation of several alkaloids. One of these, reserpine (20), obtained in 1954, was used

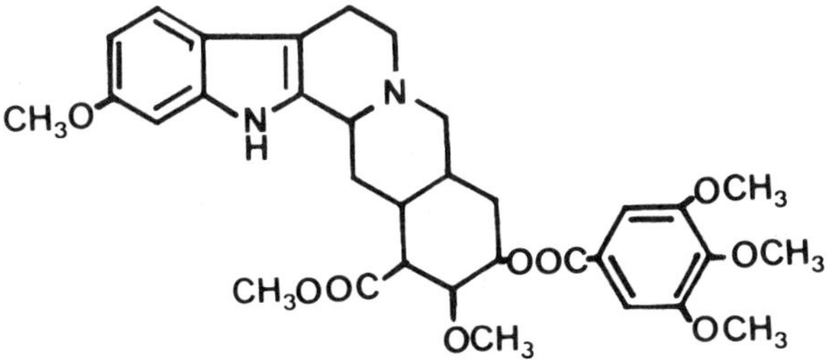

(20) Reserpine

---

*This is the usual spelling of the name of the drug in general scientific literature and in commerce. The botanical name of the genus is correctly spelled *Rauvolfia*.

widely as the first of the modern tranquilizers. Many reviews and histories have been written and details of the CNS action of reserpine may be found in any standard textbook of pharmacology [62,63].

Reserpine depletes the stores of serotonin [5-hydroxytryptamine (5-HT)], noradrenaline, and dopamine, and this is thought to cause the "tranquilized" state of indifference to external stimuli that is unaccompanied by the ataxia produced by some other sedatives such as alcohol. The mental depression brought about in some patients by reserpine has led to its being abandoned as a psychotherapeutic agent.

F. Turkestan Mint

The leaves of the Turkestan mint *Lagochilus inebrians* Bunge (Labiatae) have been used as an intoxicant by the Tatars, Turkmens, Uzbeks, and other inhabitants of Central Asia [11]. The leaves are toasted and then made into a tea. Russian workers have isolated lagochilin (21) from the plant [76] and its sedative properties have been well documented [11]. The drug is now official in the Pharmacopeia of the USSR.

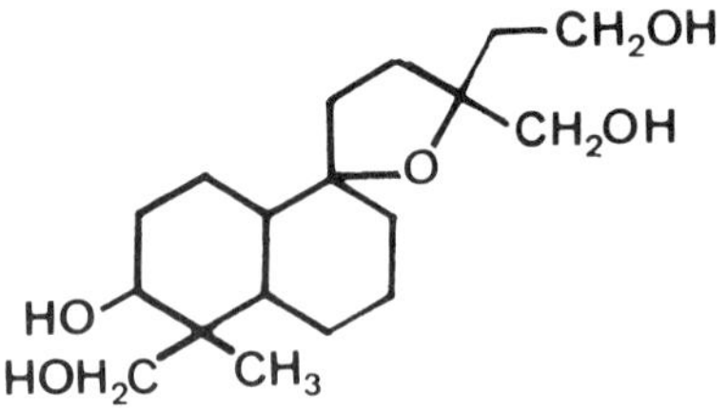

CH_2OH
CH_2OH
O
HO
HOH_2C CH_3

(21) Lagochilin

G. Other Drugs

There are a number of drugs that have a reputation in European herbal medicine as having a mild sedative action. These are listed in Table 6.1, together with the names of chemical substances isolated from them that have been shown to have pharmacological activity. In some cases, this confirms CNS activity, but in others, particularly those that contain flavonoids, much of the sedation observed may well be due to the hypotensive activity of the drugs.

In the Peoples' Republic of China over the last 30 years scientific research has been allied to Chinese traditional medicine and this combination has resulted in the introduction of several new sedative drugs in the pharmacopeia of that country [11]. These are listed in Table 6.2.

TABLE 6.1 Drugs with a Sedative Action Used in Herbal Medicine

Plant	Constituents	Comments	References
Betony (*Stachys palustris* L.)	Flavonoids	Hypotensive, spasmolytic effects	[77]
Hops *Humulus lupulus* L.)	Humulone, lupulone	Sedative, hypnotic	[78]
Lettuce opium (*Lactuca virosa* L.)	Lactucin	CNS sedative	[79]
Passion flower (*Passiflora* spp.)	Harman and related alkaloids Flavonoids	Tranquilizing effects	[80,81]
Piscidia, Jamaican dogwood (*Ichthyiomethia piscipula* P.Br.)	Piscidic acid and related compounds	Hypnotic	[82]
Pulsatilla (*Anemone pulsatilla* L.)	Anemonin	CNS depressant	[83]
Skullcap (*Scutellaria* spp.)	Flavonoids	Hypotensive, CNS action	[84]
Lime flowers (*Tilia* spp.)	Flavonoids Vanillin derivatives	Sedative, hypotensive	[85–87]
Turnera, Damiana (*Turnera diffusa* L.)	Flavones, volatile oil, caffeine		[88] [89]
Verbena (*Verbena officinalis* L.)	Iridoids: verbenalin, hastatoside	Weak parasympathetic stimulant	[90]

TABLE 6.2 Drugs with a Sedative Action Used in China

Source	Compound	Uses
Corydalis yanhusuo Hort. ex W. T. Wang (Papaveraceae), rhizome	*DL*-Tetrahydropalmatine	Analgesic, sedative
Sinomenium acutum (Thunb.) Rehd. et Wils. (Menispermaceae), root and stem	Sinomenine	Analgesic, sedative
Scopolia tangutica Maxim. (Solanaceae), root	Anisodamine, anisodine	Treatment of meningitis Treatment of migraine and cerebral vascular accident
Gastrodia elata Bl. (Orchidaceae), rhizome	Gastrodin	Sedative for treating vertigo
Daphne giraldi Nitsche (Thymeleaceae), root bark	Daphnetin	Analgesic
Loranthus parasiticus (L.) Merr. (Loranthaceae)	Tutin	Treatment of schizophrenia
Stephania dielsiana Wu (Menispermaceae), rhizome	Rotundine	Analgesic, sedative
Dactylicapnos scandens (D. Don) Hutchins. (Papaveraceae), root	*d*-Isocorydine	Analgesic
Uncaria rhynchophylla Miq. (Rubiaceae), root	Rhynchophylline	Hypotensive, sedative

Source: Ref. 41

IV. DRUGS THAT AFFECT CONSCIOUSNESS

In his seminal work on psychoactive plants, Lewin [91] classified some as "Phantastica." Under this heading, he grouped those plants that bring about evident cerebral excitation in the form of hallucinations, illusions, and visions; and the phenomena may be accompanied or followed by disturbances of consciousness or other symptoms of altered cerebral functioning.

Over the last 20 years, there has been much scientific and lay interest in these substances, as many of them have been used outside their original cultures as part of the counterculture in Western countries. Several different terms have been used to describe this type of psychoactive drug—including hallucinogen, psychotomimetic, psychodysleptic and psychedelic.

The botanical sources of these drugs are very diverse and so are the cultural groups that have used them in the past or that still do. In their original cultures, many of them are used for religious ceremonies or in shamanism, since they give an experience of "otherness" and may help in recollecting past experiences. Some of the drugs are very restricted in their use, whereas others are widely used. As well as hallucinatory experiences, these drugs often have an initial excitatory effect, followed ultimately by a depressant effect. Those that have been introduced into Western civilization are used mainly for hedonistic purposes; they are the "chemical crutches" of the young generation and replace the alcohol and tobacco of the older generation. The proponents of the counterculture have experimented with many plants in their search for hallucinatory experiences. Some of these plants mentioned below have a well-documented activity but others which have enjoyed a temporary vogue have been shown to possess no CNS activity. The more important ones of this latter class have been reviewed by Tyler [91a]. Those with genuine activity have continued to be used widely and because of this explosion in their use in the more developed countries, much research has been carried out on the major active principles of several of these drugs.

Although there is some diversity in the chemistry of the isolated active constituents, many are alkaloids and can be related to neurotransmitters known to be present in the CNS. Nevertheless, the mode of action of many, if not most, of these substances is very obscure, and it is complicated by the fact that the biochemistry of the CNS involves a delicate balance between the known, and almost certainly some as yet undiscovered, neurotransmitters. The description of ethnological hallucinogens given below follows the classification employed by Shulgin [12], but it is important to realize that, in spite of chemical resemblances to neurotransmitters, it is presumptuous to infer that specific agonism or antagonism occurs. The neurophysiological properties of many of the psychotomimetic drugs have been reviewed by Aghajanian [92].

A. Drugs with Active Principles Related to Serotonin

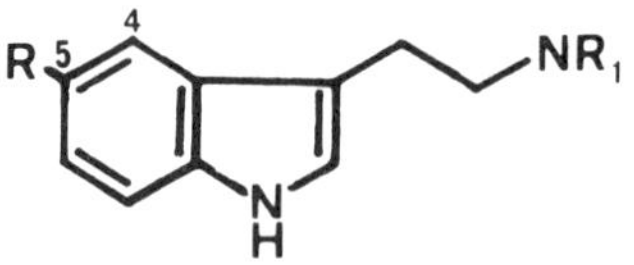

(22a) Tryptamine R = H, $R_1 = H_2$
(22b) Serotonin R = OH, $R_1 = H_2$
(22c) *N*,*N*-Dimethyltryptamine (DMT) R = H, $R_1 = (CH_3)_2$
(22d) Bufotenine R = OH, $R_1 = (CH_3)_2$
(22e) 5-Methoxy-DMT R = OCH_3, $R_1 = (CH_3)_2$

Serotin (22b) is found in the highest concentration in the CNS in the brain stem and hypothalamus. Depletion of serotonin in the brain stem leads to sleeplessness, but such depletion in the hypothalamus leads to sedation. It appears to integrate the mechanisms associated with reaction to external stimuli, particularly with regard to the response of the parasympathetic nervous system.

There are three groups of compounds found in these drugs that are structurally related to serotonin, viz. tryptamine derivatives, β-carbolines, and lysergic-acid derivatives.

1. Tryptamine Derivatives

Tryptamine (22a), when substituted in the amino function, produces compounds that are psychotomimetic when administered parenterally, e.g., by smoking, injection, or as a snuff. The most extensively studied of these compounds is *N*,*N*-dimethyltryptamine (DMT) (22c) [93]. If taken orally, they are quickly deaminated and so are not active unless administered with a monoamineoxidase inhibitor (MAOI). If the indole ring is substituted, particularly in the 4-position, with an oxygen function, the tryptamines are orally active and more potent. Similar substitution in the 5-position results in a loss of activity but a rapid onset and short cycle of intoxication when the tryptamines are taken orally. Tryptamine derivatives are found in several psychoactive preparations used in America; these are discussed below.

a. Snuffs from *Anadenanthera* species. A South American snuff called *yopo* or *cohoba* in Colombia and *vilca* in Peru is made from the powdered seeds of *Anadenanthera peregrina* (L.) Speggazini. Methods of preparation vary from one ethnic group to another, but usually alkaline plant ash and sometimes tobacco powder is added to the snuff. The snuff is blown into the nostrils by self-administration with the help of a Y-shaped tube or another person. A full account is given by Holmstedt and Lindgren [94].

The snuff has a rapid onset of action, being absorbed into the blood from the nose and then getting to the brain. Initial excitement, accompanied by micropsia, macropsia, and chromatopsia, is followed by a period of trance and unconsciousness.

The two major bases obtained from *yopo* are DMT (22c) and its 5-hydroxy analog bufotenine (22d); minor related compounds are also present [95,96]. Szara [93] has shown that the symptoms experienced on injection of DMT are very similar to those reported when *yopo* is inhaled and the action of the *yopo* may be explained largely by its DMT content. Bufotenine, however, does not seem to exert a psychotomimetic action when given on its own [97], although in admixture it may act as a synergist.

b. Snuffs from *Virola* species. In the northwestern Amazon region and the uppermost reaches of the Orinoco, species of *Virola* (Myristicaceae) are used as snuffs known as *yakee, epena,* or *parica*. The plant sources and use of these snuffs and related preparations have been reviewed by Schultes [98] and Seitz [99].

The red resin from the inner bark of *Virola calophylla* Warb., *V. calophylloidea* Markgr., or *V. elongata* (Spruce ex Benth.) Warb. is scraped off and kneaded in water and the extract thickened and then mixed with ash. It is in this form that the mixture is used. This is the most widespread method of preparation and is practiced by the Waika of the Orinoco headwaters.

A variation seen in the northwestern Amazon region of Brazil and Colombia is to dry shavings of the inner bark of *V. theiodora* (Spruce ex Benth.) Warb. over a fire and store them until required. They are crushed and mixed with the powdered fruit of *Bartholletia excelsa* Humb. et Bonpl. (Lecythidaceae), the Brazil nut tree. This mixture then has alkaline ash and powdered leaves of *Justicia pectoralis* Jacq. var. *stenophylla* Leonard (Acanthaceae) added to it.

The symptoms exhibited on taking *Virola* are very similar to those seen with *yopo*. This is not surprising in view of the chemical composition of *Virola* snuff; for Holmstedt et al. [100] and Agurell et al. [101] have shown that the major constituent is 5-methoxy-DMT (22e) and that it is accompanied by related tryptamine derivatives. Although no psychoactive substances have been detected in any of the other plant materials added to the *Virola* snuffs, recent investigations have shown that certain constituents of the *Justicia pectoralis* used may exert a synergistic effect [102].

In addition to the snuffs, oral preparations containing tryptamine derivatives are also employed. The Huitoto Indians of the Colombia-Peru border area make pellets of *Virola* resin coated with ash, and a psychoactive drink called *jurema* has until recently been used in north-eastern Brazil. *Jurema* is prepared as an infusion of the roots or bark of *Mimosa hostilis* (Mart.) Benth. (Leguminosae), a tree related to *Anadenanthera* species. DMT has been isolated from both these plants, but the reason for their activity, bearing in mind that DMT is rapidly inactivated when taken orally, is still unclear.

c. *Teonanacatl* and related fungi. Archeological evidence for the ritual use of mushrooms is found widely throughout Central America, and in the late 1930s Schultes established that the sacred mushrooms were still being used. Subsequently, the species employed were identified as belonging to the genera *Psilocybe*, *Conocybe*, and *Stropharia* (Strophariaceae). Since then, they have been the subject of much research, and compounds similar to their active principles have been found in related species and in species occurring in other parts of the world [103–108]. The hedonistic use of such mushrooms has also spread.

Teonanacatl, "Flesh of the Gods," is the name of the mushrooms still being used in magico-religious ceremonies in southern Mexico. They are eaten raw or in a dried state. Visual and auditory hallucinations are experienced and are followed by a euphoric sleep. The major active constituent isolated from *Psilocybe* species is psilocybin (23); a minor component is psilocin (24).

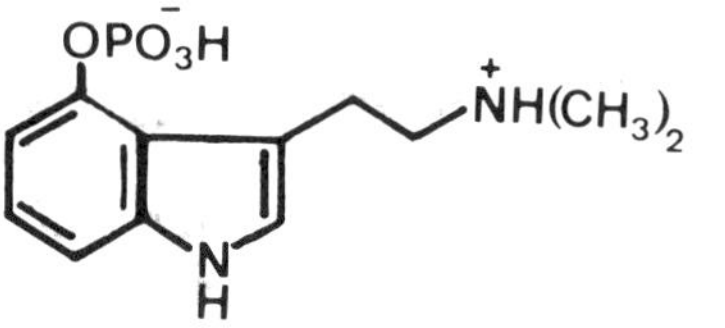

(23) Psilocybin

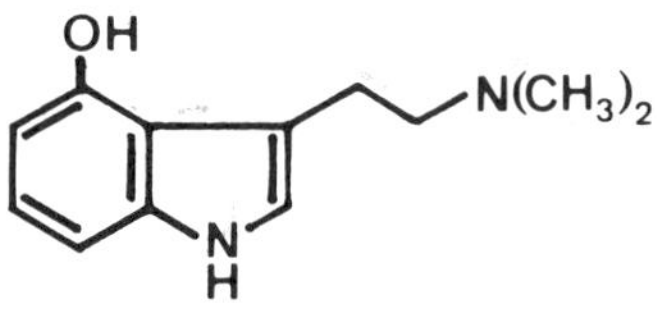

(24) Psilocin

Studies on the effects of various doses of psilocybin [103] indicate that the amount equivalent to 2 g of fungus, i.e., 4–8 mg of alkaloid, produces a feeling of relaxation and detachment from the environment followed by alterations in the perception of time, space, and oneself. There is also visual hypersensitivity and long-forgotten memories are recalled.

Wohlbach et al. [109] have compared the effects of psilocybin and psilocin with LSD-25 and mescaline. Qualitatively, the effects are similar. The actions of psilocybin and psilocin indicate an enhancement of the monosynaptic spinal reflexes and depression of motor behavior. The disappearance of slow waves in the EEG is thought to be due to inhibition of the thalamus. On isolated organs, inhibition of serotonin is detected. One feature of these compounds is their relatively low toxicity—for psilocybin, the LD_{50} in mice is 280 mg/kg.

2. β-Carboline Derivatives

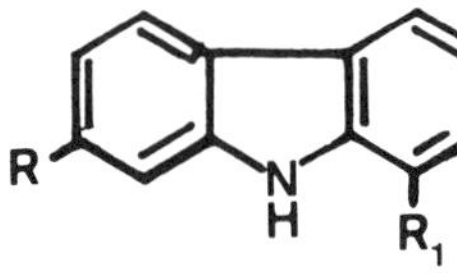

(25a) β-Carboline (Nor-harman) $R = R_1 = H$
(25b) Harman $R = H, R_1 = CH_3$
(25c) Harmaline $R = OCH_3, R_1 = CH_3, \Delta^3$ saturated

Derivatives of β-carboline (25a) can be formed in vitro by cyclization of tryptamines [110]. β-Carboline derivatives have been shown to inhibit monoamine oxidase. They are active orally, and if they accompany tryptamine derivatives in a mixture they cause these compounds to exert activity, since their inactivation is inhibited by the MAOI activity of the carbolines [111]. The only β-carboline that has been studied to any great extent in man is harmaline (25c). The carbolines are found in several plants, but it seems that only species of *Banisteriopsis* have been used as sources of psychotomimetic agents.

a. *Ayahuasca.* Details of the preparation and use of *ayahuasca*, the "Vine of the Souls," have been reviewed by Schultes [112] and Rivier and Lindgren [113]. The drug is also known as *caapi* and *yage* and it is used for medicinal, social, and shamanistic purposes throughout the western Amazon region.

Ayahuasca consists of a drink prepared by boiling the stems of *Banisteriopsis caapi* (Spruce ex Griseb.) Morton or B. *inebrians* Morton (Malpighiaceae) in water together with other plants, in particular the leaves of *Psychotria viridis* Ruiz et Pav. or *P. cathanginensis* L. (Rubiaceae). The leaves of *Diplopterys cabrerana* (Cuatr.) Gates and *Tetrapteris methystica* R. E. Schultes (both Malpighiaceae), are used as additives in Ecuador and northwestern Brazil, respectively.

The mixture is boiled for an hour and when cool enough is drunk, as it loses its potency very rapidly. Within one-half hour, the taker starts vomiting and singing, and hallucinations occur which feature bright colors and images of large animals, objects, and structures—they are often perceived simultaneously by several people in a group. If the visions experienced are terrifying, tobacco or the leaves of *Ocimum micranthum* Willd. are smoked to dispel them.

The psychoactivity of *ayahuasca* is similar to that of harmaline (25c), the major psychotomimetic agent found in *Banisteriopsis* [114]. Other alkaloids have also been obtained [115]. The two *Psychotria* species that are added to *ayahuasca* and *Diplopterys cabrerana* have been shown to contain DMT (22c), and, in view of the MAOI activity of harmaline, this tryptamine derivative can add significantly to the psychomimetic properties of the drink. Naranjo [114] has reported fully on the psychic changes associated with harmaline and some of its analogs when taken on their own.

3. Lysergic Acid Derivatives

Lysergic acid (26a) is the parent structure of the alkaloids found in the fungus ergot, *Claviceps purpurea* Tulasne (Hypocreaceae), which grows on many species of the grass family. The cereal rye is the most important host, since pharmaceutical ergot is grown on it, and although there are no indications of ergot being used deliberately as a CNS-active drug, the historical records of rural Europe contain many references to ergot poisoning through eating infected rye bread. These poisonings were sometimes accompanied by hallucinations caused by the alkaloids present. It was from an ergot derivative that the well-known hallucinogen lysergic acid diethylamide LSD-25 (26b) was synthesized, and much has been written on its psychoactive properties.

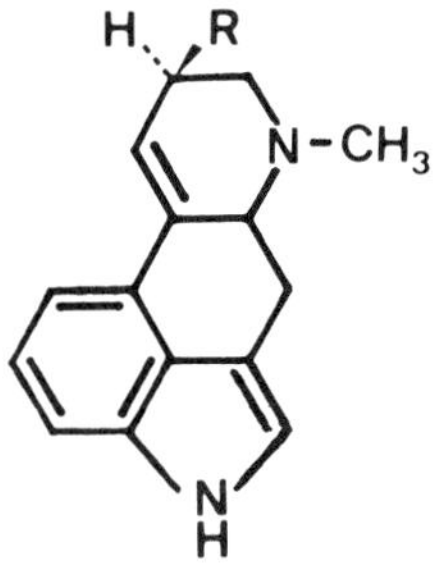

H R
N-CH_3
N
H

(26a) Lysergic acid R = COOH
(26b) Lysergic acid diethylamide R = $CON(C_2H_5)_2$

These compounds are potent at small doses and lead to a considerable modification of perception, with brilliant swirling colors, confused and wavering shapes, and a loss of sense of time and space. Often, there are strong memories from the past that may be pleasant or unpleasant [116].

a. *Ololiuqui* is the Aztec name for a hallucinogenic drug used by them. Is identity remained a mystery until Schultes [117] determined that it is the seeds of *Turbina corymbosa* (L.) Rafinesque (Convolvulaceae). A related plant, *Ipomoea violacea* L., is also used by the Zapotec Indians. The seeds may be ground and soaked in cold water and the liquid drunk or they may be eaten. Visual hallucinations occur after an initial euphoric state and the effects may last for several hours [103]. Because the seeds have a hard indigestible coat, many more seeds are required when they are to be eaten than when they are to be used for making the drink. In 1960 the active principles of *ololiuqui* were isolated and found to be amide derivatives of lysergic acid, in particular ergine (27a) and isoergine (27b) [118].

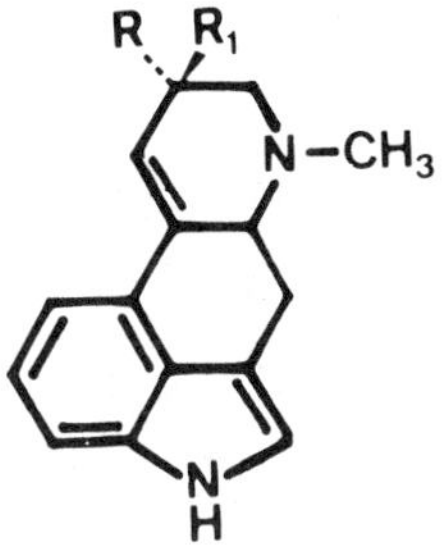

R R1
N−CH3
N
H

(27a) Ergine $R = H$, $R_1 = CONH_2$
(27b) Isoergine $R = CONH_2$, $R_1 = H$

Hofmann [119] has investigated the pharmacology of ergine and Vogel et al. [120] have obtained evidence for the psychoactivity of isoergine.

Also present are the hydroxyethylamides of lysergic acid, which may serve as metabolic precursors. These and related compounds are found in other species of Convolvulaceae—in comparatively large amounts in *Argyreia nervosa* Lour. [121].

B. Drugs with Active Principles Related to Dopamine

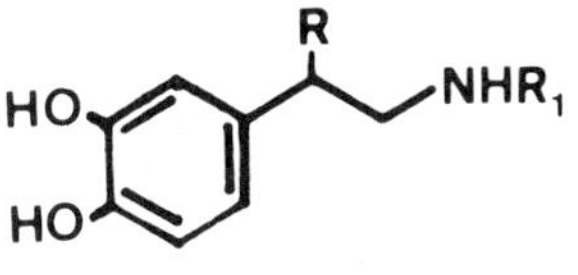

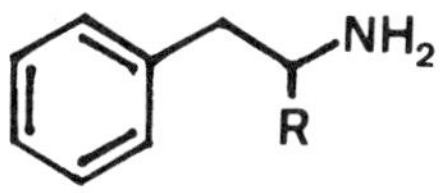

R
HO
NHR1
HO

NH2
R

(28a) Dopamine $R = R_1 = H$
(28b) Epinephrine (adrenaline) $R = OH$, $R_1 = CH_3$

(29a) Phenethylamine $R = H$
(29b) Amphetamine $R = CH_3$

Dopamine (28a) is the simplest of the catecholamine neurotransmitters found in the CNS, the best known example being adrenaline/epinephrine (28b). The related substance phenethylamine (29a) is present but the amount varies with different diseases, being decreased in depression and increased in schizophrenics [4]. It has been suggested that it may be an endogenous stimulant. The compounds occurring naturally in the body are quickly deactivated by monoamine oxidase (MAO). Extensive substitution of the aromatic ring, however, prevents this deactivation and renders a substance psychoactive if ingested. Protection from MAO activity is also afforded by substitution on the carbon next to the primary amine function, e.g., amphetamine (29b), and such compounds—the phenylisopropylamines—also have CNS activity. The activity is marked by an overall stimulant action accompanied by vivid hallucinatory effects.

1. Phenethylamine Derivatives

a. *Peyotl* and related cacti. *Peyotl* or *peyote* is the name given to the drug used by Indians in northern Mexico and the southwestern United States and obtained from *Lophophora williamsii* (Lam.) Coulter (Cactaceae). Other cacti have been used in the same area as well as in parts of South America for similar purposes. Several reviews have appeared that deal with the use and constituents of *peyotl* and related drugs [122–128].

Peyotl, thin dried slices of the cactus, may be eaten or used to make a tea and drunk. It is a central element in the rites of the Native American Church. Initial effects are nausea, anxiety, and dislocation of visual perspective. The unpleasant symptoms subside and mental stimulation ensues. This period, which lasts for about 3 h, is characterized by brilliantly colored visions involving much movement and an exaggerated sensitivity to sounds and other sensory impressions. A gradual return to normality occurs, which may be accompanied by sleep. There is excellent recall of what has been experienced during the intoxication.

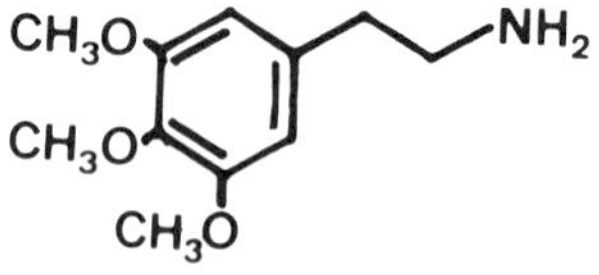

(30) Mescaline

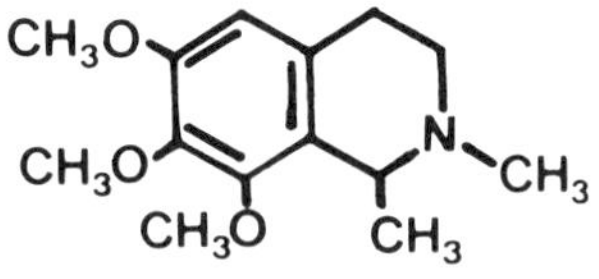

(31) Pellotine

The main substance responsible for these hallucinatory effects is thought to be mescaline (30), first isolated in 1896. Subsequently, more than 50 different alkaloids have been obtained from *L. williamsii*.

Mescaline and related compounds are found in other cacti used as hallucinogens, e.g., *Trichocereus pachanoi* Britton et Rose [125], and also in some which have no such ethnopharmacological use, e.g., *Carnegia gigantea* (Engelm.) Britton et Rose [129]. *Lophophora diffusa* (Croizat) H. Bravo, which is closely related to the *peyotl* plant, has a very limited distribution range and it contains active principles, among them pellotine (31) [130], that are sedative and hypnotic rather than hallucinogenic; this chemical disparity was a source of confusion in the early work on *peyotl*. It is not known whether *L. diffusa* has been used ritually or not.

2. Phenylisopropylamine-Related Compounds

Amphetamine (29b) and its derivatives are a large group of synthetic compounds related to phenylisopropylamine. The only naturally occurring substances connected with them are certain components of the volatile oils present in some drugs and spices which may be metabolized in vivo to phenylisopropylamines.

a. Nutmeg. Nutmeg, the dried kernel of the seed of *Myristica fragrans* Houtt. (Myristicaceae), is widely used as a spice and medicine. It came originally from the Moluccas in eastern Indonesia but is now grown extensively in other parts of the tropics. Although its psychoactivity had been described over 100 years ago by Purkinje, its psychotomimetic properties seem to have been "discovered" only recently and its consequent hedonistic use has been restricted to the "drug culture" of Western civilization and prison inmates. Its uses, chemical constituents, and pharmacology have been reviewed by Weil [131,132], Shulgin [133], Shulgin et al. [134], Truitt [135], and Kalbhen [136].

The nutmeg is grated and 5–30 g of it is stirred with water and the suspension drunk. Onset of the symptoms occurs after 2–5 hr and often only a burning thirst, severe headache, and giddiness are experienced before stupor sets in. Some subjects, however, have hallucinations of time and space rather than visual effects. A common feeling is that of floating in the air with the limbs separated from the body. Because of the unpleasant physical symptoms associated with ingestion of nutmeg, subjects often try it only once. A common effect is a lasting aversion to the taste of even small amounts of the spice.

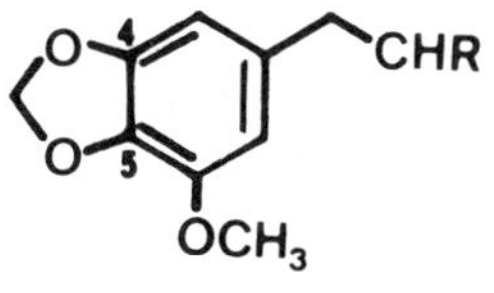

O 4 CHR
O 5
OCH_3

(32a) Myristicin R = $=CH_2$
(32b) MMDA R$=CH_3$, NH_2

The psychoactivity of nutmeg is generally considered to be due to the aromatic constituents of the volatile oil present, particularly the myristicin (32a) which is similar in structure to the amphetamine analog MMDA (32b). Shulgin et al. [137] indicate that the presence of the methylenedioxy group, instead of two methoxy groups, at positions 4 and 5 in the phenethylamines decreases the potential for visual distortion. Otherwise, the effects are the same. Following the discovery by Kawabata [138] that rats convert allylbenzene to amphetamine, Braun and Kalbhen [139] demonstrated that myristicin is converted in vitro to the corresponding amine, whereas Oswald et al. [140] showed that in vivo in rats and guinea pigs different products are formed. No metabolic studies have been carried out in humans, so that this postulated biotransformation is still unproved. An explanation for the activity of *aryl*-substituted amphetamines and other amines such as mescaline has been put forward by Snyder and Richelson [141]; it takes into account the quantitative differences in the hallucinogenic effects between different isomers. When the compounds are substituted in the 3,4,5- or 2,4,5-positions in the aromatic part of the molecule, hydrogen bonding can occur and the shape of and electron distribution in them is then comparable with that in the ring systems of hallucinogenic substances such as LSD-25.

Recent work by Sherry et al. [142] has shown that light-petroleum extracts of nutmeg bring about an increase in the duration of both light and deep sleep in young chickens. None of the phenylpropides thought to be responsible for the psychoactivity of nutmeg could be detected in the extracts. However, they were able to show that the presence of trimyristin, a glyceride, tended to increase the hypnotic effect of the extract. It seems, therefore, that the chemical basis for the CNS activity of nutmeg needs further elucidation.

C. Drugs with Active Principles Related to Acetylcholine

Acetylcholine (33) is a major neurotransmitter in both the central and peripheral nervous systems. The tropane alkaloids, e.g., scopolamine (34a) and hyoscyamine/atropine (34b), are an important chemical group of alkaloids and they exhibit a certain similarity in chemical structure to acetylcholine against which they exert a potent inhibitory action.

This well-known inhibition of acetylcholine shown by these alkaloids extends into their effects on the CNS, scopolamine (hyoscine) having the greatest central activity. These CNS effects differ in several respects from those produced by the compounds related to serotonin and dopamine discussed previously. Thus, one area of difference lies in the accompanying effects due to impairment of the peripheral parasympathetic nervous system, leading to such symptoms as pupillary dilation, dry mouth, and tachycardia. Other differences are associated more with central activity. There is often intellectual impairment and confusion—an initial violent panic and afterwards difficulty in remembering details of the experiences undergone during the intoxication.

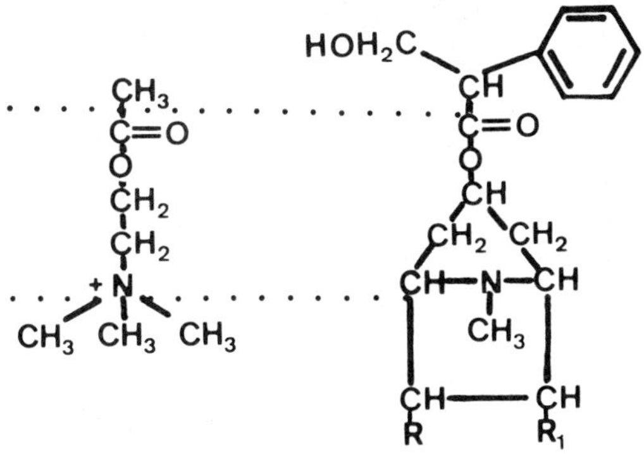

(33) Acetylcholine (34a) Scopolamine R, R_1 = —O—
(34b) Hyoscyamine (Atropine) R = R_1 = H

Historically, plants of the family Solanaceae containing these tropane alkaloids have the widest geographical distribution of any of the psychoactive drugs, although nowadays *Cannabis* is grown and used worldwide. The use and sources of these various plants are discussed briefly below, but fuller information about them can be found in the following references: Schultes and Hofmann [1], Hoffer and Osmond [5], Lewis and Lewis [8], and Lockwood [143]. In all the plants, scopolamine, and to a lesser extent, atropine/hyoscyamine are the psychoactive compounds present.

i. Pituri is the name given to a narcotic used by the Australian seminomadic tribes. The leaves and stems of *Duboisia hopwoodii* R. Br. are mixed with alkaline charcoal and chewed, sometimes also being swallowed. Although it seems mainly to be used for reducing hunger and fatigue, it is also taken as a hallucinogen and often the memory of long-term users is affected.

ii. Dhatura is the Sanskrit name for *Datura metel* L. which has long been used in India and China and during the last millenium by the Arabs. Its use now extends throughout southern Asia and into Africa. Normally, the drug is smoked; either the seeds are mixed with *Cannabis* or the leaves are mixed with tobacco.

iii. European solanaceous plants include belladonna (*Atropa belladonna* L.), mandrake (*Mandragora officinalis* L.), and henbane (*Hyoscyamus niger* L.). All still hold an important place as sources of the alkaloids used in modern medicine, but in the past these plants were surrounded by superstition. They were a constituent of drinks, "witches' brews," or of ointments made and applied to mucous membranes or the genital area. One of the sensations experienced was that of flying, and it is this which has given rise to the common picture of witches flying on broomsticks. *Hyoscyamus niger* was used in China under the name *lang tang*.

iv. Another plant, now found wild in Europe, is jimsonweed, *Datura stramonium* L. An extract of it was used by some tribes of eastern North America as an intoxicant in adolescence rites. *D. stramonium* is sometimes used in asthma cigarettes and these have been abused in North America for hallucinogenic purposes [144].

v. Toloache is the name given to Mexican solanaceous plants used for their psychoactive properties, especially *Datura innoxia* L. The roots or seeds are used in ceremonies by the Zuris, Yunans, and Yokuts, and the Tarahumaras still add the seeds to fermented maize drinks.

vi. Torna-loco, from *D. ceratocaula* L., also has powerful narcotic properties.

Johnston [145] has reported that among the Tonga in South Africa *D. fastuosa* L. is included in initiation rites for girls.

vii. In South America, several species of *Brugmansia* Pers. have long been cultivated and used as hallucinogens, particularly in the western Amazon and Pacific Coast regions. Many local names are given, including *barrachero, toa,* and *tonga*. Other uses are for the correction of unruly children and, in the past, the drugging of wives and slaves before live burial with their dead master. In several areas, special varieties are grown, e.g., in the Sibundoy valley in Colombia where aberrant forms are cultivated by medicine men and used for specific purposes. The drugs are usually taken orally as a drink made from the leaves or seeds, but sometimes the powdered seeds are added to food.

viii. Mitskyway borrachera is the closely related plant *Methysticodendron amesianum* R. E. Schultes. It also is grown in the Sibundoy valley and is reserved for very specific medicinal and narcotic use.

ix. Other members of the Solanaceae, e.g., species of *Brunfelsia, Solandra,* and *Iochroma*, have been stated to have psychoactive properties, but little work has been done on their chemical constituents.

Scopolamine in quite small doses produces depression of the cerebral cortex, expecially the motor areas, so causing drowsiness. It is extensively used for this CNS effect in preoperative medication and for the treatment of motion sickness. It is not used for its hallucinatory action.

D. Other Drugs Containing Alkaloids As Active Principles

1. Iboga

The roots of *Tabernanthe iboga* Baill. (Apocynaceae) are used in Gabon in Central Africa as a stimulant, aphrodisiac, and in larger doses as a hallucinogen known by the name *iboga*. Its use has been described by Harrison and Pope [146] and Naranjo [114].

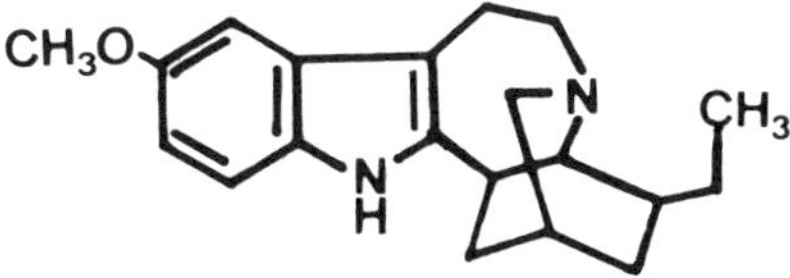

(35) Ibogaine

The major alkaloid present in *iboga* is ibogaine (35) and it is accompanied by at least a dozen other alkaloids. Its use forms the basis of the Bwiti cult, initiates allowed to enter being those who, having eaten *iboga*, "see" Bwiti in a hallucinatory experience. Visions appear for several hours and are followed by sleep, which lasts for several days. In small doses, *iboga* is taken to ensure wakefulness and stimulation of the CNS, thus enabling hunters to remain alert and motionless for hours at a time. Studies on the pure alkaloid have cast doubt on the idea that ibogaine is responsible for the hallucinogenic effect of *iboga* [114], although its role in the sedation process has been confirmed. However, Sloviter et al. [147] in a rat model have demonstrated that ibogaine is similar to proven hallucinogens such as LSD-25 and mescaline in activating the central 5-HT receptors.

2. *Nymphaea* species

Recently, there has been interest in the narcotic use of the buds of *Nymphaea* species (Nymphaeaceae), water lilies, depicted in Egyptian hieroglyphs [148,149] and in the frescoes and literature of the Mayas of Central America [150–152]. The species used were probably *N. caerulea* Sav. and *N. ampla* (Salisb.) DC., respectively. There is no evidence that their use is still current

The rhizomes of the related plant *Nuphar luteum* L. have been shown to contain a mixture of alkaloids "nupharine," one constituent of which is nupharidine (36). On testing such a mixture, no sedative action was observed; and variation in the "nupharine" content from one plant sample to another and according to season makes it difficult to draw meaningful conclusions. Alkaloidal extracts of *Nymphaea ampla*, however, have antispasmodic and sedating properties; in 1975 Diaz [153] isolated apomorphine (37) from its bulbs and roots.

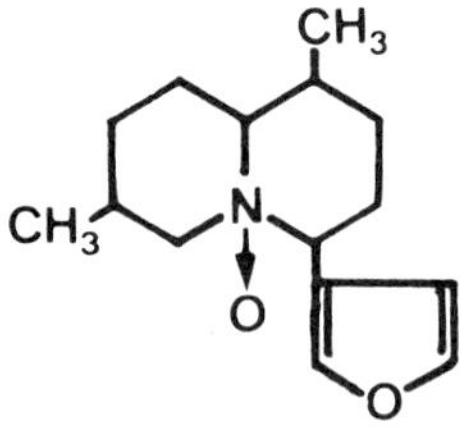

(36) Nupharidine

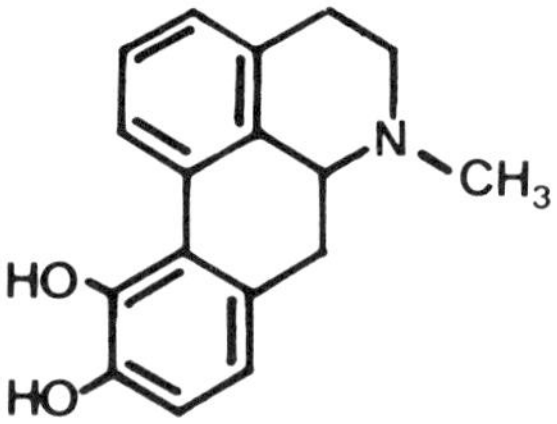

(37) Apomorphine

Diaz [151] and Tamminga et al. [154] have investigated the pharmacology of apomorphine and have demonstrated that in large doses it produces stereotyped psychotomimetic behavior because of its action on the presynaptic dopamine receptors. This behavior would be looked upon as a typical shamanistic performance and could well explain the ritual use of these water lilies. It should, however, be pointed out that the flower buds of the plant still require detailed chemical study, and reconsideration of the pharmacological basis for the reputed use of these plants could be necessary.

3. Mescal beans

The mescal bean, *Sophora secondiflora* (Ort.) Lagasca ex DC. (Leguminosae), is worn by the Indians of Peru and northern Mexico as part of their ceremonial dress, and in former days the beans were ingested as a hallucinogen in a vision-seeking dance ceremony. Studies by Hatfield et al. [155] have established that cytisine (38) is the

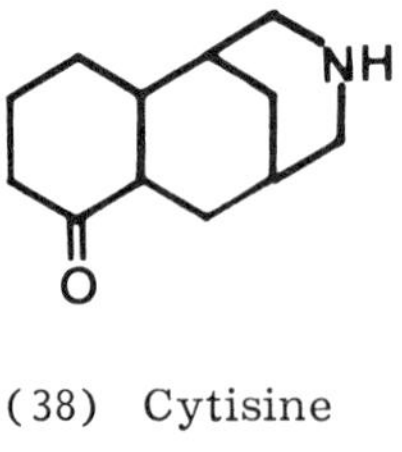

(38) Cytisine

alkaloid present in greatest amount. There are no records that cytisine has hallucinogenic properties—indeed, it is a very toxic alkaloid and

Hatfield et al. concluded that subjective reaction to the environment was the main contribution to the CNS activity in those taking part.

4. Heimia

In Mexico a hallucinatory drink called *sinicuichi* is prepared by crushing the leaves of *Heimia salicifolia* (HBK.) Link et Otto (Lythraceae) in water and allowing the juice to ferment [156]. Auditory rather than visual hallucinations are experienced and events long past are recalled. Six alkaloids have been extracted from *H. salicifolia*, the chief one being cryogenine (39).

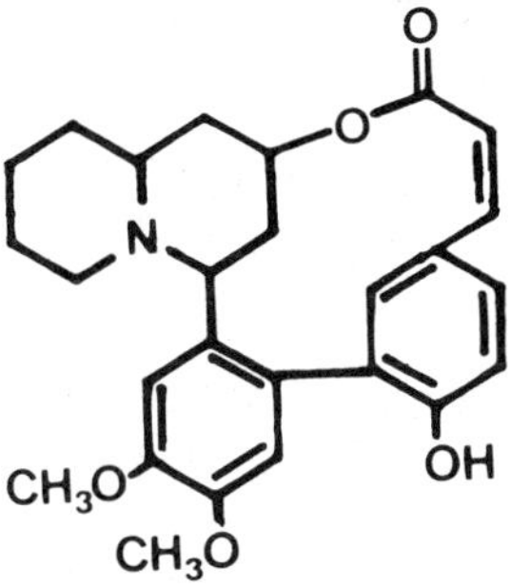

(39) Cryogenine

Some pharmacological studies on cryogenine and related bases have been carried out [157,158]. However, hallucinatory activity has not been detected, possibly because the chemical investigation was performed on the fresh, and not fermented, plant. Nevertheless, interesting evidence concerning the potential of cryogenine as a tranquilizing drug was acquired during the work.

5. Fly Agaric

Amanita muscaria (L. ex Fr.) Pers. ex Hook. (Amanitaceae), the mushroom commonly known as "fly agaric," occurs widely throughout the northern temperate zone of Eurasia and America. Wasson [159,160] has reviewed its hallucinogenic uses and he has also identified *soma*—the plant narcotic worshipped in the hymns of the ancient Indian *Rig Veda*—with it [161]. The chemistry and pharmacology of fly agaric has been discussed by Shulgin [12], Eugster [162], Waser [163], Chilton [164], and Theobald et al. [165].

The known hallucinogenic use of fly agaris is by the Uralic-speaking peoples of western Siberia and by the Paleo-Siberian Chukchi, Koryak, and Kamchadal (Itelmen) of the extreme northeastern part of Siberia. It has been used both ceremonially to commune with the spirit world and as an inebriant. The dried mushrooms are swallowed, often with fruit juices or reindeer milk. A unique feature of the use of fly agaric as an intoxicant is the drinking of the urine of people who have taken it by other people who then in turn experience its psychoactive effects. Most of the active compounds are excreted unchanged in the urine.

The activity of fly agaric is due to the presence of isoxazole compounds, particularly muscimol (40a), ibotenic acid (40b), and muscazone (41). Ibotenic acid is usually the main component.

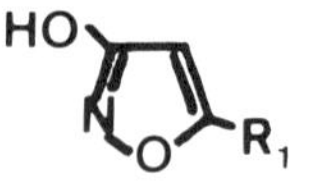

HO, N, O, R_1

(40a) Muscimol R = CH_2NH_2
(40b) Ibotenic acid R = $CH(NH_2)COOH$

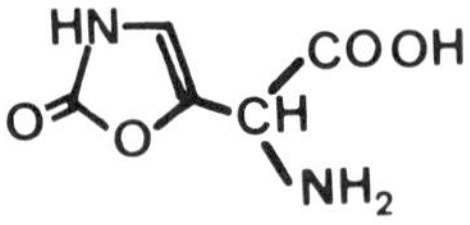

HN, O, O, COOH, CH, NH_2

(41) Muscazone

Muscimol has five times the activity of ibotenic acid. They are both potent agonists of the CNS inhibitory neurotransmitter γ-aminobutyric acid (GABA) and their central effect is thought to be due to inhibition of the motor functions of the CNS. Chilton [164] found that doses of about 100 mg of ibotenic acid produced dizziness and visual and auditory distortions followed by sedation. Ingestion of the mushrooms leads after about 20 min to an abnormal sleep from which the subject cannot be roused but during which he is aware of some of the surrounding sounds. In the course of this "sleep," which lasts for about 2 hr, some individuals experience visions that are less vividly colored than those seen with tryptamine derivatives. On waking, there is sometimes a period of elation and acts of considerable physical effort may be undertaken. Certain analogs of muscimol have been investigated as sedatives because of their GABA-agonist activity, and the cyclic analogue THIP has reached the stage of clinical testing as an analgesic agent. (See Chap. 1, pages 45 and 47.)

E. Drugs with Nonalkaloidal Active Principles

1. Cannabis

Cannabis is known by many different names, among them: Indian hemp, charras, marijuanha, ganja, bhang, dagga, hashish, and pot. There is still discussion among botanists as to whether the genus consists of a variable monotypic *Cannabis sativa* L. (Cannabaceae) or whether it is polytipic. Originally used in India and some parts of the Middle East, its use as a hedonistic drug has now spread throughout the world and many tons are grown and consumed in various ways. Its use is illegal in many countries and much smuggling goes on. The most active part of the plant is the flowering tops of the female plants—they secrete a resin containing the psychoactive compounds. The flowering tops of the male plants produce a similar resin, but since the male plants are smaller and die off quickly, they are not used as a source of the drug [168]. Among the many different ways in which cannabis is used are smoking, drinking, and eating.

In the western world, cannabis is usually inhaled by smoking a cigarette of either the dried leaves and flowering tops (a "joint") or tobacco mixed with the resin or impregnated with an alcoholic extract of the plant or resin (a "reefer").

In Eastern civilizations, cannabis has been in use much longer. It is smoked, often through a waterpipe that filters out many of the constituents of the smoke but not the lipophilic cannabinoids which are the active components. A drink is made by mixing the dried powdered herb with milk and water, while a sweetmeat is prepared by heating the herb in butter, cooling the mixture, washing it with water, and mixing it with flour and sugar.

A vast amount of scientific literature on cannabis has been published in recent years, dealing with many aspects of the chemistry, pharmacology, and sociology of the drug, e.g., Graham [166], Nahas [167], Shulgin [12], Joyce and Curry [168], Turner et al. [169], Mechoulam [170,171], Kettenes-van den Bosch et al. [172], Braude and Szara [173], and Coper [174]. Hence, only a brief summary can be given here.

As with many other psychoactive drugs, the subjective experiences of those who take cannabis is to some extent governed by their expectations and the setting in which the drug is taken. Studies indicate that regular users experience a general euphoria with a keener sense of sound, a state of relaxation, and a feeling of slowed time together with thirst and hunger. A fairly large minority suffer feelings of anxiety and other mental disturbances, such as interruptions in the euphoric state, after smoking cannabis. Large doses produce mostly pleasant hallucinations.

On a more objective level, impairment of motor function, short-term memory, concept formation, and tactile discrimination seem to be well-established effects of connabis.

The principal active constituents of cannabis are generally considered to be tetrahydrocannabinols. Unfortunately, two systems of numbering are used for the cannabinoid skeletons. The one used here is the "pyran" system, the one most widely used in the United States, according to which the two major psychoactive compounds are Δ^9- and Δ^8-trans-tetrahydrocannabinol (THC) (42a). In the alternative numbering—the "monoterpenoid" system, which is used more in Europe—the same two compounds are known as Δ^1- and $\Delta^{1(6)}$-THC (42b). Opening of the pyran ring, as in the substance cannabidiol (CBD) (43), necessitates a change of numbering for the "pyran" but not the "monoterpenoid" system. The structure-activity relationships of cannabinoids have been discussed by Mechoulam [175].

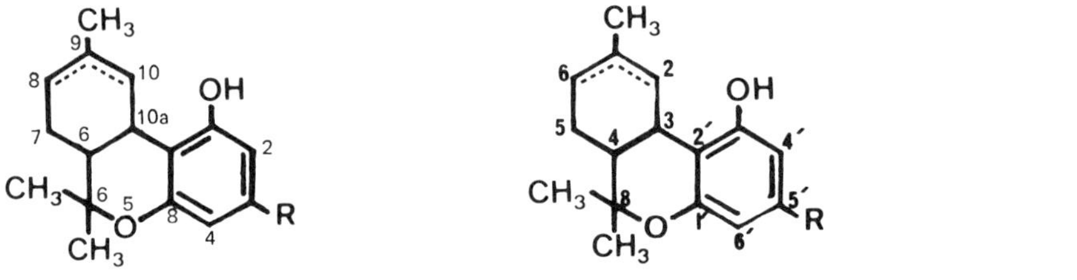

(42a)
(42b) Numbering systems of Tetrahydrocannabinol (THC) $R = C_5H_{11}$

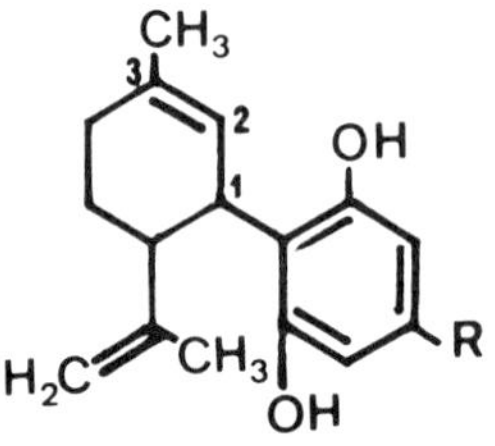

(43) Cannabidiol (CBD) $R = C_5H_{11}$

There is considerable variation in the nature of the cannabinoids present in samples of cannabis, resulting from both genetic and environmental factors. Consequently, there is variation in the CNS activity of the drug. A further source of variation in activity arises from the method of taking the drug. Smoking causes a more rapid onset of action, but the duration is shorter not only because absorption through the lungs is quicker but also because the inactive cannabinoid acids present are decarboxylated to the active neutral compounds.

The effects of cannabis and particularly THC on the CNS are little understood at the neurochemical level. THC and its analogs are lipophilic and must upset membrane equilibria. They inhibit RNA and protein synthesis and may thus affect the storage of information and distort the turnover of some neurotransmitters. Overall, the effects of cannabis are a mixture of stimulation and depression of the CNS [11].

In recent years, there has been considerable research into semisynthetic compounds based on the cannabinoid nucleus and the subject has been reviewed by Cohen and Stillman [176] and Lemberger [177] with reference their potential therapeutic use.

Although the cannabinoids have useful antiemetic, bronchodilatory, anticonvulsant, antiglaucoma, and sedative activity, their application is precluded by the associated CNS side effects. Hence, the semisynthetic derivatives have been designed to retain the useful properties while minimizing the side effects.

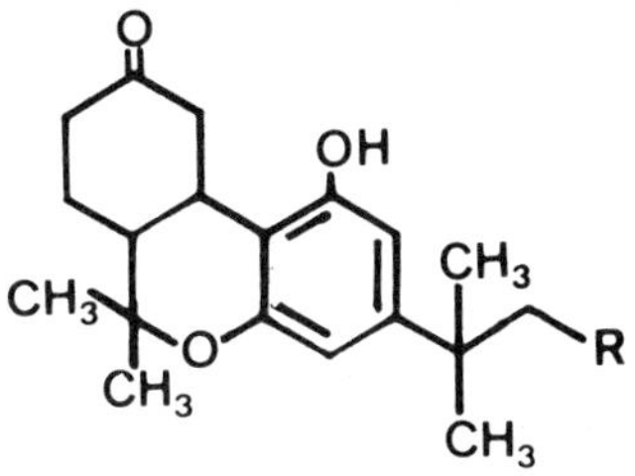

(44) Nabilone R = C_5H_{11}

Nabilone (44) is one such derivative which retains the CNS-depressant activity of Δ^9- THC and shows antianxiety activity. Since the degree of activity is not as good as that of the benzodiazepines, further development in this direction has not been pursued. However, nabilone has shown great promise as an antiemetic agent, especially in connection with the radio- or chemotherapeutic treatment of certain types of cancer. Another area where nabilone and other synthetic cannabinoids have shown promise is in treating glaucoma. The drug is effective by both systemic and topical application. One of the synthetic agents used is a *N*-containing cannabinoid analog SP1 (45).

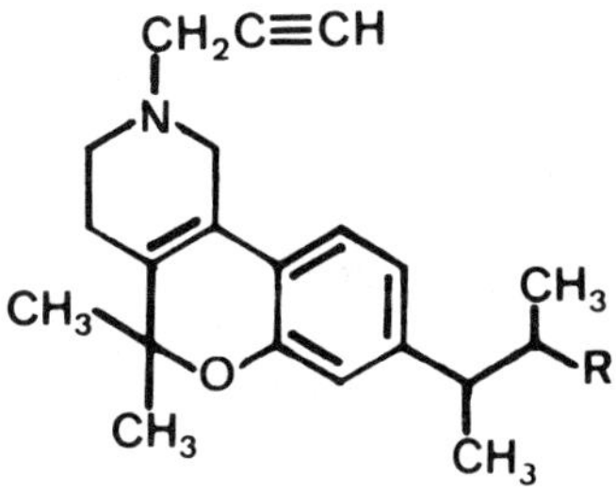

(45) SP1 R = C_5H_{11}

2. Thujone-Containing Plants

Puleo [178] has drawn attention to the psychoactive properties of plants such as European sage [*Salvia* species (Labiatae)], *Tanacetum* species (Compositae), and absinth [*Artemisia absinthium* L. (Compositae)]. All these plants contain thujone (46). It is interesting to note that the leaves of *Salvia divinorum* Epling et Jativá are crushed and used as a divinatory hallucinogen by the Mazatecs of Oaxaca, Mexico. This is thought to be the drink known as *pipiltzintzintli* to the Aztecs. No chemical constituents have yet been isolated from the plant.

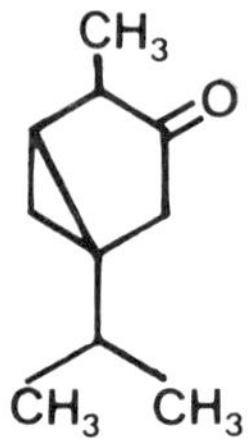

(46) Thujone

Although none of the European plants are now used for their psychoactivity, the toxic CNS effects of absinth, a liqueur made from *Artemisia absinthium*, caused great concern during the latter half of the 19th century because of its widespread consumption. The history of its use and abuse has been documented by Vogt [179]. Some of its effects are hallucinatory in character. Del Castillo et al. [180] have related the molecular geometry of thujone to that of the cannabinoids in attempting to explain the psychoactivity of absinth and other plants containing thujone.

V. THERAPEUTIC POTENTIAL OF CNS-ACTIVE PLANT SUBSTANCES

A. Psychostimulants

The widely used stimulants such as caffeine, betel nut, tobacco, and khat are likely to enjoy continued use socially on a considerable scale, although in many countries measures are being taken to reduce the consumption of tobacco because of its carcinogenic and cardiotoxic properties.

There are signs of reviving medical interest in the use of coca as distinct from cocaine, but the greater thrust seems to be toward removal of the stigma of addiction applied to those Indians in South America who use it as part of their everyday lives. The illicit trade in cocaine and its associated evils will no doubt prevent easy availability and widespread use of coca.

Most interest and development is focused on the adaptogen ginseng, from both *Panax* and *Eleutherococcus*. And although its therapeutic value is well established in the Far East and USSR, it has not yet been accepted by the medical establishment in the West. It is, however, sold and purchased in quite large amounts—world trade is estimated to be about 2000 tons annually [181]—and further appraisal of its reputed properties under conditions acceptable to orthodox medicine is needed.

The greater part of research and development on naturally occurring drugs is carried out in parts of the world other than the industrialized

West and significant advances may well come from China and other countries where this type of research is encouraged.

B. Psychodepressants

Because of the widespread use of the cheap tranquilizers such as diazepam, interest is concentrated on less potent "natural" alternatives and more satisfactory antiepileptic drugs. Most claims for the vegetable drugs reputed to have sedative activity have been substantiated by chemical and pharmacological investigation. The plants thus comprise a reservoir of chemical structures that could be further studied to determine with greater precision the essential chemical parameters and so could well lead to the development of new sedative drugs.

Most current research in the West in this field is directed toward the goal of finding nonaddictive analgesics comparable with morphine or is concerned with the sedative drug valerian which is widely used in continental Europe.

C. Drugs that Affect Consciousness

The bulk of the interest in many of these drugs has had a social rather than medical basis. There is limited interest in some compounds such as lysergic acid derivatives and mescaline for the treatment of psychoses and as tools to help the psychiatrist enter into the experience of psychosis.

With the drugs used illicitly on a large scale, in particular cannabis, much research has been aimed at their detection and at the assessment of their damaging effects, and the mood concerning the introduction of these drugs into medicine is very cautious.

REFERENCES

1. R. E. Schultes and A. Hofmann, *The Botany and Chemistry of Hallucinogens*, 2nd ed., Charles C. Thomas, Springfield, Illinois, 1980.
2. D. H. Efron (Ed.), *Ethnopharmacologic Search for Psychoactive Drugs*, Public Health Service Publication No. 1645, U.S. Department of Health, San Francisco, 1967.
3. R. E. Schultes, in *Principles of Psychopharmacology* (W. G. Clark and J. del Guidice, Eds.), Academic, New York, 1978, p. 41.
4. W. A. Emboden, *Narcotic Plants*, Studio Vista, London, 1979.
5. A. Hoffer and H. Osmond, *The Hallucinogens*, Academic, New York, 1967.

6. J. L. Diaz, *Ann. Rev. Pharmacol. Toxicol.*, 17:647 (1977).
7. J. M. Watt, *Lloydia*, 30:1 (1967).
8. W. H. Lewis and M. P. F. Lewis, *Medical Botany*, Wiley, New York, 1977, p. 377.
9. R. E. Schultes, *Ann. Rev. Plant Physiol.*, 21:571 (1970).
10. R. E. Schultes and N. R. Farnsworth, *Bot. Mus. Leafl. Harvard Univ.*, 28:123 (1980).
11. V. E. Tyler, *Lloydia*, 29:275 (1966).
12. A. T. Shulgin, in *Psychopharmacological Agents* (M. Gordon, Ed.), Vol. 4, 1976, p. 59.
13. F. Hoffmeister and G. Stille (Eds.), *Psychotropic Agents*, in *Handbook of Experimental Pharmacology*, Vol. 55/III, Springer Verlag, 1982.
14. C. J. Estler, in *Handbook of Experimental Pharmacology* (F. Hoffmeister and G. Stille, Eds.), Vol. 55/III, Springer Verlag, 1982, p. 369.
15. R. M. Gilbert, in *Research Advances in Alcohol-Drug Problems* (R. J. Gibbus, Y. Israel, H. Kalart, R. C. Popham, W. Schmidt, and R. G. Smart, Eds.), Wiley, New York, 1976, p. 49.
16. O. Eichler, *Kaffee und Coffein*, 2nd ed., Springer, Berlin, Heidelberg, New York, 1976.
17. W. H. Calhoun, in *Pharmacological and Biophysical Agents and Behavior* (E. Furchgott, Ed.), Academic, New York, London, 1971, p. 181.
18. A. Getahun and A. D. Krikorian, *Econ. Bot.*, 27:353 (1973).
19. A. Getahun and A. D. Krikorian, *Econ. Bot.*, 27:378 (1973).
20. O. Wolfes, *Arch. Pharm. (Berlin)*, 268:81 (1930).
21. H. Hofmann, K. Optiz, and H. J. Schnelle, *Arzneimittel-Forschung*, 5:367 (1955).
22. R. L. Baxter, L. Crombie, D. J. Simmonds, and D. A. Whiting, *J. Chem. Soc., Chem. Commun.*, 465 (1976).
23. R. L. Baxter, L. Crombie, D. J. Simmonds, D. A. Whiting, O. J. Braerder, and K. Szendrei, *J. Chem. Soc., Perkin II*, 2965 (1979).
24. R. L. Baxter, W. M. L. Crombie, L. Crombie, D. J. Simmonds, D. A. Whiting, and K. Szendrei, *J. Chem. Soc. Perkin II*, 2982 (1979).
25. X. Schorno and E. Steinegger, *Experientia*, 35:572 (1979).
26. D. W. Peterson, C. K. Maitai, and S. B. Sparker, *Life Sci.*, 27:2143 (1980).
27. S. Qedan, *Planta Med.*, 21:410 (1972).
28. World Health Organization Document WHO/APD 127 Rev 1, 8-1-64. Cited in ref. 23
29. F. Robicsek, *The Smoking Gods. Tobacco in Maya Art, History and Religion*, University of Oklahoma Press, Norman, Oklahoma, 1978.

30. O. Janiger and M. Dobkin de Rios, *Econ. Bot.*, 30:149 (1976).
31. M. J. Plotkin, R. A. Mittermeier, and I, Constable, *J. Ethnopharmacol.* 2:295 (1980).
32. J. Wilbert, in *Flesh of the Gods. The Ritual Use of Hallucinogens* (P. T. Furst, Ed.), Praeger, New York, 1972, p. 55.
33. B. Holmstedt and G. Lindgren, *Ann. N.Y. Acad. Sci.*, 142:126 (1967).
34. E. H. Poindexter and R. D. Carpenter, *Phytochemistry*, 1:215 (1962).
35. A. K. Nadkarni, *Indian Materia Medica*, 3rd ed., Vol. 1, Dhootapapeshwar Prakashan, Panvel, 1954.
36. E. M. Holmes, *Pharm. J.*, 77:621 (1907).
37. S. Suwanlert, *Bull. Narcotics*, 27 (3):21 (1975).
38. E. J. Shellard, *Bull. Narcotics*, 26 (2):41 (1974).
39. K. S. Grewal, *J. Pharmacol. Exptl. Therap.*, 46:251 (1932).
40. E. Macko, J. A. Weisbach, and B. Douglas, *Arch. Internat. Pharmacodynam. Therap.*, 198:145 (1972).
41. Xiao Peigen, *Proc. 2nd International Meeting on Medicinal and Aromatic Plants*, Citta di Castello, September 1981 (publ. 1983), p. 179.
42. F. Khuong-Huu-Lainé, J. P. Leforestier, G. Maillard, and R. Goutarel, *C. R. Acad. Sci., Paris*, 270 (C):2070 (1970).
43. I. I, Brekhman and I. V. Dardymov, *Lloydia*, 32:46 (1969).
44. I. M. Popov and W. J. Goldwag, *Am. J. Chin. Med.*, 1:263 (1973).
45. K. Karzel, *Proc. 1st Ginseng Symposium, Seoul*, 1974, p. 69.
46. Hu Shiu-Yung, *Amer. Chin. Med.*, 5:1 (1977).
47. H. Saito, *Proc. 2nd Internat. Ginseng Symposium*, Korea Ginseng Research Institute, Seoul, 1978, p. 109.
48. Hyo-Won Bae (Ed.), *Korean Ginseng*, 2nd ed., Korean Ginseng Research Institute, Seoul, 1978.
49. I. I. Brekhman, *Proc. 2nd Internat. Pharmacol. Meeting, Prague 1963*, Vol. 7, Pergamon Press, Oxford, 1965, p. 97.
50. S. Fulder, *New Scientist*, 87:576 (1980).
51. W. Petkov, *Arzneimittel-Forschung*, 9:305 (1959).
52. R. M. Baxter, P. C. Dandry, S. I. Kandel, A. Okany, and G. C. Walker, *Nature*, 185:466 (1960).
53. J. Vrkoc, V. Herout, and F. Sorm, *Coll. Czech. Chem. Commun.*, 26:3183 (1961).
54. R. T. Martin, *Econ. Bot.* 24:422 (1970).
55. R. Ashley, *Cocaine. Its History, Uses and Effects*, St. Martins Press, New York, 1975.
56. L. Grinspoon and J. B. Bakalar, *J. Ethnopharmacol.*, 3:149 (1981).
57. B. Holmstedt and A. Fredga, *J. Ethnopharmacol.*, 3:113 (1981).
58. A. T. Weil, *J. Ethnopharmacol.*, 3:367 (1981).

59. C. Andrews and D. Solomon (Eds.), *The Coca Leaf and Cocaine Papers*, Harcourt Brace Jovanovich, New York and London, 1975.
60. T. Plowman, *J. Ethnopharmacol.*, 3:195 (1981).
61. L. Volicer, I. Janku, O. Motl, and Z. Jiricka, in *Pharmacology of Oriental Plants* (K. K. Chen and B. Mukerji, Eds.), *Proc. 2nd Internat. Pharmacol. Meeting, Prague 1963*, Vol. 7, Pergamon Press, 1965, p. 29.
62. *Martindale, The Extra Pharmacopoeia*, 27th ed., Pharmaceutical Press, London, 1977, p. 951.
63. L. S. Goodman and A. Gilman, *The Pharmacological Basis of Therapeutics*, 6th ed., MacMillan, New York, 1980.
64. R. R. Arndt and P. E. J. Kruger, *Tetrahedron Lett.*, 3237 (1970).
65. F. Keller and M. W. Klohs, *Lloydia*, 26:1 (1963).
66. L. D. Holmes, in *Ethnopharmacologic Search for Psychoactive Drugs* (D. H. Efron, Ed.), Public Health Service Publication no. 1645, U.S. Department of Health, San Francisco, 1967, p. 107.
67. M. W. Klohs, in *Ethnopharmacologic Search for Psychoactive Drugs* (D. H. Efron, Ed.), Public Health Service Publication no. 1645, U.S. Department of Health, San Francisco, 1967, p. 126.
68. H. J. Meyer, in *Ethnopharmacologic Search for Psychoactive Drugs* (D. H. Efron, Ed.), Public Health Service Publication no. 1645, U. S. Department of Health, San Francisco, 1967, p. 133.
69. J. P. Buckley, A. R. Furgiuele, and M. J. O'Hara, in *Ethnopharmacologic Search for Psychoactive Drugs* (D. H. Efron, Ed.), Public Health Service Publication no. 1645, U.S. Department of Health, San Francisco, 1967, p. 141.
70. A. T. Shulgin, *Bull. Narcotics*, 25 (2):59 (1973).
71. P. W. Thies, *Tetrahedron Lett.*, 1163 (1966).
72. H. Hikino, Y. Hikino, H. Kobinata, A. Aizawa, C. Konno, and Y. Ohizumi, *Shoyakugaku Zasshi* 34:19 (1980).
73. H. Wagner, K. Jurcic, and R. Schaette, *Planta Med.*, 39:358 (1980).
74. R. B. Arora and C. K. Arora, in *Pharmacology of Oriental Plants* (K. K. Chen and B. Mukerji, Eds.), *Proc. 2nd Internat. Pharmacol. Meeting, Prague 1963*, Vol. 7, Pergamon Press, 1965, p. 51.
75. A. Raison, *Scient. Orient.*, no. 7, p. 1 (1977).
76. O. S. Chizhov, A. V. Kessenlileh, I. P. Yakovlev, B. M. Zolotarev, V. A. Petukhov, and N. D. Zelinskii, *Tetrahedron Lett.*, 1361 (1969).
77. R. V. Telyateva and N. K. Fruentov, *Vopr. Farm. Dal'nem Vostoka*, 1:136; cited from: *Chem. Abstr.* 83:756 (1975).
78. L. Bravo Diaz, J. Cabo Torres, A. Fraile-Ovejero, and J. Jumenez, *Boll. Chim. Farm.*, 113:310.

79. A. W. Forst, *Arch. Exptl. Pathol. Pharmakol.*, 195:1 (1940).
80. J. Lutomski, B. Maleb, and L. Rybacka, *Planta Med.*, 27:112 (1975).
81. J. Lutomski, E. Segie, K. Szpunar, and K. Goisse, *Pharm. Unser. Zeit*, 10 (2):5 (1981).
82. E. G. Auxense, *Econ. Bot.*, 7:270 (1953).
83. Raymond-Hamet, *Bull. Sci. Pharmacol.*, 34:143 (1927).
84. R. A. Akundov, A. A. Nasudari, and A. V. Reish, *Azerb. Med. Zh.* 54 (3):15 (1977); cited from: *Chem. Abstr.* 87:96 003 (1977).
85. M. R. Zub, *Farm Zh. (Kiev)*, 27 (5):86 (1972); cited from: *Chem. Abstr.* 78:40 406 (1978).
86. L. Cina and G. Fassina, *Arch. Ital. Sci. Farmacol.*, 11:288 (1961).
87. J. P. Theallet, *Prod. Pharm.*, 18:12 (1963).
88. X. A. Dominguez and M. Hinojosa, *Planta Med.*, 30:68 (1976).
89. E. V. Vieira, F. J. A. Matos, G. S. G. Barros, M. P. Souza, and M. C. Madeiros, *Rev. Brasil. Farm.*, 49:67 (1968); cited from: *Chem. Abstr.*: 69:95 034 (1968).
90. H. Rimpler and B. Schaefer, *Tetrahedron Lett.*, 1463 (1973).
91. L. Lewin, *Phantastica. Narcotic and Stimulating Drugs. Their Use and Abuse*, Kegan Paul, London, 1931.
91a. V. E. Tyler in *Natural Products as Medicinal Agents* (J. L. Beal and E. Reinhard, Eds.), Hippokrates Verlag, Stuttgart 1981, p. 339.
92. G. K. Aghajanian, in *Handbook of Experimental Pharmacology* (F. Hoffmeister and G. Stille, Eds.), Vol. 55/III, Springer Verlag, Berlin, Heidelberg, New York, 1982, p. 89.
93. S. Szara, *Experientia*, 12:441 (1956).
94. B. Holmstedt and J. E. Lindgren, in *Ethnopharmacologic Search for Psychoactive Drugs* (D. H. Efron, Ed.), Public Health Service Publication no. 1645, U.S. Department of Health, San Francisco, 1967, p. 339.
95. M. S. Fish, N. M. Johnson, and E. C. Horning, *J. Am. Chem. Soc.*, 77:5892 (1955).
96. G. Legler and R. Tschesche, *Naturwissenschaften*, 50:94 (1963).
97. W. J. Turner and S. Merks, *Arch. Neurol. Psychiatr.*, 81:121 (1959).
98. R. E. Schultes, *J. Ethnopharmacol.*, 1:211 (1979).
99. G. J. Seitz, in *Ethnopharmacologic Search for Psychoactive Drugs* (D. H. Efron, Ed.), Public Health Service Document no. 1645, U.S. Department of Health, San Francisco, 1967, p. 315.
100. B. Holmstedt, W. J. A. Vandenheuvel, W. L. Gardner, and E. C. Horning, *Anal. Biochem.*, 8:151 (1964).
101. S. Agurell, B. Holmstedt, J. E. Lindgren, and R. E. Schultes, *Acta Chem. Scand.*, 23:903 (1969).
102. R. Prentis, Ph. D. Thesis, University of London, 1982.
103. A. Hofmann, *Bull. Narcotics*, 23 (1):3 (1971).

104. R. G. Wasson, *Bot. Mus. Leafl. Harvard Univ.*, 20:25 (1962).
105. R. G. Wasson, *The Wondrous Mushroom*, Harcourt Brace Jovanovich, New York, 1980.
106. G. M. Hatfield, L. J. Valdes, and A. H. Smith, *Lloydia*, 41:140 (1978).
107. R. A. Weeks, R. Suger, and W. L. Hearn, *J. Nat. Prod. (Lloydia)*, 42:469 (1979).
108. P. A. Cox, *J. Ethnopharmacol.*, 4:115 (1981).
109. A. B. Wohlbach, E. J. Miner, and H. Isbell, *Psychopharmacologia*, 3:219 (1962).
110. L. L. Hsu and A. J. Mandell, *J. Neurochem.*, 24:631 (1975).
111. K. J. Keller, G. R. Elliot, J. V. Holman, and J. D. Barclay, *J. Pharmacol. Exptl. Therap.*, 198:619 (1976).
112. R. E. Schultes, *Bot. Mus. Leafl. Harvard Univ.*, 18:1 (1957).
113. L. Rivier and J. E. Lindgren, *Econ. Bot.*, 26:101 (1972).
114. C. Naranjo, *The Healing Journey: New Approaches to Consciousness*, Pantheon Press, New York, 1973.
115. V. Deulofeu, in *Ethnopharmacologic Search for Psychoactive Drugs*, (D. H. Efron, Ed.), Public Health Service Publication no. 1645, U.S. Department of Health, San Francisco, 1967, p. 393.
116. R. G. Wasson, A. Hofmann, and C. A. P. Ruck, *Road to Eleusis: Unveiling the Secret of the Mysteries*, Harcourt Brace Jovanovich, New York, 1978.
117. R. E. Schultes, *A Contribution to our Knowledge of Rivea Corymbosa the Narcotic Ololiuqui of the Aztecs*, Thesis, Harvard University, 1941, p. 15.
118. A. Hofmann and H. Tscherter, *Experientia*, 16:414 (1960).
119. A. Hofmann, *Bot. Mus. Leafl. Harvard Univ.*, 20:194 (1963).
120. W. H. Vogel, R. A. Carapellotti, B. D. Evans, and A. Der Marderosian, *Psychopharmacologia*, 24:238 (1972).
121. J. Chao and A. H. Der Marderosian, *J. Pharmacol. Sci.*, 67: 588 (1973).
122. J. G. Bruhn and C. Bruhn, *Econ. Bot.*, 27:241 (1973).
123. R. A. Bye Jr., *J. Ethnopharmacol.*, 1:23 (1979).
124. R. E. Schultes, *Bull. Narcotics*, 22 (1):25 (1970).
125. M. Dobkin de Rios, *Econ. Bot.*, 22:191 (1968).
126. J. L. McLaughlin, *Lloydia*, 36:1 (1973).
127. G. J. Kapatia and M. B. E. Fayez, *Lloydia*, 36:9 (1973).
128. A. T. Shulgin, *Lloydia*, 36:46 (1973).
129. J. G. Bruhn, *Econ. Bot.*, 25:320 (1971).
130. J. S. Todd, *Lloydia*, 32:395 (1969).
131. A. T. Weil, in *Ethnopharmacologic Search for Psychoactive Drugs* (D. H. Efron, Ed.), Public Health Service Publication no. 1645, U.S. Department of Health, San Francisco, 1967, p. 188.

132. A. T. Weil, *Bull. Narcotics*, 18 (4):15 (1966).
133. A. T. Shulgin, *Nature*, 210:380 (1966).
134. A. T. Shulgin, T. Sargent, and C. Naranjo, in *Ethnopharmacologic Search for Psychoactive Drugs* (D. H. Efron, Ed.), Public Health Service Publication no. 1645, U.S. Department of Health, San Francisco, 1967, p. 202.
135. E. B. Truitt, in *Ethnopharmacologic Search for Psychoactive Drugs* (D. H. Efron, Ed.), Public Health Service Publication no. 1645, U.S. Department of Health, San Francisco, 1967, p. 215.
136. D. A. Kalbhen, *Angew. Chem.*, 10:370 (1971).
137. A. T. Shulgin, T. Sargent, and C. Naranjo, *Pharmacology*, 10:12 (1973).
138. H. Kawabata, *J. Pharm. Soc. Japan*, 65:9 (1945).
139. U. Braun and D. A. Kalbhen, *Pharmacology*, 9:312 (1973).
140. E. O. Oswald, L. Fishbein, B. J. Corbett, and H. P. Walker, *Biochim. Biophys. Acta*, 244:322 (1971).
141. S. H. Snyder and E. Richelson, in *Psychopharmacology* (D. H. Efron, Ed.), Public Health Service Publication no. 1836, Washington, 1968, p. 1199.
142. C. J. Sherry, L. E. Ray, and R. E. Herron, *J. Ethnopharmacol.*, 6:61 (1982).
143. T. E. Lockwood, *J. Ethnopharmacol.*, 1:147 (1979).
144. J. M. Gowdy, *J. Am. Med. Assoc.*, 221:585 (1972).
145. T. F. Johnston, *Econ. Bot.*, 26:340 (1972).
146. G. P. Harrison and H. G. Pope, *Econ. Bot.*, 23:174 (1969).
147. R. S. Sloviter, E. G. Druit, B. P. Damano, and J. D. Connor, *J. Pharmacol. Exptl. Therap.*, 214:231 (1980).
148. W. A. Emboden, *Econ. Bot.* 32:395 (1980).
149. W. A. Emboden, *J. Ethnopharmacol.*, 3:39 (1981).
150. W. A. Emboden, *J. Ethnopharmacol.*, 5:139 (1982).
151. J. L. Diaz, *Ann. Rev. Pharmacol. Toxicol.*, 17:647 (1977).
152. M. Dobkin de Rios, *Current Anthrop.*, 15:147 (1974).
153. J. J. Diaz, *Ethnofarmacologia de Plantas*, Centro de Estudios en Farmacodependencia, Mexico D.F., 1975, p. 174.
154. C. A. Tamminga, M. H. Scheffer, R. C. Smith, and J. M. Davis, *Science*, 200:567 (1978).
155. G. M. Hatfield, L. J. J. Valdes, W. J. Keller, W. L. Merrill, and V. H. Jones, *Lloydia*, 40:374 (1977).
156. R. E. Schultes, *Bull. Narcotics*, 21 (4):15 (1969).
157. R. C. Robichaud, M. H. Malone, and A. E. Schwarting, *Arch. Internat. Pharmacodynam. Therap.*, 150:220 (1964).
158. H. R. Kaplan and M. H. Malone, *Lloydia*, 29:348 (1966).
159. R. G. Wasson, in *Ethnopharmacologic Search for Psychoactive Drugs* (D. H. Efron, Ed.), Public Health Service Publication no. 1645, U.S. Department of Health, San Francisco, 1967, p. 405.

160. R. G. Wasson, *Bull. Narcotics*, 22 (3):25 (1970).
161. R. G. Wasson, *SOMA. Divine Mushroom of Immortality*, Harcourt Brace Jovanovich, New York, 1969.
162. C. H. Eugster, in *Ethnopharmacologic Search for Psychoactive Drugs* (D. H. Efron, Ed.), Public Health Service Publication no. 1645, U. S. Department of Health, San Francisco, 1967, p. 416.
163. P. G. Waser, in *Ethnopharmacologic Search for Psychoactive Drugs* (D. H. Efron, Ed.), Public Health Service Publication no. 1645, U.S. Department of Health, San Francisco, 1967, p. 419.
164. W. S. Chilton, *McIlvainia*, 2:17 (1975).
165. W. Theobald, O. Buchi, H. A. Kurz, P. Krupp, E. G. Stenger, and H. Heimann, *Arzneimittel-Forsch.*, 18:311 (1968).
166. J. D. P. Graham (Ed.), *Cannabis and Health*, Academic, London, 1976.
167. G. G. Nahas (Ed.), *Marihuana—Chemistry, Biochemistry and Cellular Effects*, Springer Verlag, New York, 1976.
168. C. R. B. Joyce and S. H. Curry (Eds.), *The Botany and Chemistry of Cannabis*, Churchill, London, 1970.
169. C. E. Turner, M. A. Elsohly, and E. G. Boeren, *J. Nat. Prod.*, 43:169 (1980).
170. R. Mechoulam, *Marihuana*, Academic, New York, 1973.
171. R. Mechoulam, in *Handbook of Experimental Pharmacology* (F. Hoffmeister and G. Stille, Eds.), Vol. 55/III, Springer Verlag, Berlin, Heidelberg, New York, 1982, p. 119.
172. J. J. Kettenes-van den Bosch, C. A. Salemink, J. van Noordwijk, and I. Khan, *J. Ethnopharmacol.*, 2:197 (1980).
173. N. C. Braude and S. Szara (Eds.), *Pharmacology of Marihuana*, Raven Press, New York, 1976.
174. H. Coper, in *Handbook of Experimental Pharmacology* (F. Hoffmeister and G. Stille, Eds.), Vol. 55/III, Springer Verlag, Berlin, Heidelberg, New York, 1982, p. 135.
175. R. Mechoulam, N. K. McCallum, and S. Burstein, *Chem. Rev.*, 76:75 (1976).
176. S. Cohen and R. C. Stillman (Eds.), *The Therapeutic Potential of Marihuana*, Plenum, New York, 1976.
177. L. Lemberger, *Ann. Rev. Pharmacol. Toxicol.*, 20:151 (1980).
178. M. A. Puleo, *Econ. Bot.*, 32:65 (1978).
179. D. D. Vogt, *J. Ethnopharmacol.*, 4:337 (1981).
180. J. del Castillo, M. Anderson, and G. M. Rubottom, *Nature*, 253:365 (1975).
181. Dr. A. Smith, Tropical Products Institute, Culham, Abingdon, personal cummunication.

Index

A

Absinth, 323
Acanthaceae, 307
Acanthopanax senticosus, 292
Acepromazine, 177
Acetyl choline (*see also* anti-cholinergics)
  blockade by neuroleptic drugs, 176-178
  chemical structure, 315
  drugs related to, 314-316
Acetylenic GABA (*see* Gamma-acetylenic GABA)
Acromegaly, 266-267
Acupuncture
  relief of pain, 16-17
Adaptogens
  stress-adaption drugs (anti-fatigue) such as ginseng and eleutherococcus, 292, 324
Adenyl cyclase
  neuroleptic drug action on, 161-162
Adrenaline (*see* epinephrine)
Adrenocorticotropin (ACTH)
  opiate antagonist, 44
Affective (disorders) (*see* Depression)
Aizoaceae, 297, 298
Alchornea floribunda, 291
Alchorneine
  chemical structure, 291
  excitory sympathetic component of niando, 291
Alcohol (ethyl alcohol), 284, 287, 305
Alfentanyl
  chemical structure, 33
  narcotic analgesic, congener of fentanyl, 32
Alphaprodine
  opioid agonist analgesic, 4
Alphapyrones, 299
Alprazolam
  antidepressant properties of, 130
  pharmacokinetics, 129
  triazolo benzodiazepine, 127
Amanitaceae, 319
Amanita muscaria, 319
Amantadine
  hydrochloride, in treatment of Parkinson's disease, 271
Amenorrhea, 263, 265

Amineptine
  antidepressant, 94
Aminobytyric acid (*see* Gamma-aminobutyric acid)
Aminoglutethimide
  adrenal inhibitor used in treatment of Cushing's syndrome, 267
Aminooxyacetic acid
  GABA-T inhibitor, as analgesic, 45
Amitriptyline
  antidepressant, 72, 79, 82, 84, 86, 88, 112
  chemical structure, 78
  ECG effects, 81
Amobarbital
  chemical structure, 137
Amoxapine
  antidepressant, 94
Amphetamine
  antagonism by asarone, 293
  antidepressant properties, 72, 86, 108-109, 112
  chemical structure, 311
  derivatives in hallucinogenic herbs, 288
  treatment of hyperkinesia in children, 109 (*see also* Introduction)
Anadenanthera sp, 307, 308
  peregrina, 307
Analgesia
  definition, 27
  non-opioid, 26, 30
  stimulation produced, 16
Analgesics
  centrally acting, 1
  from opium, 296-297
  limitations in therapy of pain, 17-25
  mode of action, 26-29
  models for testing, 26-29
  needs and criteria for new drugs, 25-26
  newer synthetic opioids, 32-36
Analgesics (continued)
  non-opioid, 42, 44, 46
  sites and mechanism of action, 29-30
Anemonin, 303
Anileridine
  opioid agonist analgesic, 4
Anisodamine, 304
Anisodine, 304
Anti-anxiety agents (*see* anxiolytics)
Anticholinergic(s)
  alkaloids, from solanaceae, 314-316
  properties of
    antidepressants, 80, 88, 112
    neuroleptics, 176-178
  treatment of Parkinson's disease, 270
Anticonvulsant(s)
  barbiturates, 138-139 (*see also* benzodiazepines and seizures)
Antidepressants, 71
  classes of drugs, 76-77, 112
  "second generation," 93-106, 112
  tricyclic, 76-88
    antagonism of effects of reserpine, 81-84, 87
    anti-anxiety (anxiolytic) properties, 72, 80, 86, 88, 93, 100
    biogenic amine involvement and mode of action, 84-88
    efficacy, 77
    mode of action, 81-86
    pain, treatment of, 15-16
    pharmacokinetics, 79-80
    side-effects, 80-81
Antihistamine
  property of phenothiazine neuroleptics, 176
Antipsychotics (*see* neuroleptics)
Anxiety
  classes of, 130 (*see also* 73)
  treatment with
    antidepressants, 73, 88, 104

Anxiety (continued)
  treatment with (continued)
    benzodiazepines, 123, 128-131
Anxiolytics (anti-anxiety agents)
  antidepressants, 72, 80, 86, 93, 104, 106, 112
  benzodiazepines, 123, 141
  choice of, 130
  non-benzodiazepine, 123, 141
  partial agonist properties of newer, 142-143
  selective, 142
Aphrodisiac, 317
Apocynaceae, 301, 317
Apomorphine
  chemical structure, 318
  dopamimetic alkaloid from Nymphaea, 318
  locomotor inhibitory properties at low dose, 157
  treatment of Parkinson's disease, 271
Aquifoliaceae, 286
Araliaceae, 292
Areca catechu L, 290
Arecoline
  chemical structure, 290
  psychostimulant component of Betel, 290
Argyreia nervosa, 311
Artemisia absinthium, 323
Asarone
  chemical structure, 293
  constituent of calamus, 293
Atropa belladonna, 315
Atropine
  chemical structure, 313
  psychoactive anticholingeric, 314-315
Ayahuasca, 309, 310

B

Baclofen
  analgesic properties of, 45
Banisteriopsis, 309, 310
  caapi, 309
  inebrians, 309
Barbital
  chemical structure, 137
  sleeping time lengthening by dihydromethysticin, 299
Barbiturates, 123
  adverse-effects, 140-141
  chemical structure of, 137
  chemistry, biotransformation, and pharmacokinetics, 136-138
  drug interactions, 141
  history, 136
  lipid solubility, 136-137
  mechanism of action, 139-140
  structure-activity relationships, 136
  tolerance, 141
  treatment of seizure disorders, 138-139
Barrachero, 316
Bartholletia excelsa, 307
Belladonna (*see* atropa belladonna and atropine)
Benperidol, 154
Benzamide(s)
  substituted derivatives as neuroleptics agents, 156-157
Benzomorphans
  opioid mixed agonist-antagonist analgesics, 9-10
Benzodiazepines, 123
  adverse-effects, 135-136
  assessment of efficacy, 130-131
  chemical structures, 125
  chemistry, biotransformation, and pharmacokinetics, 124-128
  drug interactions, 128
  hepatic biotransformation, 127-128
  history, 124
  lipophilicity and distribution, 127
  mechanism of action, 133-135

Benzodiazepines (continued)
1,4-benzodiazepines, 124, 125
receptors, 133-135 142
tolerance to, 132, 135
treatment
of anxiety, 128-131
of insomnia, 131-132
of seizure disorders, 132-133
triazolo-1,4-, 124, 125
Benztropine, 275
mesylate, 270
Beta-carboline, 306
chemical structure, 309
from tobacco, 289
psychomimetic derivatives from plants, 309-310
Betel
nut, 324
psychostimulant, 289-290
Betony, 303
Bhang (*see* cannabis)
Binodaline
antidepressant, 98
Biogenic amine, 84
Biperiden, 270
Breast
treatment of benign disease of, 265-266
Bremazocine
narcotic analgesic, 35
Bromocryptine
treatment of,
acromegaly, 267
breast pain, 266
Cushing's syndrome, 267
hyperprolactinaemia, 264
Parkinson's disease, 272
PCO syndrome, 272
Bromperidol, 154
Brugmansia, 316
Brunfelsia, 316
Bufotenine, 307
chemical structure, 306
Buprenorphine
chemical structure, 10
limitations in therapy of pain, 24-25
Buprenorphine (continued)
opioid mixed agonist-antagonist analgesic, 9, 13
Bupropion
antidepressant, 95, 100, 109
Butabarbital
chemical structure, 137
Butaclamol
neuroleptic drug, 163
Butaperazine
neuroleptic drug, 206
Butorphanol
chemical structure, 10
limitations in therapy of pain, 23-24
opioid mixed agonist-antagonist analgesic, 9, 12
Butryptyline
chemical structure, 78
tricyclic antidepressant, 100
Butyrophenones
neuroleptic drugs, 154
treatment of,
Huntington's disease, 276
pain, 14

C

Caapi (*see* ayahuasca)
Cactaceae, 312
Cade, J.F.J.
lithium therapy in mania, 106-107
Caffeine, 284, 324
containing drugs, 285-287
psychopharmacology of, 286-287
Calamus
stimulant used by Cree Indians of Alberta, 293
Calcitonin
peptide, analgesic properties, 44
Calmodulin
modulation of effects by neuroleptic drugs, 161, 162

Cannabaceae, 320
Cannabidiol, 321
  chemical structure, 322
Cannabinoids
  active components of cannabis, 321
Cannabis, 284, 315, 320-323, 325
  sativa, 320
Carbamazepine
  treatment of seizures, 138
Carbidopa, 271
Carnegie gigantea, 313
Caroxazone
  antidepressant, 98, 105-106
  Type B selective MAO inhibitor, 92
Catalepsy
  side effect of neuroleptic drug therapy, 157
Catechol-O-methyl-transferase (COMT)
  detoxification of extraneous primary amines, 88-89
Catha edulis, 287
Cathedulins
  sesquiterpine alkaloids from Khat, 288
Cathinone
  active stimulant constituent of Khat, 288
  chemical structure, 288
Cecropia sciadophylla, 294
Celastraceae, 287
Charras (*see* cannabis)
Chat (*see* Khat)
"Cheese syndrome"
  MAO inhibitors side effect, 89-90, 100
Chlopenthixol, 155
Chlopimozide
  neuroleptic drugs, 154
Chloral hydrate, 123
Chlordiazepoxide (Librium®*)
  anti-anxiety agent, 124
Chlordiazepoxide (continued)
  chemical structure, 125
  pharmacokinetics, 127, 129
Chlorgyline (*see* clorgyline)
Chloride
  ionophores and channels, in modes of action of benzodiazepines, 134
Chlorimipramine (clomipramine)
  analgesic, 15
  antidepressant, 79, 82, 85, 88
  chemical structure, 78
Chlorophenoxamine, 270
Chlorpromazine (CPZ)
  chemical structure, 153
  Huntington's disease, treatment of, 276
  metabolites, 181
  neuroleptic agent, 149, 152
Chlorprothixene
  chemical structure, 155
  neuroleptic drugs, 155
Chlothiapine
  neuroleptic drug, 155
Chocolate
  from cocoa, 285-286
Cholecystokinin (CCK)
  interaction with striatal dopamine, 182, 242
  peptide, analgesic properties of, 44
Ciclazindol (WY-23409)
  antidepressant, 98-99
Cimoxatone
  Type A selective MAO inhibitor, 92
Ciramidol
  narcotic analgesic, 34
Citalopram
  antidepressant, 97, 100
  analgesic, 15
Clebopride, 192
Clomiphene, 269

---
* ® Registered Trademark.

Clonazepam
chemical structure, 125
treatment of seizure disorders, 132-133
Clonidine, 174
analgesic properties of, 46
Clorazepate
chemical structure, 125
pharmacokinetics, 129
Clorgyline
chemical structure 90
Type A selective MAO inhibitor, 91-92
Clozapine
agranulcytosis properties, 156
anticholinergic properties, 218
atypical neuroleptic drug, 156, 171-173, 217, 222, 242, 264
chemical structure, 155
neuroleptic drug, 155-156
CL-218872
chemical structure, 142
recognition of benzodiazepine receptor sub-types, 142
Coca, 284 (*see also* cocaine);
psychostimulant effects of, 294-295
reviving medical interest, 324
Cocaine
chemical structure, 295
principal active constituent of coca, 284, 294-295, 324
Cocoa
psychostimulant containing caffeine and theobromine, 285-286
Codeine
analgesic from opium and morphine, 296
chemical structure, 5, 297
limitations in therapy of pain, 19-20
opioid agonist analgesic, 3, 4, 7-8
Coffee
psychostimulant, seeds containing caffeine, 285
Cognition
depression of by barbiturates, 140-141
disorders (*see* Introduction)
Cohoba (*see* yopo)
Cola
nitida L, 286
nuts, psychostimulant, source of caffeine, 286
Compositae, 323
Convolvulaceae, 311
Convulsive (disorders) (*see* seizures and epilepsy)
Corydalis yanhusuo, 304
Cryogenine
chemical structure, 319
major alkaloid from Heimia, 319
Cushing's syndrome (disease), 267-268
CU 32-085, 267
Cyclazocine, 12
Cyclorphan, 12
Cycrimine, 270
Cyproheptadine
serotonin antagonist in treatment of Cushing's syndrome, 267
Cytisine
chemical structure, 318
major alkaloid from mescal beans, 318-319

D

Dactylicapnos scandens, 304
DADL (*see* enkephalin)
Dagga (*see* cannabis)
Damiana (*see* Turnera)
Dammarane
triterpenoids, 292
Danazol, 266
Daphne giraldi, 304
Daphnetin, 304
Datura
ceratocaula, 316
fastuosa, 316

Datura (continued)
innoxia, 316
stramonium, 316
Dependence
on,
analgesics, 17-25, 297
barbiturates, 141
benzodiazepines, 136
Khat, 289
psychostimulants, 285
Deprenyl
chemical structure, 90
treatment of Parkinson's disease, 91, 271
Type B MAO inhibitor, 91-92
Depression, 71
alternatives to drug treatment, 111
classification, 73-75, 110, 111
current research into, 110-111
diagnostic rating scales, 74
drug induced, 296
epidemiology, 72-73
etiology, 75-76
treatment of, 75-76
Desimipramine (desipramine)
antidepressant, 79-80, 86
chemical structure, 78
Dexamethasone
suppression test for diagnosis of endogenous depression, 111
Dextromoramide, 14
Dextropropoxyphene
chemical structure, 5
hydrochloride, 4, 20
limitations in therapy of pain, 20-21
napsylate salt, 4
comparison with hydrochloride, 20
opioid analgesic, 4, 8-9
Dezocine
narcotic analgesic, 34
Dhatura
metel, 315
Diazepam (Valium*®)
chemical structure, 125, 142
pharmacokinetics, 127, 129
treatment of,
anxiety, 130
status epilepticus, 132
Dibenzapines
tricyclic antidepressants, 79
Dibenzocycloheptadienes
tricyclic antidepressants, 79
Dihydrocodine
opioid agonist analgesic, 4
Dihydrokawain
chemical structure, 299
Dihydromethysticin
effect on barbital induced sleeping time, 299
Dihydromorphine
opioid agonist analgesic, 4
tritiated; ligand for μ-opiod receptor, 2, 29
Dihydropicrotoxin
convulsant, inhibition of binding by barbiturates, 140
Dimethyltryptamine (NN) (DMT)
chemical structure, 306
Diphenhydramine, 270
Diphenylbutylpiperadine
derivatives, as neuroleptic drugs, 154
Diplopterys cabrerana, 309, 310
Diprenorphine
opioid antagonist, 3
DN-1417,
peptide TRH analogue as antidepressant, 100
Domperidone, 272
tritiated ligand, 163
Dopa (L)
treatment of,
hyperprolactinemia, 264
Parkinson's disease, 271

*®Registered Trademark.

Dopamine
agonist and antagonist ligands (tritiated), 163
chemical structure, 311
drugs related to, 311-314
potentiation of effects by antidepressants, 84, 100, 103, 109
receptors,
blockade by neuroleptic drugs, 150, 157, 247
classification, 186-202
definition of D-1 and D-2, 187, 188
displacement of ligands by neuroleptic drugs, 162-167
multiple locations of, 184-185
supersensitivity, 224
schizophrenia, hypothesis of, 150-151, 245-248
Doxapram, 25
Doxepin
antidepressant, 72, 82, 84, 86, 88, 112
chemical structure, 78
ECG effects, 81
Doxpicomine
narcotic analgesic, 34
Droperidol
neuroleptanalgesic, 14
Drugs
of ethno-origins, 283
classification, 284
drugs which affect consciousness, 305-324, 325
psychodepressants, 296-302, 325
psychostimulants, 285-296, 324-325
reviews on, 283-284
Duboisia hopwoodii, 315
Dynorphin
des-tryosine derivative, opioid antagonist, 44
endogenous opioid, 30
Dyskinesia
drugs reported to be beneficial in the treatment of, 239, 273-275
tardive, side effects of neuroleptic drug therapy, 149, 152-152, 224, 239, 248-249

E

Effects of drugs (adverse, *see* side-effects)
on consciousness, 305
Electrocardiogram (ECG)
produced by tricyclic antidepressants, 81
Electroconvulsive therapy (ECT)
treatment of depression, 71, 107-108, 111
Electroencephalography (EEG)
role in discovery and clinical evaluation of antidepressants, 101, 106, 112
Eleutherococcus, 292
senticosus, 292
Eleutheroside-B (*see also* eleutherococcus)
chemical structure, 292
Endocrine
disturbances, treatment with CNS active drugs, 263-270
Endorphin(s)
endogenous opioids, 30-31
Enkephalin(s)
biosynthetic origins and digestion, 31
chemical structure, 31
derivatives, as analgesics, 38-42
leucine and methionine-, as endogeneous opioids, 30-31
tritiated ligands, 2, 29
Enkephalinase inhibitors
analgesics, 37-38

Epena (*see* yakee, 307)
Epilepsy
  treatment with,
    benzodiazepines, 128, 132-133
    diazepam, 132
    drugs from Kava, 299
Epinephrine (adrenaline)
  chemical structure, 311
Ergine
  chemical structure, 311
Ergot
  hallucinogenic drugs from, 283
  treatment of migraine (*see* Introduction)
Erythroxylum
  coca, 294
  novogratense; var, truxillense, 294
Ethoheptazine
  opioid agonist analgesic, 4
Ethno-origins (*see* drugs of ethno-origins)
Ethyl alcohol (*see* alcohol)
Ethylketocyclazocine
  tritiated ligand for kappa-opioid receptor, 29
Etoperidone, 97, 100
Euphorbiaceae, 291
Extra-pyramidal
  assessment by inducing supersensitivity, 217
  side effects of neuroleptic drugs, 151, 160, 245, 249

F

Femoxetine (FG-4963)
  analgesic, 15
  antidepressant, 96
Fentanyl (citrate)
  neuroleptanalgesic, 14
  opioid agonist analgesic, 32
FK 33-824
  chemical structure, 39
  synthetic enkephalin analogue as analgesic, 38-40
FLA-336
  chemical structure, 90
  Type A MAO selective inhibitor, 91, 92
FLA-788
  desmethyl metabolite of FLA-336, 91, 92
Flavokuwins
  from Kava, 299
Flavonoids
  sedatives, 302-303
"Flesh of the Gods" (*see* Teonanacatl)
Flunitrazepam
  chemical structure, 125, 142
  non-sedating anti-anxiety agent, 142
Fluoxetine
  analgesic, 15
  antidepressant, 96, 100, 104, 110
  chemical structure, 102
  selective 5-HT uptake inhibitor, 100, 104, 112
Flupenthixol
  chemical structure, 155
  decanoate, as depot neuroleptic drug, 155
  displacement of [^{3}H]trifluoperazine from calmodulin, 162
  neuroleptic drug, 155
Fluphenazine
  decanoate and enanthate esters as depot drugs, 154, 155
  neuroleptic drug, 154
  treatment of Gilles de la Tourette Syndrome, 275
Flurazepam
  chemical structure, 125
  treatment of insomnia, 131

Fluspirilene
neuroleptic drug, 154
Fluvoxamine
antidepressant, 96, 100, 112
Fly Agaric (*see* amanita muscaria)
FS-32 (*see also* FS-37);
potent inhibitor of DA uptake, 95
FS-37, 95, 100
FW 34-569
analgesic, 40

G

GABAergic agents (*see also* Gamma-aminobutyric acid (GABA))
analgesics, 45
Galactorrhea, 263, 265
Gamma-acetylenic GABA
GABA-T inhibitor, as analgesic, 45
Gamma-aminobutyric acid (GABA)
agonists, 45, 47, 320
inhibitory neurotransmitter, role in,
analgesia, 45
mode of action of benzodiazepines, 133-135; and barbiturates, 140
interaction with neuroleptics, 178-179
Gamma-vinyl GABA
GABA-T inhibitor, as analgesic, 45
Ganja (*see* cannabis)
Gastrodia elata, 304
Gastrodin, 304
Gilles de la Tourette Syndrome, 275
Ginseng
"adaptogen" activity, 292-293, 324
Siberian, 292
Glycosides
active components of ginseng and eleutherococcus, 293
Guarana
psychostimulant containing caffeine, 286

H

Halazepam, 127
chemical structure, 126
Hallucinogen, 305, 306
Haloperidol
chemical structure, 153
decanoate, 154
neuroleptanalgesic, 14
neuroleptic, 154, 173
treatment of,
Gilles de la Tourette Syndrome, 275
Huntington's disease, 276
Hamilton Depression Rating Scale, 74, 104, 105 (*see also* Depression)
Harmaline
chemical structure, 309
psychotomimetic alkaloid, 309-310
Harman, 303
chemical structure, 309
Hashish (*see* cannabis)
Hastatoside, 303
Heimia, 319
salicifolia, 319
Henbane (*see* hyoscyamus niger)
Heroin
opioid agonist analgesic, 4, 297
Himmelsbach
point system for evaluation of abstinence syndrome of centrally acting analgesics, 17, 20, 24
Histamine
blockade of effects by neuroleptics, 176

Homobaldrinal
  chemical structure, 300
  sedative degradation product from European valerian, 300-301
Hops, 303
HRP-197
  potent inhibitor of NA and DA uptake, 95
HRP-459, 99
Humulone, 303
Humulus lupulus L, 303
Huntington's disease (chorea), 275-276
Hydergine (*see* Introduction)
Hydrocodone (*see* dihydrocodeine)
Hydromorphine (*see* dihydromorphine)
Hydroxy-tryptamine (5) (Serotonin)
  antidepressants, role in action of, 81-88, 100, 104, 105, 110-112
  chemical structure, 306
  drugs related to, 306
  lack of involvement in action of neuroleptics, 175-176
Hydroxytryptophan (5)
  analgesic, 16
Hyoscine (*see* scopolamine)
Hyoscyamine (*see* atropine)
Hyoscyamus niger, 315, 316
Hyperprolactinaemia, 263-265
Hypnotics (*see* sedative-hypnotics, insomnia, benzodiazepines, and barbiturates)
Hypotension
  orthostatic, 14, 15

I

Iboga, 317
Ibogaine
  alkaloid present in psychoactive iboga from central Africa, 317
Ibotenic acid
  chemical structure, 320
Icthyiomethia piscipula P.Br., 303
Ilex paraguensis L, 286
Imipramine
  analgesic properties, 15
  antidepressant, 72, 79, 80, 82, 85, 88
  chemical structure, 78
  effect on model of learned helplessness, 111
  metabolism, 79-80
  pharmacokinetics, 79-80
Incazan (*see* Metraindole)
Indalpine
  antidepressant, 97, 100
Indeloxazine
  antidepressant, 99
Indian hemp (*see* cannabis)
Infertility, 268-269
Insomnia, 141
  rebound, 132
  treatment by benzodiazepines, 128
Insulin
  shock therapy of depression, 108
Iochroma, 316
Ipomoea violacea, 311
Iprindole
  antidepressant, 83, 99, 110
Iproniazide
  chemical structure, 90
  MAO inhibitor antidepressant, 89
Iridoids
  verbenalin and hastatoside stimulants from Verbena, 303
Irwin
  swimming rat test for antidepressants, 111

Isocarboxazid
MAO inhibitor, 92
Isocorydine(d), 304
Isoergine
chemical structure, 311
Isoniazid
chemical structure, 90
MAO inhibitor antidepressant, 89

J

Jamaican dogwood (*see* Piscidia)
Jatamansone
chemical structure, 301
tranquillising sesquiterpine, 301
Jimson weed, 316
Jurema, 308
Justicia pectoralis, 307, 308

K

Kanna
South African hallucinogen, 297-298
Kava
psychodepressant from South Pacific, 298-300
Kawain
chemical structure, 299
major component of Kava, 299
Kessyl alcohol
from valerian, chemical structure, 300
Khat (chat)
psychostimulant, 287-289, 324
Kratom
stimulant from South-East Asia, 290-291
Kuhn
demonstration of clinical antidepressant effects of imipramine, 72

L

Labiatae, 302, 323
Lactuca virosa L, 303
Lactucin, 303
Lagochilin
sedative, chemical structure, 302
Lagochilus inebrians, 302
Lang tang, 316
Laudanum
tincture of opium, 297
"Learned helplessness"
response to stress in etiology and tests of depression, 111
Lecythidaceae, 307
Leguminosae, 308, 318
Levallorphan, 23
Levorphanol
opioid agonist analgesic, 4
Lignocaine
local anaesthetic, chemical structure, 295
Lilly-51641
Type A MAO selective inhibitor, 92
Lime flowers, 303
Lisuride
treatment of,
acromegaly, 267
hyperprolactinaemia, 264
Parkinson's disease, 272
Lithium (salts), 72
bromide, 106
carbonate, in treatment of mania, 107
chloride, 106
intoxication, 107
prophylactic management of manic-depression, 106
treatment of mania, 106-107, 112
Lophophora
diffusa, 313
Williamsii, 312

Loranthaceae, 304
Loranthus parasiticus, 304
Lorazepam
  chemical structure, 126
  pharmacokinetics, 129
Loxapine
  chemical structure, 155
  neuroleptic drug, 155
LR-5182
  potent inhibitor of NA and
    DA uptake, 95, 100
LSD-25 (*see* lysergic acid)
Lupulone, 303
LY-141685
  selective dopamine D-2
    agonist, 189
Lysergic acid
  chemical structure, 310
  derivatives, 306, 310-311, 325
  diethylamide (*see* LSD-25)
  LSD-25, 175, 308
    chemical structure, 310
Lythraceae, 319

M

Magnoliaceae, 295
Malpighiaceae, 309
Mandragora officinalis, 315
Mandrake, 315
Maprotiline
  antidepressant, 94, 103-104
  chemical structure, 102
Marijuanha (*see* cannabis)
Maté
  psychostimulant, source of
    caffeine, 286
MD-780515
  Type A selective MAO
    inhibitor, 92
Medazepam
  chemical structure, 126
Melatonin
  pineal, implication in depression,
    111
Memory (*see also* Introduction);
  enhancing drugs (*see* HRP-459,
    Indeloxazine)
  loss, with ECT in depression,
    108
Menispermaceae, 304
Mental Disorders
  diagnostic and Statistical
    Manual of (DSM-111), 130
Meperidine
  limitations in therapy of pain,
    18-19
  opioid agonist analgesic, 4, 7
Mephobarbital
  chemical structure, 137
Meptazinol
  narcotic analgesic, 34
Mescal beans, 318-319
Mescaline
  active principal of hallucinogenic
    cacti Peyotl (Peyote), 312
  antagonism of effects by asarone,
    293
  chemical structure, 312
  comparison with other hallucino-
    gens, 308-309
Mesembrine
  chemical structure, 298
  chief alkaloid constituent of
    Kanna, 298
Mesembryanthemum, 297
  expansum L, 297
  tortuosum L, 297
Mesoridazine
  neuroleptic drug, 153
Methadone
  opioid agonist analgesic, 4
  prolactin release, evaluation of,
    364
Metharbital
  chemical structure, 137
Methedrine, 288
Methixene, 177
Methotrimeprazine
  phenothiazine derivative, use in
    treatment of pain, 14

Methoxy-DMT (5), 307
  chemical structure, 306
Methyl dopa (alpha)
  stimulation of prolactin release, 264
Methyl phenidate (*see also* Introduction);
  psychostimulant, 296
Methysticin
  chemical structure, 299
  protection against strichnine convulsions, 299
Methysticodendron amesianum, 316
Metkephamid (LY 127623)
  analogue of [met]-enkephalin, analgesic, 38, 40-42
  chemical structure, 39
Metoclopramide, 174
  antiemetic properties, 156
  chemical structure, 156
  displacement of 3H-sulpiride binding, 170
Metopon
  opioid agonist analgesic, 4
Metraindole (Incazan)
  antidepressant, 99
Metyrapone
  steroid synthesis inhibitor in treatment of Cushing's Syndrome, 267
Mianserin
  antidepressant, 72, 93, 97, 101-102, 106, 110, 112
  chemical structure, 102
Mimosa hostilis, 308
Mitragyna speciosa Korth, 290
Mitragynine
  chemical structure, 291
  principal alkaloid of Kratom, 291
Mitskyway borrachera, 316
MMDA, 314
  chemical structure, 313
Moclobemide (RO-111163)
  Type A selective MAO inhibitor, 92
Monoamine oxidase inhibitors (MAO-inhibitors), 306
  antidepressants, 71-72, 77, 88-93
  beta carbolines, 309-310
  chemical structures, 90
  history, 88-89
  selectivity towards Type A and B MAO, 91-93, 112
Moraceae, 294
Morphine, 1, 5, 325
  chemical structure, 5, 297
  elevation of prolactin release, 264
  from papaver somniferum, treatment of acute severe pain, 296
  limitations in therapy of pain, 18, 297
  opioid agonist analgesic, 4, 5-6
Motor
  effects of neuroleptic drugs, 157-160 (*see also* extra-pyramidal)
Moxefensine
  antidepressant, 94, 100
Muscazone
  chemical structure, 320
Muscimol
  active constituent of amanita muscaria, 320
  chemical structure, 320
Myristicaceae, 307, 313
  fragrans, 313
Myristicin
  chemical structure, 313
  role in hallucinogenic activity of nutmeg, 313-314

N

Nabilone
  Δ^9-THC derivative,
    antiemetic agent in cancer chemotherapy, 323

Nabilone (continued)
chemical structure, 323
Nalbuphine
chemical structure, 10
limitations in therapy of pain, 22-23
opioid mixed agonist-antagonist analgesic, 9, 11-12
Nalorphine, 12
Naloxazone
irreversible μ-opioid antagonist, 41
Naloxone
antagonist of stimulation produced analgesia, 16, 17
opioid antagonist, 3, 9, 40
treatment of ON-OFF syndrome and dyskinesias induced by L-DOPA treatment of Parkinson's disease, 273
tritiated, ligand for μ-opioid receptors, 2, 29
Naltrexone
opioid antagonist, 3, 11
Napactadine
antidepressant, selective 5-HT uptake inhibitor, 100
Narcotics (*see* analgesics)
Nardostachys jatamansii DC, 301
Nefopam
new analgesic, 36
Neuroleptanalgesia, 14
Neuroleptic(s)
action of atypical drugs, 167-173
actions on,
adenyl cyclase, 161-162
brain dopamine function, 157-173, 245
multiple sites within striatal complex, 183-205
non-dopamine systems, 173-183
agents, 152
classes, 152-157
Neuroleptic(s) (continued)
dopamine receptors,
adaptation to administration of, 205-244
displacement of ligands by, 162-167
motor inhibitory properties of, 157-160
side effects of, 149-150
treatment of,
schizophrenia, 149
pain, 14-15
Neurotensin
interaction with striatal dopamine, 182
peptide, analgesic properties, 44
Niando
stimulant/depressant from Zaire, 291
Nicotine
active component of tobacco, 289
chemical structure, 289
Nitalapram (*see* Citalopram)
Nitrazepam
chemical structure, 126
treatment of insomnia, 131
Nitrous oxide
anaesthesic properties, 15
analgesic properties, 44-45
Nomifensine
antidepressant, 72, 93, 94, 100, 102-103, 109, 112
chemical structure, 102
Noradrenaline (NA) (*see* norepinephrine)
Nordiazepam
metabolite of diazepam and metabolic precursor to oxazepam, 128
Norepinephrine (*see also* Noradrenaline (NA) *passim*);
acute action on, by neuroleptic drugs, 173-175

Norepinephrine (continued)
potentiation of effects by tricyclic antidepressants, 81, 84-88
Norharman (*see* beta-carboline)
Nor-pseudoephedrine (d)
chemical structure, 288
constituent of Khat, 288
Nortriptyline
chemical structure, 78
ECG, 81
tricyclic antidepressant, 79, 88
Nor-Zimelidine (*see also* zimelidine)
long-acting antidepressant, 96, 100, 104
Nupharine, 317
Nupharidine, 317
chemical structure, 318
Nupar luteum, 317
Nutmeg, 313
Nymphaea
ampla, 317, 318
caerulea, 317
species, source of nupharine and apomorphine, 317-318

O

Ocimum micranthum, 310
Ololiuqui, 311
Opiate
definition, 2
Opioid(s)
definitions of, 2–3
endogenous, 30-32, 45
mixed agonist-antagonist analgesics, 2, 9-13, 25
multiple receptors, mu, kappa, delta, etc., 3, 26, 38, 40-42, 47-48
newer synthetic, 32-36
non-analgesic uses, 48
peptidal antagonists, 44
peptides, 36-42
Opipramol
chemical structure, 78
metabolism, 79
tricyclic antidepressant, 78
Opium, 1, 284, 296-297
lettuce, 303
source of narcotic analgesics morphine and codeine, 5, 296
Orchidaceae, 304
Org-2305, 98
Org-3770, 98
Org-6582
analgesic, 15
antidepressant, 97, 100
Oripavine, 13
Orthostatic hypotension (*see* hypotension)
Oxaprotiline
antidepressant, 94
Oxazepam
chemical structure, 126
pharmacokinetics, 129
Oxiperomide, 154
atypical neuroleptic, 160
Oxycodone
opioid agonist analgesic, 4
Oxymetazoline, 174
Oxymorphone
opioid agonist analgesic, 4

P

Pain, 1
definition, 26-27
threshold, alteration by morphine, 5
treatment with,
acupuncture, 16
analgesics, 1
antidepressants, 15
neuroleptics, 14
Palmae, 290
Panax
ginseng C, 292
japonicum C, 292

Panax (continued)
  notoginseng, 292
  quinquefolium L, 292
Papaveraceae, 296, 304
Papaver somniferum, 296
Pargyline
  chemical structure, 90
  MAO inhibitor antidepressant, 89, 92
Parica (*see* yakee)
Parkinson's disease, 270-273
Passiflora spp, 303
Passion flower, 303
Paullinia
  cupana L, 286
  yoco L, 286
Pellotine, 313
  chemical structure, 312
Penfluridol
  neuroleptic drug, 154
Pentabarbital
  chemical structure, 137
Pentazocine
  chemical structure, 10
  limitations in therapy of pain, 21-22
  opioid mixed agonist-antagonist analgesic, 9, 10-11
Peptides
  derivatives as analgesics, 38-45
  effects on, by neuroleptics, 179-182
  endogenous opioid substances, 30-32
  TRH analogues as antidepressants, 99-101, 110-111
Pergolide
  treatment of,
    acromegaly, 267
    hyperprolactinemia, 264
    Parkinson's disease, 272-273
Perlapine, 155
Perphenazine
  neuroleptic drug, 153
Pethidine (*see* Meperidine)
Peyote (*see* peyotl)
Peyotl, 312, 313
Phantastica, 305
Phencyclidine
  receptors, relationship with sigma opioids, 47
Phenelzine
  antidepressant MAO inhibitor, 89, 90, 92, 112
  chemical structure, 90
Phenobarbital
  chemical structure, 137
  treatment of seizures, 139
Phenoperidine, 14
Phenothiazine(s)
  derivatives as neuroleptic drugs, 152-154
  treatment of,
    Huntington's disease, 276
    pain, 14
Phentolamine, 174
Phenylalanine
  D-isomer, analgesic effects, 37
Phenylethylamine
  chemical structure, 311
  derivatives, 312-313
  MAO-inhibiting properties of, 91, 92
Phenylisopropylamine
  related compounds, 313-314
Phenytoin
  treatment of seizure disorders, 138
Pholcodine
  opioid agonist analgesic, 4
Physostigmine, 275
Picenadol
  narcotic analgesic, 35
Piflutixol
  tritiated dopamine antagonist, 163
Piminodine
  opioid agonist analgesic, 4
Pimozide
  chemical structure, 153
  neuroleptic drug, 154
  treatment of Gilles de la Tourette syndrome, 275

Piper
  betle L, 290
  methysticum L, 298
Piperaceae, 290, 298
Piperacetazine
  neuroleptic drug, 153
Piperazinyldibenzoxazepine
  derivatives, as neuroleptic agents, 155-156
Pipiltzintzinli, 323
Pirandamine
  antidepressant, 95, 100
Pirazol (*see* pirlindole)
Pirlindole
  antidepressant, 98
Piscidia (Jamaican dogwood), 303
Piscidic acid, 303
Pituri, 315
PK-8165
  chemical structure, 142
  quinoline derivative as selective antianxiety agent, 142
PK-9084
  selective antianxiety agent, 142
Polycystic ovarian syndrome (PCO), 268-269
Pot (*see* cannabis)
Prazepam, 127
Pre-proenkephalin (*see* proenkephalin)
Pridefine
  antidepressant, 98
Procyclidine, 270
Proenkephalin
  protein precursor of enkephalins, 31
Prolactin
  effect on levels by neuroleptics, 167, 215, 222
  serum levels in hyperprolactinemia, 263
Promazine
  neuroleptic drug, 153
Pro-opiomelanocortin
  source of β-endorphin, 31
Propiram
  narcotic analgesic, 36
Propoxyphene (*see* dextropropoxyphene)
Propyl benzilyl choline mustard (tritiated)
  cholinergic ligand for central receptor assay, 81, 178
Propyl-norapomorphine (N,n), 157, 197
  treatment of Parkinson's disease, 271
Protopanaxadiol (*see also* ginseng);
  chemical structure, 292
Protopanaxatriol, 293 (*see also* ginseng);
  chemical structure, 292
Protriptyline
  chemical structure, 78
  tricyclic antidepressant, 79, 82, 88
Psilocin, 308
  chemical structure, 308
Psilocybin, 308
  chemical structure, 308
Psychodepressants
  from drugs of ethno-origins, 296-304, 325
Psychostimulants (*see also* stimulants);
  ethno origins of, 285-296
  therapeutic potential of, from plants, 324-325
Psychotria, 310
  catharginensis, 309
  viridis, 309
Pulsatilla, 303
  anemone, 303

Q

Quinuclidinyl benzylate
  tritiated, ligand for central anticholinergic activity, 178

R

Rauwolfia (Rauvolfia), 284, 301-302 (*see also* reserpine)
  serpentina L, 301
Reserpine
  antagonism of effects by antidepressants, 81-84
  chemical structure, 301
  CNS depressant alkaloid from Rauwolfia, 301-302
  stimulation of prolactin release, 264
  treatment of tardive diskinesia, 274
Rhynchophylline, 291, 304
Rotundine, 304
Rubiaceae, 285, 290, 304, 309
RX-77368
  peptidal TRH analogue, 99-100

S

Salvia, 323
  divinorum, 323
Sapindaceae, 286
Sarpagandha (*see* Rauwolfia)
Sceletium, 297
Schizandra chiensis
  psychostimulant from Far East, 295
Schizandrine
  chemical structure, 296
  crude extract from schizandra chiensis, pharmacology of, 295-296
  methylphenidated like activity, 296
Schizophrenia
  dopamine hypothesis of, 150-151, 245-248
  treatment by neuroleptic drugs, 149, 224
Scopolamine
  chemical structure, comparison with acetyl choline, 315
  psychoactive anticholinergic drug, 275, 284, 314
Scopolia tangutica, 304
Scutellaria spp., 303
Secobarbital
  chemical structure, 137
Sedative-Hypnotics, 123
  barbiturates, 136, 138, 139
  benzodiazepines, 131-132
Seizure (disorders), 141 (*see also* epilepsy);
  sub-types, 132, 138
  treatment, 123, 132-133, 138-139
Serotonin (*see* hydroxytryptamine (5))
Side-effects
  of,
    analgesics, 17-26, 38, 46
    barbiturates, 140-141
    benzodiazepines, 135-136, 141
    ECT treatment of depression, 108
    MAO inhibitors, 89-90
    neuroleptics, 149-150
    psychostimulants, 285
    tricyclic antidepressants, 77, 80-81
Sigg, E.B.
  effects of tricyclic antidepressants on central adrenergic neurons, 84
Sinicuichi, 319
Sinomenine, 304
Sinomenium acutum, 304
SKF 38393
  selective dopamine D-1 agonist, 189, 190
Skullcap, 303
Sleep (disorders), 131 (*see also* insomnia)
  R.E.M. sleep, 132
Solanaceae, 304, 315, 316
Solandra, 316

Somatostatin
  peptide, analgesic properties, 44
Sophora secondiflora, 318
Spiperone
  neuroleptic drug, 175
  tritiated, 163, 193
Spiroperidol (*see* spiperone)
SP1
  chemical structure, 323
  N-containing cannabinoid analogue, 323
Stachys palustris L, 303
Stephania dielsiana, 304
Sterculiaceae, 285, 286
Sternbach, L.H.
  structure-activity relationships of 1,4-benzodiazipines, 124
Stimulants
  antidepressants, 109
  masticatory, property of cola nuts, 286; of Khat, 287
  psycho, 285-296
Stimulation produced analgesia (SPA) (*see* analgesia)
Strychnine
  convulsions, protection by methysticin, 299
Substance-P, 179
  antidepressant properties, 111
  peptide, analgesic properties, 44
Sufentanil
  chemical structure, 33
  narcotic analgesic, congener of fentanyl, 32
Sulpiride
  atypical neuroleptic drug, 167-171, 217, 242
  chemical structure, 156
  neuroleptic drug, 175
Sulser, F
  correlation of antidepressant activity with down-regulation (subsensitivity), 110
Sultopride
  chemical structure, 156
  neuroleptic agent, 156
Sympathomimetic amine, 84

T

Tabernanthe iboga, 317
Tamoxifen, 266
Tanacetum sp, 323
Tandamine
  antidepressant, 95
Tardive dyskinesia (*see* dyskinesia)
Tea
  psychostimulant, leaves containing caffeine, 285
Teflutixol, 206, 208, 211
Temazepam
  chemical structure, 126
  metabolite of diazepam, 128
  treatment of insomnia, 131
Teonanacatl, 308
Tetrabenazine
  antagonism of depressant effects by tricyclic antidepressants, 81
Tetrahydrocannabinols (THC)
  chemical structure, 322
  principle active constituents of cannabis, 321
  semi-synthetic analogues, 323
Tetrahydropalmatine, 304
Tetrapteris methystica, 309
Theaceae, 285
Thea sinensis (*see* Tea)
Thebaine
  from *papaver bracteatum* and conversion to codeine, 297
Theobroma cacao
  seeds; source of cocoa, chocolate, caffeine and theobromine, 285
Theobromine
  alkaloid from higher plants, 285
  chemical structure, 285

Theobromine (continued)
  diuretic properties, 286
Thiamylal
  chemical structure, 137
Thiethylperazine, 174
Thiobarbiturates
  lipid solubility, 136-137
  pharmacokinetics compared with oxybarbiturates, 137 (*see also* thiopental)
Thiopental
  chemical structure, 137
Thioridazine
  anticholinergic activity, 153, 160
  antihistaminergic activity, 176
  chemical structure, 153
  metabolites, 180
  neuroleptic drug, 153
Thiorphan
  chemical structure, 38
  enkephalinase-A inhibitors, analgesic properties of, 37
Thioxanthene
  derivatives, as neuroleptic drugs, 154-155
Thioxene
  neuroleptic drug, 155
THIP
  analgesic properties, 45, 47
Thujone
  chemical structure, 324
  principle of several pyscho-stimulant plants, 288, 323-324
Thymeleaceae, 304
Tiapride
  atypical neuroleptic, 160
  chemical structure, 156
  treatment of dyskinesias, 157
Tifluadom
  agonist analgesic, 35
Tilia spp, 303
Timostenil (*see* Caroxazone)
Toa (*see* barrachero)
Tobacco, 284, 305, 324
  source of,
    nicotine, 289
    β-carbolines such as harman and nor-harman, 289
Toloache, 316
Toloxatone
  antidepressant, 96
  Type A selective MAO inhibitor, 92, 96
Tonga (*see* barrachero)
Torna-loco, 316
Tourette (Gilles de la) (Syndrome), 275
Tranylcypromine
  chemical structure, 90
  MAO inhibitor, 92
Trazodone
  antidepressant, 72, 93, 97, 104-105, 112
  anxiolytic properties, 104
  chemical structure, 102
Triazolam
  treatment of insomnia, 131
Trichocereus pachanoi, 313
Tricyclics (antidepressants), 72, 76-88, 112 (*see also* antidepressants)
Trifluoperazine
  chemical structure, 153
  neuroleptic drug, 227
  tritiated ligand, 163
Trifluopromazine
  neuroleptic drug, 153
Trifluperidol, 154
Trihexphenidyl, 270
Trimipramine
  chemical structure, 78
  tricyclic antidepressant, 78
Tripelennamine
  abuse in combination with pentazocine, 22
Tropane alkaloids
  antagonists of side effects of acetyl choline, 314-315
Tryptamine
  chemical structure, 306

Tryptamine (continued)
- derivatives, 306-310

Tryptophan
- L-isomer as potential antidepressant, 100

Turbina corymbosa, 311
Turkestan mint
- intoxicant from Central Asia, 302

Turnera (Damiana), 303
- diffusa L, 303

Tutin, 304

U

U-50488
- Kappa opioid agonist analgesic, 35

Uncaria, 291
- rhynchophylla, 304

V

Valepotriates, 300-301
Valeranone (*see* Jatamansone)
Valerian
- sedative from valeriana officinalis, 300-301, 325

Valeriana
- officinalis, 300
- Wallichii, 300

Valerianaceae, 300
Vallillin
- derivatives from Tilia spp, 303

Valtrate
- chemical structure, 300

Verbena
- officinalis L, 303

Verbenalin, 303
Vilca (*see* Yopo)
Viloxazine
- antidepressant, 99, 100, 103, 109
- chemical structure, 102

"Vine of the Souls" (*see* Ayahuasca)
Virola, 307
- calophylla, 307
- calophylloidea, 307
- elongata, 307
- snuffs, 308
- theiodora, 307

Vitamin(s)
- C, content in Maté, 286
- in coca, 294

X

Xanthine(s)
- parent ring system of caffeine, 285

Y

Yage (*see* Ayahuasca)
Yakee, 307
Yangonin
- chemical structure, 299

Yohimbine, 291
Yopo, 307

Z

Zimelidine
- analgesic properties of, 15
- antidepressant, 96, 104, 110, 112
- chemical structure, 102